"Few authors today are more trusted by natural parents than Sarah Buckley. *Gentle Birth, Gentle Mothering* is an exceptional book that gives families the confidence they need to follow their own instincts."

—Peggy O'Mara, editor and publisher of *Mothering* magazine

"I love this book. It is one of the most important and unique works of the new millennium. In it, Dr. Buckley helps to return birth—as opposed to "delivery"—to its rightful place as the center of the family, the cornerstone of the human race."

—Jay Hathaway, director of The Bradley Method® and co-author of *Children at Birth*

"*Gentle Birth, Gentle Mothering* has the potential to give us unprecedented insight into the mysteries and wonders of birth—and into its resulting impact on our world."

—Gail J. Dahl, author of *Pregnancy and Childbirth Secrets* and executive director of the Canadian Childbirth Association

"*Gentle Birth, Gentle Mothering* is the book Hygieia College can fully endorse. Sarah Buckley is a true birthkeeper. As a mother, she knows what having two hearts feels like. Yet as a birthkeeper, she has *soul*. I am honored to be Sarah's colleague."

—Jeannine Parvati Baker, midwife and author of *Prenatal Yoga and Natural Childbirth*

"Sarah Buckley is precious, because she is bilingual. She can speak the language of a mother who gave birth to her four children at home. She can also speak like a medical doctor. By intermingling the language of the heart and scientific language she is driving the history of child birth towards a radical and inspiring new direction."

—Michel Odent, MD, surgeon, author, and natural birth pion

"Sarah Buckley is one of the few people in this world telling the about pregnancy and birth."

—Jan Tritten, midwife and editor of *Midwifery Today*

"Sarah Buckley marries the medical mind and the birthing woman's body wisdom. Her writing comes from the unique perspective of a holistic integration of these often-poles-apart realities. Unfortunately, this combination is very rare in modern obstetrics. Her writing opens up new possibilities for those lucky enough to imbibe."

> —Gloria Lemay, midwifery educator and contributing editor of *Midwifery Today*

"Dr. Buckley's book offers parents and practitioners outstanding resources and references to make informed decisions regarding pregnancy, birth, and neonatal care. Dr. Sarah's unique writing style combines science, clinical expertise, and parental experience, creating a comprehensive compilation with tremendous value. I envision this book to have a major impact on the future shift in consciousness about birthing."

> —Jeanne Ohm, DC, International Chiropractic Pediatric Association executive coordinator

"This book challenges the medical model of childbirth on its own terms, drawing on a vast range of research to help women and practitioners understand why we have got birth wrong, and how to get it right. It is a lifeline for women who want to give birth rather than be delivered, and for practitioners who want to nurture rather than control them."

> —Mary Nolan, National Childbirth Trust senior tutor

"A thoughtful discussion of the central issues in today's childbirth in industrialized countries. I have not seen a more penetrating analysis with thorough documentation from the scientific literature. I would wish this book would be read by every obstetrician, family physician, midwife, and obstetric nurse. In addition, this book would be a wonderful primer for women and families searching for a better childbirth."

> —Marsden Wagner, MD, perinatologist and former WHO regional director, Ohio

gentle birth, gentle mothering

Dr. Sarah Buckley

Foreword by
INA MAY GASKIN,
CPM

A Doctor's Guide to Natural Childbirth
and Gentle Early Parenting Choices

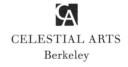

CELESTIAL ARTS
Berkeley

For mothers, babies, fathers,
and families everywhere.

Published in the United States by Celestial Arts,
an imprint of the Crown Publishing Group,
a division of Random House, Inc., New York.
www.crownpublishing.com
www.tenspeed.com

Celestial Arts and the Celestial Arts colophon are
registered trademarks of Random House, Inc.

A version of chapter 1 was previously published
in *The Age*, Melbourne, Nov 29, 1996; a version
of chapter 2 was previously published as "A
Vision of Birth" in *Midwifery Today*, number
68, Winter 2003; a version of chapter 3 was previously published in *Living Now*, Winter 2002,
supplement *Women Now*; versions of chapter 5
were previously published in *Mothering* no. 102,
Sept-Oct 2000 and in Nexus, vol 9, no. 6, Oct-Nov
2002; versions of chapter 6 were first published
in *Journal of Prenatal and Perinatal Psychology
and Health* 17(4) Summer 2003 and in *MIDIRS
Midwifery Digest*, Jun and Sept 2004, Vol 14 (2),
pp 203–209 and Vol 14 (3), pp 353–359; a version
of the essay "Emma's Birth—Sweet and Oceanic" was first posted at www.birthlove.com; a
version of the essay "Maia's Birth—A Family
Celebration" was previously published in *Midwifery Today Birthkit*, Winter 2001; an expanded
version is posted at www.sarahjbuckley.com; a
version of chapter 7 was previously published
in *Mothering* no. 133, Nov-Dec 2005, as "The
Hidden Risks of Epidurals"; a version of chapter 8 was first published in *Lotus Birth*, Shivam
Rachana, Greenwood Press 2000; a version of the
essay "Jacob's Waterbirth" was published in *Australia's Parents Pregnancy*, winter 1999; a version

of the essay "Jacob's Placenta" was published
as "The Amazing Placenta" in *Mothering* no.
131, Jul-Aug 2005; the material in chapter 9 was
originally written as a background briefing for
Queensland Members of Parliament on behalf
of the Maternity Coalition; a version of chapter
10 was originally written as a fact sheet for the
Brisbane Home Midwifery Association (Queensland, Australia, 2003); a version of chapter 12
was first published in the *Courier Mail* (Brisbane,
Australia), 7 May 1998, as "Breastfeeding and
Bonding"; a version of the essay "Bees, Baboo
and Boobies: My Breastfeeding Career" was first
published as "My Breastfeeding Career" in *The
Mother* (UK) 2004, no. 10; a version of "Ten Tips
for Safe Cosleeping" was previously published in
Natural Parenting no. 4, Spring 2003.

Library of Congress Cataloging-in-Publication
Data
Buckley, Sarah J.
Gentle birth, gentle mothering : a doctor's guide
to natural childbirth and gentle early parenting
choices / Sarah Buckley ; foreword by Ina May
Gaskin.
        p. cm.
1. Natural childbirth. 2. Newborn infants—
Care. I. Title.

RG661.B83 2009
618.4'5--dc22
                                    2008043685

ISBN-13: 978-1-58761-322-7 (pbk.)

Printed in the United States of America

Cover and text design by Toni Tajima

        18th Printing

First Edition

CONTENTS

Foreword by Ina May Gaskin / 2

Introduction / 4

Part 1 Gentle Birth

1. Reclaiming Every Woman's Birth Right / 8
2. Vision and Tools for Instinctive Birth / 12
   Emma's Birth—Sweet and Oceanic / 20
3. Healing Birth, Healing the Earth / 25
   Zoe's Birth—Challenge and Transformation / 32
4. Your Body, Your Baby, Your Choice: A Guide to Making Wise Decisions / 37
5. Ultrasound Scans: Cause for Concern / 78
6. Undisturbed Birth: Mother Nature's Blueprint for Safety, Ease, and Ecstasy / 95
   Maia's Birth—A Family Celebration / 128
7. Epidurals: Risks and Concerns for Mothers and Babies / 132
8. Leaving Well Enough Alone: Natural Perspectives on the Third Stage of Labor / 154
   Jacob's Placenta / 185
9. Cesarean Surgery: The Whole Story / 193
10. Choosing Homebirth / 204
    Jacob's Waterbirth—Perfect Timing / 212

Part 2 Gentle Mothering

11. Love, Attachment, and Your Baby's Brain: How Gentle Early Parenting Promotes Lifelong Well-Being / 217
12. Breastfeeding: The Gift of a Lifetime / 234
    Bees, Baboo, and Boobies: My Breastfeeding Career / 241
13. Babies, Mothers, and the Science of Sharing Sleep / 247
    Ten Tips for Safe Sleeping / 263

Epilogue: Becoming a Parent / 267
Resources / 273
Acknowledgments / 279
Notes / 281
Index / 342

FOREWORD

HOORAY FOR Sarah Buckley! Her broadly informed, authoritative voice is sorely needed in these trying times when there is so much fear, ignorance, and confusion surrounding childbirth and the decision-making and organization of maternity care. Never has there been so much at stake for women giving birth, in terms of age-old knowledge and wisdom that may be lost for decades or longer if current trends continue unabated. In many countries, it is only the middle-aged and the elderly who remember the time when only four or five women out of every hundred had their babies by cesarean. How will people of the future even know that un-interfered-with birth is safer than surgical birth? Will feminists of the future believe today's birth activists, or will they believe the obstetricians who are far more comfortable with surgery than with physiological processes that have their own timing?

Fear can make for irrational decision-making, and here we have a good example of this phenomenon at work. In many areas of the world, women have become sufficiently afraid of nature's plan for labor and birth that they are literally clamoring for surgical birth when there is no medical reason to justify the added risk such surgery poses to them and their babies. There is no historical precedent for a phenomenon such as this. We have mass hysteria spreading over the planet—a rather strange development after the second wave of the women's movement, since it involves women being afraid of their own wombs. Ironically, this widespread fear leads countless women to agree to deliberate injury of their uteri by cesarean section, although we don't commonly speak of these acts in such stark language. Women, like most of the rest of our society, are not given the information necessary to fully understand the risks of many of the decisions they are called upon to make around the time of birth. While all this happens, the confusion grows even deeper, and it becomes ever more difficult for young women to learn about the gifts and capacities of their bodies.

Horrible birth stories can now be sent around the world at lightning speed via satellite television and movies, with the result that uninformed attitudes (many of which arose originally in the United States) that promote ever more routine medical intervention in birth for healthy women

2

are threatening to make the ancient way of birth viewed as a selfish or irresponsible act on the part of the woman who wishes to make this choice.

Most women have little awareness of how important an autonomous midwifery profession is when it comes to retaining age-old wisdom of women's true capacities in labor and birth. When midwives no longer have the ability to honor women's right to labor as long as they are willing to continue, when their and their babies' vital signs are good, in the birth site of their choice; when hospital-based midwives are forced to split their attention among several laboring women in a busy maternity unit; when student midwives and physicians are no longer assured the chance of witnessing the normal physiological process of labor during their training; we lose the meaning of birth, step by step, and myths take further precedence over physiological realities.

Here's what makes Sarah Buckley's writing so authoritative and compelling. She knows medicine because of her years of medical training and experience. But unlike 99 percent of her medical colleagues in the wealthy countries, she also knows unmedicated birth in a way that only one who has experienced it can. She has lived her education in the most real way possible—by giving birth at home four times. That fact alone speaks volumes.

Her knowledge is in her bones, but she also knows where it is corroborated by scientific research that you can rely upon. You'll find rich resources in this book on each subject discussed in relation to pregnancy, giving birth, breastfeeding, mother-infant attachment, and cosleeping.

Young feminists, are you listening? Remember, here we have a physician who knows more, and has a broader range of experience, than those of her profession who disagree with her, those who have never tried out the birth-giving capacities of their bodies. Feminism is about courage and strength and celebration of feminine power. True feminism does not disrespect the woman who finds power in giving birth without medication or unnecessary interference. Few women who have such an experience will come away from birth subscribing to a belief in a creator who, some maintain, deliberately created women's bodies to be poorly designed for giving birth. Rather, they are far more likely to gain new respect for the heretofore hidden powers of their bodies.

—Ina May Gaskin, CPM

INTRODUCTION

THE SEEDS FOR *Gentle Birth, Gentle Mothering* were sown in the blissful days and weeks following the birth of my son, Jacob Patrick. Jacob's birth, my third at home, had been intense and yet ordinary, challenging but joyous, and ultimately ecstatic and fulfilling. Holding my new baby in my arms, I wished that every family could be so blessed by birth.

In the years that followed Jacob's birth, I took an extended break from my work as a family physician, gaining more opportunities to explore my path as a mother and to write about my experiences. I became especially interested in exploring the nexus between biomedical perspectives and gentle approaches in birth and mothering.

I was excited to discover that many birth and parenting practices that I had instinctively chosen—for example, homebirth, bed sharing, and child-led breastfeeding—were well supported by evidence from science, anthropology, psychology, and medicine. I felt strongly that parents deserve to know this, so that they can distinguish cultural disapproval from genuine risks when they evaluate birth and parenting choices.

Through my research and writing, I also learned about the evolutionary wisdom of bed sharing and long-term breastfeeding, and the positive impact of secure attachment on lifelong mental health. I came to see—from my reading, my observations, and my own experiences—just how profound is the imprint of birth and early mothering on child development and family relationships.

With the birth of my fourth baby, Maia Rose, in 2000, I experienced giving birth as our foremothers may have: birth as pure instinct and pleasure. This amazing experience inspired me to look at the ecstasy of birth from a scientific perspective, and I began to develop the material on ecstatic and undisturbed birth that you will read here, first published in *Mothering* magazine.

"Gentle Birth," the first part of *Gentle Birth, Gentle Mothering*, focuses on gentle approaches to pregnancy and birth, and includes a wealth of scientific evidence about current maternity-care choices. These chapters are relevant to women giving birth in any setting, with information that will also help partners and family to understand and trust the natural processes of labor and birth.

"Gentle Birth" includes my own experiences in pregnancy and birth, including the homebirths of Emma, my first child, who was born almost a month early; Zoe, who was born on her due date and, like Emma, emerged posterior (facing up); Jacob, my third child, who was born in the water almost three weeks past his original due date; and the unassisted (and also surprising) semi-water birth of my fourth baby Maia. "Gentle Birth" also features a chapter called "Vision and Tools for Instinctive Birth," which offers many ideas and tools to help prepare for birth. In the chapter called, "Healing Birth, Healing the Earth," one of my most popular writings, I share my own inspiration for birth.

Other chapters in this first part review pregnancy and birth choices from medical and scientific perspectives. My personal belief is that women are the experts in their own bodies and babies, and that, given full information, they will make the choices that are right for themselves and their babies, whether or not these choices are in agreement with current medical or cultural beliefs. I also encourage all prospective parents to be attentive to their instincts and intuition, beyond previous ideas, ideals, or political correctness, so that they can be truly responsive and responsible. I believe that fathers can have an important role in decision making about their own babies, if they choose to accept this, and that they also need to receive support and understanding during these times.

I have included a chapter about ultrasound, because I feel that parents are generally not given sufficient accurate information to make an informed choice about this technology. Chapter 4 introduces the "BRAN" approach to decision-making, and uses this model to look at three common pregnancy choices: testing for gestational diabetes; screening and antibiotics for group B strep; and induction for "going overdue." The centerpiece of this part, and of the book as a whole, is my article "Undisturbed Birth: Mother Nature's Blueprint for Safety, Ease, and Ecstasy." This expansion of my ecstatic birth material, previously published in *Mothering* magazine, features a wealth of scientific research that supports the ecstasy and the evolutionary wisdom of gentle birth. I also detail some of the possible consequences of disturbing birth with intense monitoring and with medical interventions. The power of this chapter is in the extensive material (and I am always finding more to add!) and its resonance with many women's cellular memories of giving birth and with the experiences of those who support undisturbed birth.

Chapter 8, "Leaving Well Enough Alone," explains the natural processes of the third stage of labor and explores the impact of early cord clamping (including cord blood banking), which can have a major impact on the health of mother and baby. The chapters on epidurals (also first published in *Mothering* magazine) and cesareans give important information to help parents make informed choices, with information covering vaginal birth after cesarean (VBAC) and suggestions for having a good cesarean, when necessary. This section concludes with a review of the scientific evidence on the safety of homebirth, along with some practical guidance for those who make this responsible choice.

The second part of the book, "Gentle Mothering," covers gentle parenting choices. New parents will enjoy information on the science of attachment, the benefits of breastfeeding, and the safety of bed sharing; experienced parents can feel supported by the medical information that validates these often-instinctive choices. You can also read about my journey—sixteen years, in total—as a breastfeeding mother, and the benefits of breastfeeding past the first year for mother and child.

Many of these chapters were featured in the first (Australian) edition of *Gentle Birth, Gentle Mothering*, published in 2005, and it has been a pleasure to have the opportunity to update the scientific studies for wider distribution. I have especially enjoyed documenting the solid science that supports attachment-style parenting and bed sharing and other styles of cosleeping, so that you too can feel confident about these sometimes-misunderstood choices.

Birth and mothering have blessed me, and I am passing that blessing on to you through this book. May you be inspired, informed, and supported by what you read, and may your parenting benefit from a firm and gentle foundation, based on instinct, wisdom, and love.

Part 1

gentle birth

chapter 1

RECLAIMING EVERY WOMAN'S BIRTH RIGHT

In our culture childbirth has been seen as a medical procedure, with the majority of public discussion concerned with safety and statistics, as defined by physicians, and with little room for debate and dissension—especially from those who are at the center of the process: women themselves. This chapter balances this medical perspective with the personal impact of birth for mothers, babies, fathers, and families, and calls for a more comprehensive approach that acknowledges the power of birth and its centrality in the social and emotional lives of families.

Birth is a women's issue, birth is a power issue; therefore birth is a feminist issue. My logic may be correct, but the issue of birth has been at the bottom of the feminist agenda in western countries for some years[1]—well behind matters such as equal opportunity, sexual harassment, bedroom politics, abortion, and body image, to name but a few.

Feminism has championed many other women's health issues and resisted the medicalization of the other major women's rite of passage in our culture—menopause; however, there seems to have been no equivalent, large-scale analysis of birth in feminist thinking. Yet most women in our culture will give birth at some time in their lives, and for the majority it is their first experience as a hospital patient, with the loss of autonomy implied in that role. Many will feel the conflict between their own desires, needs, and ways of knowing, and the technology-does-it-better approach that the medicalization of birth has produced.

This medical approach—founded on the assumption that every birth is potentially high-risk, and endorsed by our culture's infatuation with technology[2]—has not benefited the healthy majority of mothers and babies in the United States and other westernized countries.

Although the United States spends more on health care than any other Organization for Economic Cooperation and Development (OECD) country,[3] its high infant mortality rate ranks the United States twenty-sixth among thirty industrialized countries—equivalent to Poland and worse than Hungary—in terms of infant survival. Of equal concern, maternal mortality in the United States has been rising in recent years,[4] which may be linked to escalating rates of cesareans. In 2006, 31.1 percent of U.S. women gave birth by cesarean[5] (the comparable figure for 2005–2006 in Canada was 26.5 percent of births,[6] and in England, 23.5 percent[7]). Compare this with 10.5 percent in the United States in 1970[8] and with World Health Organization recommendations of no more than 10 to 15 percent.[9]

But it is not only mothers who undergo cesareans who feel the impact of these extreme intervention rates. The 2002 Listening to Mothers (LTM) Survey found "virtually no natural childbirth" among the 1,583 women surveyed.[10] In a repeat survey published in 2006, 94 percent of those women who gave birth vaginally had routine electronic fetal monitoring, 86 percent used pain-killing drugs, 80 percent were administered IV fluids, and 76 percent had epidural analgesia. In total, 41 percent of LTM respondents reported that their caregiver had tried to induce labor.[11] All of this in an extremely healthy population, among whom at least 70 to 80 percent could give birth without drugs or intervention, according to some estimates.

As a family physician and a mother I ask myself why women are tolerating this situation. Why are educated, articulate women, who are prepared to battle for their rights in their personal and professional lives, so accepting of the high intervention rates that characterize this group in particular?[12]

I ask why we are not at least advocating for our babies at a time when science is discovering what mothers have known for years: that a newborn baby is a highly sentient being, exquisitely sensitive to its emotional and physical environment, and that a baby's experiences during labor and birth—for example, exposure to some drugs—can have lifelong consequences.[13]

Perhaps there is a perception among women that there have been improvements in maternity care. In many places, choices may seem greater, with birth centers available for low-risk women. However, birth centers are politically precarious in almost every setting with many free-standing centers closing in recent years. A woman who chooses to give birth there has a high chance of being transferred to a hospital at some stage of labor, especially first-time mothers. Birth center options also may be limited by externally dictated policies and politics, especially if a birth center is physically contained within a hospital setting.

Labor and delivery rooms are looking more comfortable and homey, with fathers' presence being allowed—even expected—during labor and birth. However, cosmetic changes do not guarantee a low-technology philosophy, and fathers may be reluctant participants, unprepared for the intensity of labor and birth and feeling distressed and frightened at seeing their partner in the endorphin-altered state that is natural for a laboring woman. It has even been suggested that the increased use of epidurals for pain relief parallels the advent of fathers in the labor room, perhaps reflecting a subtle pressure on women to behave more normally in labor. Clearly, men need more support in this role.

Perhaps the lack of birth activism, individually and collectively, also reflects our small families and our busy working lives, which give each of us less motivation to lobby for improvements. A bad birth experience can be forgotten in the intensity of the early months, and then we go back to our careers, where we feel safe and life is more predictable.

Yet I feel that there is an enormous amount of disappointment and hurt around giving birth. As a pregnant woman I noticed that other women told me almost exclusively negative stories about their own birth experiences. I wonder, too, about depression and distress after birth, which affect up to one in five women, and which have been linked in some studies to forceps and cesarean births[14, 15] and early separation of mother and baby.[16]

However, I am not advocating one particular type of good birth, nor even birth without intervention. A woman's satisfaction with her birth experience is related more to her involvement in decision-making than to the outcome.[17] But women need the information necessary to make informed choices and decisions, and this requires that doctors, nurses, and midwives take time to listen and explain, and that women and their partners take their share of responsibility.

This is also a prescription for lower rates of litigation, which at present are frightening obstetricians into defensive and often interventionist practices, which ultimately benefit neither doctors nor women.

This informed-choice approach also implies that parents can be trusted to make good decisions; this is a radical departure from the paternalistic approach that has been prevalent in obstetrics. It is also welcome because many current obstetric practices are not supported by evidence of effectiveness or cost-benefit. For example, an evidence-based analysis, reflecting the best of international research, shows that models of care that prioritize women's choices—such as home birth[18] and continuity of care with midwives[19]—are at least as safe as conventional obstetric care, with higher rates of satisfaction.

Consumers now have access to evidence-based information through the work of the UK-based Cochrane Collaboration. This group produces the regularly updated book, *A Guide to Effective Care in Pregnancy and Childbirth*,[20] and their information is also available on the Cochrane Collaboration website,[21] which is freely accessible in many countries. Both resources provide an excellent base from which to assess birth choices.

Perhaps the most exciting aspect of evidence-based obstetrics is the implied possibility for institutional change. Murray Enkin, one of the authors of *A Guide to Effective Care in Pregnancy and Childbirth*, states that "The only justification for practices that restrict a woman's autonomy, her freedom of choice, or her access to her baby, would be clear evidence that these restrictive practices do more good than harm."[22]

If all involved in birth were to take these premises seriously, profound changes would take place in the birth room.

Birth is women's business; it is the business of our bodies. And our bodies are indeed wondrous, from our monthly cycles to the awesome power inherent in the act of giving birth. Yet in our culture I do not see respect for these extraordinary functions: instead we diet, exercise, abuse, conceal, and generally punish our bodies for not approximating an unrealistic and unobtainable ideal. This lack of trust in and care for our bodies can rob us of confidence in giving birth. Conversely, an experience of the phenomenal capacity of our birthing body can give us an enduring sense of our own power as women. Birth is the beginning of life; the beginning of mothering, and of fathering. We all deserve a good beginning.

chapter 2

VISION AND TOOLS FOR INSTINCTIVE BIRTH

Giving birth is an innately instinctive act, hardwired into our brains and bodies through millions of years of mammalian evolution, and designed to ensure the best possible outcomes for mothers and babies. In this chapter I ask, "How can we optimize our instincts to enhance ease, pleasure, and safety for ourselves and our babies?" This chapter also contains suggestions and resources for natural, instinctive birth.

A vision of Birth came to me in the months after I gave birth to Zoe, my second baby. As I meditated on the challenges that I had encountered during my labor I began to see my experience, and Birth herself, as a huge multifaceted crystal. I saw that the different aspects of Zoe's birth, like facets of a crystal, would not add up to one clear picture but would reflect at many different angles.

For me, each of these exquisite facets was worthy of many months of meditation; alternatively, I could stand back and appreciate the beauty and wholeness of Birth and of my own experience. I also saw that, to paraphrase poet Walt Whitman, "Birth can contradict herself because she is vast, she contains multitudes," and that I could not expect rationality or even consistency as I worked to integrate my experience.

This vision comes back to me when I think about some of the more complex and controversial aspects of birth. I see all of us, with our unique experiences, beliefs, and skills, as different parts—facets if you like—of this Birth crystal. Although we may not share the same angle on birth, our differences are necessary and our dialogues essential.

Birth as an Instinctive Act

When I think of instinctive birth, I imagine myself as occupying one or more facets of this birth crystal. From my perspective as a family physician and writer on gentle and undisturbed birth, I can say that birth is essentially an instinctive act; that is, "an elaborate pattern of actions occurring as a whole in response to stimuli . . . ."

As a physician I know that important hormones—such as oxytocin, the hormone of love; endorphins, hormones of pleasure and transcendence; epinephrine/norepinephrine (adrenaline/noradrenaline), hormones of excitement; and prolactin, the mothering hormone—are produced deep within the brain of the laboring female, and mediate the "elaborate pattern of actions" of birth and of instinctive mothering behavior in humans as well as in our mammalian cousins (see chapter 6).

Like other mammals, human mothers, also need a safe and private space so that our labor and birth instincts can unfold with ease. Sometimes I imagine how difficult it would be for a pregnant cat or ape to give birth in a large, brightly lit room, surrounded by strangers, as most laboring women do today. The excellent outcomes at Michel Odent's clinic in Pithiviers, France, where women gave birth in quiet, semidark, and private conditions highlight the importance of an undisturbed environment.[1] In these circumstances, a laboring woman can let down her guard, switching off her rational brain and opening to the "unreasoned impulse" of her instincts.

But if I look from another angle, I could also ask, "Is birth any less instinctive than, for example, eating or making love?" We are all hardwired to perform these enjoyable activities, but our hardwiring does not guarantee easy digestion, ecstatic sex, or instinctive birth. And there are many women who have had ideal environments—at home with loving support, for example—who have still encountered difficulty and needed assistance in birth. (This may also reflect our negative cultural beliefs and our lack of exposure to normal birth, over several generations.) So even as I state from one perspective that birth is instinctive, I find contradictions.

Helping Our Instincts

I can imagine myself in a dialogue with my friend, Wintergreen, body worker and developer of The Pink Kit,[2] who has another valuable perspective. Wintergreen would tell me that birth may be an instinct, like sex, but we can learn to give birth just as we can learn to be good lovers.

She might agree that it is important to look at the external circumstances of birth, but she would also say that we can influence our internal circumstances by learning to work with our birthing bodies. She might mention the importance of the internal work of The Pink Kit—a multimedia kit that takes us into our own body knowledge, teaching us to map and work with our anatomy, to massage ourselves internally in preparation for birth, and to feel inside our own vaginas during late pregnancy and labor.

These tools are immensely valuable, helping us to be in touch with our own bodies—which, even in birth, may be seen as the province of professionals—and assisting us to birth instinctively in whatever birth setting we choose.

I see that there are other levels to be cleared in order to be able to birth instinctively. This facet of birth—which I could ascribe to my friend, director of the International College of Spiritual Midwifery Shivam Rachana,[3] and which has been validated through many women's experiences—looks at our past experiences and beliefs, all of which are stored in our bodies, and concentrates on freeing us up emotionally, physically and spiritually for birth.

Here, like women in many cultures, we can use movement, counseling/psychotherapy, rebirthing, bodywork, yoga, and other therapies to clear out all the emotional and psychological issues that can arise for us in labor and birth. For example, I found the Osho meditation CD, *Chakra Breathing*, to be superb preparation for birth.

Counseling/psychotherapy was my ally when giving birth to my first baby, Emma. Clearing out was a very powerful facet for me with Zoe's birth, and I realized, in retrospect, how much my own childhood experience of being displaced by the birth of my younger sister had affected this birthing.

Connecting with the Earth

We are also creatures of the Earth, and our bodies need the Earth's nourishment to work efficiently in any instinctive behavior. Good nutrition is a very important aspect of instinctive birth, as any animal breeder will affirm.

Australian naturopath and author Francesca Naish ascribes much of our modern difficulties in labor and birth to poor nutrition, and it is certainly true that our modern western diets are generally not wholesome or replete with all the nutrients that our bodies and our babies need. Her work, published in the United States as *Healthy Parents, Better Babies*,[4] contains valuable information to help us enhance our birth experience, and the long-term health of our babies, through optimal nutrition.

There are also deeper levels to our connection with the Earth. For some women, pregnancy brings an urge to garden or to go walking, to hike or just to gaze at the scenery of earth and sky. All of these activities help align us with the Earth, our great Mother, and teach us respect and love for the natural order.

If we want to birth instinctively, we can prepare ourselves by beginning to live more instinctively. We can, for example, make an effort to live less by the clock, which British birth activist Sheila Kitzinger calls "an unevaluated technological intervention that has major impact on the conduct of birth."[5] When we live without a clock—or simply stop wearing a watch—we can more easily tune into our own instinctive and earth-based rhythms, which are much gentler on mothers and babies.

Spiritual beliefs and practices are another important facet of pregnancy and birth. In a practical sense, having faith helps us to believe in our bodies and in birth, and prayer is a beautiful way to prepare for birth and motherhood.

Belief systems that venerate the feminine as well as the masculine principle have a special place in my heart, as I see, from a spiritual perspective, that much damage can been done to women when religions fail to honor the female body and feminine authority. Through the ages we have also had our birthing goddesses and saints, from Artemis to Mary (who gave birth unassisted and surrounded by mammals), to remind us that birth is a natural and instinctive act for all women.

Using Our Bodies

What about the ways in which we use our bodies? Can we really birth instinctively if we cannot use our bodies freely? If we cannot squat, if our back muscles are weak from too much sitting, and if our babies are not optimally positioned because of our lifestyle and the ways we habitually misuse our bodies, can we then expect birth to be straightforward?

Physical preparation is a very important facet of preparing for instinctive birth, helping us to open to the "specified reactions" of our instincts through, for example, different postures and positions. For example, Janet Balaskas's Active Birth exercises,[6] optimal fetal positioning,[7] The Pink Kit, and prenatal yoga are all excellent tools for this. These forms of birth preparation have similarities to bodywork; when we stretch our bodies, we are also stretching our internal beliefs and feelings, because our bodies and our minds are inseparable.

It can be hard, outside the birth room, to realize how deeply we can go into our bodies during birth. For me this was one of the most powerful realizations after I gave birth to my first baby, Emma, and I was very thankful for my yoga practice, which had so beautifully taught me to "yoke" my body and mind (as the word yoga translates).

Treating our bodies gently in all that we do, talking kindly to our bodies, and navigating, as best we can, the negative attitudes about women's bodies that are so common in our culture—these simple practices will help us to keep faith in our ability to give birth instinctively, sustaining us in pregnancy and during the challenging times of labor.

Going Within

During pregnancy we are called to go deeper into our minds, our bodies, and our spirits than ever before. We may find that memories, attitudes, and experiences that were previously outside our awareness will surface. This can be confusing and challenging. Fortunately, these will usually arise gradually during pregnancy, giving us the time we need to contemplate, digest, and process. Taking time for our internal work during pregnancy is important, as it will leave us much clearer for labor and birth.

This internal work can be as simple as writing in a journal, creating time for reflection about our emotional states. Dreams can also be an invaluable resource for our inner life, and our pregnancy dreams may be especially vivid and accurate. I recommend writing down and reflecting on any memorable dreams; you can even elaborate on them with fantasy (making up a story, or "dreaming on" further with the dream) or draw, paint, or sculpture them. A Jungian perspective is to take each dream element, from animate to inanimate objects, and ponder what aspect of your self is represented by each element.

As well as our solitary internal work, we may also need to check in regularly with our partner, if appropriate, to keep in tune and in harmony.

A partner can give us valuable support and feedback—and sometimes a very useful reality check! A close friend, therapist, or midwife can offer similar support or, if we are so lucky, a circle (or workshop) with friends or wise women can give us the space to share and experience our deepest feelings.

I also used artwork in my pregnancy with Zoe, filling five books with huge pastel mandalas (drawings based on a circle). These are now a wonderful record, and Zoe can see the pictures that I drew of her in my belly, which are a more personal—and more colorful—record than a photo from an ultrasound scan. It is amazing to compare the drawings I made of my four babies and to see how my simple pictures were often accurate reflections of their nature and development. For example, I found myself drawing Maia, my fourth baby, with an elaborate heart in early pregnancy, around the time when her physical heart was developing.

You can read more about this approach in the wonderful book *Birthing from Within*,[8] and there are also some beautiful and inspiring pregnancy journals available. I suggest that you avoid books with factual accounts of your body and baby, and see how it feels to explore—and learn to rely on—your own inner knowing.

Instinct and Energy

There are many wise women (and men) who have observed that our relationships with our loved ones are potent factors, and facets, at birth. Ina May Gaskin, for example, believes, "If a woman doesn't look like a Goddess in birth, someone isn't treating her right." Her book, *Spiritual Midwifery*,[9] has many stories about midwives acting to change the energy, often between the baby's mother and father, to help the processes of labor and birth.

Another of Ina May's insights, in terms of birthing energy, is that the energy that gets the baby in, can help to get the baby out. We can use her wisdom and allow ourselves free expression of emotion, especially loving and sexual feelings, with our partners in labor, if it feels right. As I describe in chapter 12, giving birth and making love both involve the release of large quantities of oxytocin, the hormone of love, and this hormone (and the feel-good things we can do to release it) can certainly pick up a slow or stuck labor.

The other major relationship that can affect birth energy, and our ability to birth instinctively, is the relationship between mothers and daughters, especially if the mother is present at the birth. I have heard women say that they could not give birth until their mother had left the room—and there are others for whom the opposite is true.

Finally, in her book, *Prenatal Yoga and Natural Childbirth,*[10] Jeannine Parvati Baker advises us to choose our helpers carefully because giving birth will not be easy, she cautions, unless every person present in the birth room has faith in the ability of the birthing woman.

Trusting Our Instincts

I experienced another powerful facet of instinctive birth through birthing my fourth baby unassisted, and this is a perspective that I see reflected in stories of both attended and unattended (unassisted) birth. During my labor with Maia, I had an exquisite awareness of her body inside me and of exactly where I was in labor. For me, this instinct was heightened because I had no observers or assistants, and because I had worked to trust my own instincts and body knowledge.

Many other women have similar stories about following their instincts and intuition when there was no help available. For example, Laura Shanley's pregnancy dream told her how to birth her footling breech without assistance;[11] and Leilah McCracken's son was stuck at his shoulders for several minutes, but then was born easily with one enormous contraction.[12]

Conversely, women have told me, sometimes many years later, that they wish they had acted on their instincts in pregnancy and birth, instead of going along with expert opinion. The decision to prioritize external advice above their instincts has had dire consequences for some of these women, and I conclude that, just as we have been naturally selected for our physical ability to birth, we—and all our foremothers—have been selected for our accurate instincts and intuition in birth.

This makes birth as safe as possible, and also tells us, as caregivers, that we should listen carefully to women's gut feelings in pregnancy, labor, and birth. This intuitive aspect of birth is easily clouded, especially when we are conditioned to favor information from the outside—medical and technological tests—over our own internal knowledge.

We are also more able to respond to our body's instincts when we fully inhabit our bodies. This can be challenging in our overly intellectual culture; however, the simple realization that we possess these intuitive capacities can bring a huge awakening in our instincts and intuition.

The Dance of Birth

Birth is also an instinctive act for all mammalian babies: in other words, our babies know how to get themselves born. This is true for babies in all positions, whose active participation in the birth process is amazing to witness. For example, in *Breech Birth Woman Wise*,[13] New Zealand midwife and author Maggie Banks includes photos of a breech baby, born to the waist, making cycling movements between his mother's contractions, which bring him down steadily and easily.

My third baby, Jacob, at age two, showed me how he pushed with his legs to "born myself [in the] water." Some people have called this "the dance of birth," and it reminds us that there are two partners, both instinctively primed for birth, and both moving together in this most exquisite of dances.

We can also bear in mind that "birth is as safe as life gets" and that there is nothing, whether total instinct or total reliance upon technology, that can guarantee a perfect outcome, a perfect dance, for every mother and baby. Tragedy and grief are also major facets of birth, as we know intuitively. We acknowledge this with our birth rituals, which, like those of all cultures, are designed to contain our natural and appropriate fear of these extraordinary and supernatural processes.

Finally . . .

Birth is vast and multifaceted; radiant and mysterious. Birth contains multitudes, and through her we birth our multitudes. We give birth to our hopes and our fears, to our ecstasies and our agonies, to our joy and our disappointments. We give birth to our babies, each one perfect and radiant. We give birth through our instincts, and we give birth to our instincts. We give birth to our capacity for instinct, which will match us perfectly with our babies, who are, and always will be, instinctive creatures.

May we all be blessed through instinctive birth.

Emma's Birth—Sweet and Oceanic

The birth of a first baby marks an initiation, and its importance cannot be overrated. I chose to have my first baby at home because I felt that this pivotal event was more likely to be gentle and easy, for both me and my baby, in familiar surroundings.

I would encourage all parents to make careful choices about this first birth, which is the most likely to involve maximum intervention in a standard setting—as Emma's birth might have, in other circumstances. I suggest, especially for this birth, committing time and money toward gentle birth choices; choosing skilled and considerate caregivers; trusting your instincts and your body; and maintaining awareness of the baby's perspective, so that your child also has a joyful initiation into family life.

Giving birth to Emma, my firstborn, was a pivotal experience in my life. Not only did she initiate me into motherhood, but she also taught me how immense and exciting birth can be, igniting an enduring passion for birth and mothering.

Emma was conceived in March 1990, a few months after Nicholas, my beloved, and I were married. This was our exact intention. I was challenged by nausea right through my pregnancy—in retrospect I think that my busy working life was a major factor—but it didn't stop me from relishing my pregnancy and the amazing changes that my body was going through. I was also nourished by my ongoing yoga practice, and I read every book I could find by Sheila Kitzinger, whose gentle approach to birth was inspiring and easy to absorb.

We chose to give birth at home, and found a midwife and doctor to help us without difficulty. I had attended many women in the hospital during my training as a family physician, and I had also been privileged to support two friends giving birth at home. I had seen a huge difference in the quality of experience between hospital and home birth. Also, Nicholas's sister Sue (who features in the story) was a homebirth midwife, and we were lucky to be influenced by her wisdom and experiences.

Another major influence at this time was my ongoing commitment to Jungian psychotherapy, where I had the opportunity to explore, at a deep level, my attitudes towards mothering, my early experiences of being mothered, and my relationship with my own mother. Working with my therapist on these issues during my pregnancy, often through dreams, brought me to a place of ease and helped me to make the transition to motherhood smoothly and gracefully.

I was certain of the date of Emma's conception and knew, without an ultrasound scan, that she was due in early December. In late October we were surprised to discover that our baby was already deeply engaged—her head was very low in my pelvis—and we wondered if we might have an early birth. I finished work in early November, expecting to have a month of resting and nesting . . . but this was not to be.

The weekend that Emma was born, around four weeks before her due date, Nicholas's sister Sue (the midwife) was staying in Melbourne, where we lived. (She was en route from her home in New Zealand to Hobart, an hour south by plane, where John, their father, was ill with cancer.) On that Sunday morning I was enjoying a leisurely backyard chat with Sue about birth. She told me that, in her experience, having a lot of support people at the birth could make the labor slower. This was important information; I already had four friends, plus my sister from New Zealand, enlisted as support people, although with the proviso that I might not call them all. Around the same time I began to notice that my usual pattern of mild tightenings was more pronounced, and that I had a little red discharge. In the afternoon, as we drove Sue across town to her friend's place, I timed my contractions—they were regularly ten minutes apart and on arrival I had a more obvious show of blood.

Sue suggested that we abandon our plan for a walk on the beach and have a quiet night instead. Back home I settled myself on the sofa, discovering that whenever I walked about the contractions became stronger. Nicholas cooked me a plate of delicious scrambled eggs and we talked about calling Chris, our midwife. I was reluctant—in denial, really—but eventually it became clear that we needed to talk to her. She came around about 10:00 P.M., examined me, and told me I was in early labor. Even though it was obvious to everyone else, I was still shocked to hear this. She advised us to have an early night and call her in the morning, when she expected labor to get going properly.

At 10:30 Nicholas and I were lying in bed together, coming to terms with this new development. I still had baby clothes to wash and sort, and hadn't put the second coat of paint in the spare room . . . but here was our baby, eager to come. So, as I lay down on the bed, Nicholas sorted the clothes and we realized that nothing else mattered. Our task was to accept this time, this labor, in the present moment.

With this surrender, labor really began for me. At first I found that moving around during contractions was most helpful; hanging off the closet door felt good too! I used the clock to help me in early labor, discovering that the most challenging part of my contractions lasted only about half a minute; after this, my body would come down off the wave, and I used my yoga training for deep relaxation in between. At the peak, breathing and, later, sound were my allies. As labor strengthened I rocked and circled with my pelvis, moaning and moving in synchrony.

It was a sweet and intimate space; the house was dark and quiet and, although I didn't want Nicholas to touch me (I found it too distracting), I felt held by his love and presence. There was an oceanic feeling; I felt like I was riding the waves, challenged but exhilarated as I came down each time. At one point Nicholas had tears in his eyes: "It's hard to see you in so much pain," he said. "I'm fine," I replied, "I get a good break in between, and I can really relax."

After a few hours, I said, "We need to call Chris." Nicholas was reluctant: "We are having such a beautiful time with the two of us . . . ." I agreed, but my instinct was still to call her.

He also called Sue, again rather reluctantly, but I was sure that I wanted her. In the half hour or so that it took for Chris to arrive, I began to feel a catch in my throat and a mild urge to push with each wave. Nicholas began to move the furniture around, as we had planned, putting our bed into the lounge, which could be easily heated for the birth.

A little after two in the morning, Chris came walking down the corridor and Nicholas said, "She's pushing." Chris turned around and went back out to get her birth equipment! By this time I was on all fours on the bed. I knew that my baby would be born soon, and I held some fears. She was early and little: would it be all right? I still remember the reassurance that I felt as I looked into Chris's eyes: I trusted her and knew that everything would be okay.

The pushing was the least enjoyable part of this labor for me—the rock-hard feeling of her head in my vagina, which I wanted to hold against—but every fiber of my body was pushing and pushing with each wave. Like the ocean, my body's instincts were immense and unstoppable.

My baby's watery sac was bulging and I agreed for Chris to break it. Soon after, she suggested that I roll onto my side, which felt good. I wanted things to be fast and they were. Within a few pushes, her head was born—face-up (posterior) to our surprise. Nicholas took a few amazing photos as her body was born. At the same time, Peter, our family physician, arrived, which was wonderful timing. It was

2:50 A.M. Chris caught her and put her on my belly, warm and wet. We discovered her sex straight away: "Oh, Emma!" I said. She was tiny and scrawny, like a little bald rabbit. We covered her—the hat we had was several sizes too big—and I held her tenderly. After five or ten minutes, her cord had stopped pulsating and Chris clamped and cut it. Her placenta came easily, twelve minutes after her birth and just before Sue arrived.

I was elated, amazed, and a bit shocked; it had been so fast and unexpected. We made phone calls a few hours later, waking my mother in New Zealand, who said sleepily: "That's nice, dear." When I rang her back later that day, she told us she hadn't believed me! Although small—in fact, at 5 pounds 1 ounce (2.25 kg) she was the smallest baby that either Chris or Peter had attended at home—Emma was alert and fed well.

In the days that followed we lavished our special care on her, checking her temperature regularly and dutifully recording her feeding and eliminating patterns. Her first pee, twelve or so hours after birth, was especially important as it indicated that she was being well fed from my early milk and didn't need supplementary feeding. Later she became moderately jaundiced and we used home phototherapy—a few minutes in the sun and sleeping her under the window.

Sue provided wonderful support and breastfeeding help, and Chris or Peter visited us twice daily for a week. Also friends (and the birth supporters whom we hadn't called) brought us meals and did our shopping. Emma and I stayed cocooned at home, venturing tentatively out to the corner store a week later with her snuggled in the front carrier. The shopkeeper said, "I thought you had a doll in there!" Nicholas had two weeks off work, and we had a peaceful and nourishing new-family baby moon.

When Emma was three weeks old my sister Louise arrived (as originally planned for the birth), giving us lots of help and support. Fortunately she was staying on with us when Nicholas was suddenly called to be with his dying father, and she later helped me to fly to Tasmania for the funeral. It was a blessing for Betty, Nicholas's mother, to have her newest grandchild in her arms, and there was a rightness to it for us too. As we had written in our wedding ceremony, we were ". . . part of the endless cycle of birth and death which, with its joys and sorrows, involves all of us."

I have many things to be grateful for in Emma's birth. I especially appreciate my caregivers—midwife extraordinaire Christine Shanahan and the wonderful Dr. Peter Lucas—who trusted that, early as we were, birth and baby would still be safe at home. I know, from training and experience in hospital obstetrics, how differently we would have fared in the hospital.

I am grateful also for the help and support of friends and family, who formed an outer circle which held us at this time. I am thankful, too, for the synchronicity that put Emma's birth several weeks ahead of Nicholas's father's death, and that gave me my sister's support at that difficult time. Finally, my deepest gratitude goes to Emma herself who, in her soul's wisdom, chose us as her parents and gave us a sweet and oceanic birth that set us joyfully on the path to parenting.

chapter 3

HEALING BIRTH,
HEALING THE EARTH

Childbirth is more than an individual, isolated event concerning a mother and her baby. Birth is a culturally and politically powerful act, whose domination represents domination of the feminine principle. This chapter asks us to consider Birth as a living entity whose survival is threatened, and inspires us to contribute our passion, love, surrender, and power toward her recovery, so that, as the late Jeannine Parvati Baker wished, we can heal the Earth by healing Birth.

Birth, she is dying.

This primal and unspeakably powerful initiation, the only road to motherhood for our ancestors, has been stripped of her dignity and purpose in our times. Birth has become a dangerous medical disease to be treated with escalating levels and types of technological interventions.

What is worse perhaps is that the ecstasy of Birth—her capacity to take us outside (*ec*) our usual state (*stasis*)—has been forgotten, and we are entering the sacred domain of motherhood postoperatively, even posttraumatically, rather than transformationally.

These deviations from the natural order, whose lore is genetically encoded in our bodies, have enormous repercussions.

We live in a society where new mothers experience unprecedented levels of distress and depression and our babies also show significant signs of stress, through colic, reflux, and sleep problems. We live in a society where depression and anxiety are among the largest burdens of disease worldwide, according to the World Health Organization; where children as young as four are being diagnosed with these conditions; and where young people, at the prime of their lives, are choosing in large numbers to opt out of reality with mind-altering drugs, or to opt out of life permanently through suicide.

More than this, we have set ourselves as a species on the road to self-destruction through our despoiling of our collective mother, the Earth. The havoc that we wreak through waste and greed has many parallels with our treatment of mothers and babies and of our primal environment—our mother's womb.

And just as we have pitted ourselves against the Earth, forgetting that we are interdependent, so too have we begun to pit the rights of the baby against the rights of the mother, imagining a separation, a competition, that does not and cannot exist.

The wounds of Birth and of the Earth are severe but, as the Goddess Hygieia tells us, "The wound reveals the cure."[1] My belief is that we are suffering in birth from lack of passion, of love, of surrender, and from a misunderstanding of our own power, and I believe that these qualities can provide us with a way of healing Birth and, at the same time, healing the Earth.

Passion

We all began our lives in a passionate act. Our human bodies crave the intensity and pleasure that sex brings, and many cultures have recognized the capacity for healing that is inherent in the sexual act. Why is sex so powerful? As well as giving us the potential to create new life—the ultimate power—sex involves peak experiences, and peak hormone levels, of love, pleasure, excitement, and tenderness. These hormones (our bodies' chemical messengers) and their actions are exactly the same as those of birth.

In other words, giving birth is, inherently and hormonally, a passionate and sexual act. From the perspective of hormone activity in both mother and baby, we could say that birth is the most passionate experience that we will ever have.

Oxytocin, the hormone of love, builds up during labor, reaching peak levels at the moment of birth and creating loving, altruistic feelings between mother and baby. Endorphins, hormones of pleasure and transcendence, also peak at birth, as do the hormones epinephrine and norepinephrine (adrenaline and noradrenaline). These fight-or-flight hormones protect the baby from lack of oxygen in the final stages of birth and ensure that mother and baby are both wide-eyed and excited at first contact. Prolactin, the mothering hormone, helps us to surrender to our babies, giving us the tenderest of maternal feelings as our reward.

But these passionate hormones are not just feel-good add-ons. They actually orchestrate the physical processes of birth (and sexual activity) and enhance safety, ease, and pleasure for both mother and baby. This hormonal cocktail also rewards birthing mothers with the experience of ecstasy and fulfillment, making us want to give birth again and again. All mammals share virtually the same hormonal crescendo at birth, which is a necessary prerequisite for mothering in most species and switches on instinctive maternal behavior.

Birthing passionately does not necessarily mean birthing painlessly (although this may happen for some women). Giving birth is a huge event, emotionally and physically, and will make demands on the body equivalent to, for example, running a marathon. But when a woman feels confident in her body, well supported, and able to express herself without inhibition, the pain that she may feel can become bearable and just one part of the process. She can then respond instinctively with her own resources, including her most basic and accessible tools: breath, sound, and movement.

The problem in our times is that the passion of birth is neither recognized nor accommodated. Birth has become a dispassionate medical event, usually occurring in a setting that discourages emotional expression. If we are to reclaim our birthing passion, we must give ourselves permission to birth passionately, and we must choose our birth setting and birth attendants with this in mind. Birth in these circumstances will be more straightforward, with enhanced hormonal flow and less need for interventions, helping us to step into new motherhood with confidence and grace.

Passion, to my mind, is an opposite of despair and depression and an antidote for both conditions. This is clear physiologically and hormonally. If we give birth, and are born, in passion, how different will our primal emotional imprint be? And what about our brain chemistry, which is being set even as we are born? Some studies have linked exposure to drugs and medical procedures at birth with an increased risk of drug addiction, suicide, and antisocial behavior in later life, and other commentators have suggested that contemporary problems such as learning disorders and ADHD may also be linked to drugs and interventions at birth.

As a birthing mother I have both witnessed and experienced the enormous passion that can be unleashed at birth and that can fuel both passionate motherhood and a lifetime's work on behalf of mothers, babies, and the Earth. I ask: "Can we afford, as a species, to be born—and to give birth—dispassionately?"

Love

Passion and love are as powerful a combination at birth as they are in sexual activity. And in birth, as in sex, we release oxytocin, the hormone of love, in huge quantities from deep inside our brain. Here again, our hormones are directing us toward optimal and ecstatic experiences, yet this system is also extremely vulnerable to interference.

For example, a laboring woman's production of oxytocin is drastically reduced by the use of epidural pain relief—this is why epidurals prolong labor. And even when an epidural has worn off, the woman's oxytocin peak, which causes the powerful final contractions that are designed to birth her baby quickly and easily, will still be significantly lessened, and she is more likely to have her baby pulled out with forceps as a result.

The drug Pitocin (Syntocinon), which has been called the most abused drug in obstetrics, is also implicated. A synthetic form of the hormone oxytocin, it is used for induction and for augmentation (or acceleration) of labor. The majority of women giving birth in the United States receive large doses of this drug in labor for one of these reasons.

When a laboring woman has Pitocin administered intravenously for many hours, her body's oxytocin receptors will lose their sensitivity and ability to respond to this hormone. We know that women in this situation are vulnerable to hemorrhage after birth, and even more Pitocin becomes necessary to counter that risk. (See chapter 6.)

We do not know, however, what the long-term consequences of interference with the oxytocin system may be for mothers and babies and for their ongoing relationship. Animal models suggest that hormonal interference close to birth may produce lifelong deviations in hormones and behavior.

I had a very powerful experience of oxytocin as the hormone of love while laboring with my fourth baby, Maia Rose. As the waves of labor strengthened I found myself looking into the eyes of my beloved, telling him "I love you, I love you, I love you . . ." as each wave of labor washed over me. This ecstatic experience has created more love in my heart, in our relationship, and in our family, and has taught me, in a very physical way, that giving birth is also making love.

Surrender

Surrender is not a popular virtue in the West. In fact, surrender is often seen as a weakness in our culture; we are instead encouraged to be active and in control of our lives. This very yang, masculine attitude may serve us in some circumstances, but we cannot birth our babies through sheer force of will. We need to learn the more subtle—yet equally powerful— path of surrender.

I sense that, for modern women, difficulty with surrender can reflect a lack of confidence in our female bodies. This is not surprising when our society is distrustful of the natural order in general and women's bodies in particular. This view is further reinforced by the obstetric model, with its long lists of all that can possibly go wrong with our birthing bodies, and its myriad of technological fixes, designed to rescue us from these exaggerated dangers.

Surrender can be particularly problematic for women who have experienced some form of violation or abuse in the past, especially sexual abuse. Women with this history need particularly sensitive and supportive care in labor and birth, so that they can feel safe enough to surrender.

Along with this forgetting of the awesome but natural power of our female bodies, we have also lost our birthing patrons: the goddesses and saints who have, for millennia, guided women through this transition, where the veil between life and death is at its thinnest. Today this guidance is available to us, when and if we need it, in the living form of a midwife: a woman who has pledged to be with (*mid*) women (*wyfe*) in birth. A good midwife can remind us by her presence that we genetically carry the birthing successes of all our foremothers and that we already know how to give birth.

As midwife and author Jeannine Parvati Baker reminds us, giving birth is women's spiritual practice, requiring "purity in strength, flexibility, health, concentration, surrender and faith."[2] It has also been said that to be consciously present at birth is equivalent to seven years of meditation. When we birth consciously, putting our great rational mind on hold and allowing our instinctive nature to dominate, we can access the wisdom that all spiritual traditions teach: that the ego is our servant, not our mistress, and that our path to ecstasy and enlightenment involves surrendering our egoistic notions of control. This level of surrender will also serve us well through our many years of motherhood.

When we surrender conscious control, we also allow our deeper innate rhythms to surface: this can be a profound experience for a birthing woman. In allowing her labor to go at its own pace, without hurry or interference, a woman learns to trust her own, and her baby's, natural rhythms. Such trust is another gift; another way that Mother Nature ensures optimal mothering and maximum survival for our young.

In surrendering to birth, we also learn about our role on the Earth: we are neither the rulers nor the architects of creation. Life comes through us, simply and gracefully, when we allow it.

Power

It is easy to say that our problems in birth stem from the excessive power of the medical system and its agents, and a lack of power for the birthing woman. However, a deeper analysis is necessary, I believe, because the time has come to dispel the idea of a power imbalance and to assert our innate authority in birthing.

We live in a culture that prizes, and puts its faith in, technology. We reward those, such as physicians, who are masters of technology—and indeed we are fortunate to have their skills available to us when we need them. And even though we may want less technology in birth, we are witnessing more and more litigation against obstetricians, almost all of which blames them for not using enough technology.

Along with technology, we also prize information. In pregnancy and birth, becoming informed is equated with being responsible, both of which are strongly encouraged culturally; yet there is also a price to pay. We may have all of the information in the world, but we cannot predict our experiences in birth. And we diminish our own authority in birthing and in mothering—we disempower ourselves—when we put more faith in information from the outside (tests, scans, others' opinions) than our own internal knowing of our bodies and our babies.

The truth is that our babies are constantly informing us of their needs and desires and how we can best care for them. This is a physiological reality—the baby's placenta is in constant communication with our bodies, transferring blood and nutrients and generating the placental hormones that organize our bodies and our psyches for the optimal and specific mothering that this baby requires. In the same way, our cravings, yearnings, dreams, and inclinations in pregnancy can be communications from our babies, showing us the deeper ways of knowing that are richer and more true, even if less numerical or detailed, than information from the outside, such as medical tests.

In fact, from the very beginning, when we first suspect that we are creating new life in our womb, we can use this ancient system and allow our bodies, rather than a pregnancy test, to inform us. Often the truth will unfold gradually, allowing us the space to learn and adapt at our own pace, and giving us opportunities for reflection and dreaming.

When we choose this path, the path of our foremothers, we can both discover and reinforce an inalienable trust and power in ourselves and in our female bodies. This deep faith is the best preparation possible for birth and is also, to my mind, the basis of true responsibility; we are able to respond with our own truth. We also become able to use the medical system, if we choose, without giving away our power.

Beyond this, when we tap into women's ways of knowing, we can open channels of communication with our babies, enhancing the psychic powers of communication that Mother Nature intends for mothers of all species. Mothering can become a meditation, a deep mindfulness that is satisfying spiritually as well as physically and emotionally. I believe that this is nature's intent and a possibility for all of us.

How would it be to live in a society where we are all, through giving birth or being born, in possession of our own power and our own deep knowing? Where science and technology are our tools, rather than our masters? How differently would we treat our babies? How differently would we treat each other? How differently would we treat the Earth?

Birth is dying, but, like cells in her body, we each have the power to enliven her and to resurrect her in all her glory. What is needed, I believe, is the collective passion, love, surrender, and power that we pour into the ether as we birth our babies.

And in healing Birth, we are healing ourselves, our babies, and the Earth.

Zoe's Birth–Challenge and Transformation

Each birth is a unique event, an alchemical reaction between the deepest, truest, and most acute energies of mother and baby, father, family, friends, and caregivers. And birth, like chemistry, creates more than the sum of its parts: mother, father, baby can be permanently transformed in these few hours. Of my four births, Zoe's birth, my second, was my most challenging but also the most transformative. Zoe's birth changed me in ways I still do not understand, reflecting the ultimate mystery of birth and its perfection in making me the mother that Zoe needs me to be. With this birth, I was grateful to be at home, where I could own the issues confronting me, and not have them overlaid by medical drugs and intervention. Through giving birth to Zoe, I was privileged to learn more about the capacity of my birthing body and to expand my faith in my ability to surrender: capacities that have served me well in subsequent births and through my many years of mothering.

Every year, on my children's birthdays, I tell them their birth stories. Although these stories are repeated year after year, the birthday child is each time engrossed by the drama, the circumstances, and the roles of all players in their first entrance into the world.

But it's not always the same story. My version of the story changes as we—both mother and child—discover more about ourselves and each other. And my children's memories of birth, sharp and potent in the early years, tend to fade with time, so their input also is different every year.

The story of Zoe's birth, told most recently to her fourteen-year-old self, is perhaps the most elusive and mysterious. Like Zoe, this story is quixotic; indefinable; difficult to summarize, categorize, or title. But time has unfolded more of its riches, its exquisite texture and teaching, and I have come to understand more of its importance and its role in making me the mother that Zoe needed—and still needs—me to be, for her own beautiful unfolding.

The story begins, naturally, with her conception. After six months of "trying to conceive," I spent five transformative days in a Women's Mysteries workshop,[1] menstruating during that time and conceiving Zoe soon after returning home. Several tired and nauseated weeks followed, and I yearned to be alone, out in the forest somewhere, rather than in a hot Australian summer with a houseful of Christmas holiday guests.

During this time, I had several days of aching in my pelvis, and felt concerned that I could miscarry. My instinctive response was to dance, using Brazilian rhythms and hip swirls to spiral this ambivalent baby deeper into my pelvis and anchor her into my womb. (My personal belief is that our babies choose whether to stay or go, but I felt some room for influence here.) At three months, while on holiday in New Zealand, I dreamed that I miscarried a tiny baby, with no cord. Understanding the meaning, I focused on connecting with this new soul, despite my fears about displacing my precious Emma, just two.

Once I had committed to my baby and to this journey, there seemed so much inner work to do; more than I had ever attempted, and probably more than I have since needed to do. From before conception, I drew large pastel mandalas—pictures based on circles—of my journey, and later embarked on bodywork and rebirthing. I also took Sunrider Chinese herbs through the pregnancy, which soothed my nausea, and I began a delicious and long-term habit of regular massage.

I was drawn to water, and I swam during this pregnancy, partly as a substitute for the yoga that my chiropractor advised me to stop (although with more expert advice, I could likely have modified my practice to care for my delicate sacroiliac joints). I also booked my baby-to-be into baby swim classes and, with some trepidation, resigned from my steady family practice job. I agreed to fill in for my colleague, a family physician who was attending homebirths, and committed to bring my new baby along to work in his small solo family practice from three to eight months postpartum.

Within all of this exploration and change, I saw (and drew) myself as a bright butterfly, emerging from a cocoon. My baby was always green, filled with life, as the Greek name Zoe means. I also drew some rich pictures of her in-womb placenta, reflecting my growing awareness of and respect for this organ, which we had chosen to honor through lotus birth, or non-severance of the cord. (See the story "Jacob's Placenta," page 185, for more about lotus birth, in which the umbilical cord is not clamped or cut.)

With a mixture of arrogance and ignorance, I presumed that my butterfly-like emergence—my baby's birth—would be easy and smooth, perhaps even easier than the five-hour "sweet and oceanic" birth I had enjoyed with my first baby (see the story "Emma's Birth, page 20). However, as my doctor warned me when I confided my prediction that my lively green baby would be born on the first day of spring, "These things keep us humble."

I was prepared well in advance of my "due date" with this pregnancy because of my previous month-early birth. I relished the last heavy weeks that I had missed with Emma, enjoying rest, massage, walks, and even joyous dancing with my family at our community bush dance.

In the week preceding labor, I had several episodes of nighttime contractions, all subsiding by morning. After a few tiring nights, my midwife suggested I take some homeopathic caullophyllum to encourage this "false labor." I wondered how deeply into myself this baby might take me.

At 7:00 A.M., exactly on my "due date," I had a sudden powerful contraction while breastfeeding Emma. "This is how real labor feels," I remembered, and with that labor began. I called my midwife Christine and birth support Ginny, warning them that they might need to come over later in the day. Chris came quickly, thinking that it might be a fast and easy birth.

But this was not to be. Contractions were regular and painful through the morning, and I was loved and supported by Nicholas and Emma, who massaged my shoulders. Aromatherapy—a gorgeous blend of rose and jasmine oils—also helped me through some slow patches. Late in the morning I cocooned myself in the bedroom, away from the growing company, to focus on my labor. From this point, perhaps, the birth could have been quick but in my heart I wasn't ready to meet my baby.

One important photo shows me lying on my back, the only time I did this during labor, to hug with Nicholas and Emma, as a last "happy family." In this position, I felt my baby move; only later did I realize that she had turned posterior, making contractions slower. Although this shift made my labor more difficult and painful, it also gave me the time that I needed and perhaps also served Zoe, who later told me she hadn't wanted to come down.

Although my baby was now posterior, I did not experience back pain, and we figured out her position only when progress was slow and more painful in the early afternoon. Chris examined me and found her to be posterior, with a rim of cervix—an "anterior lip"—preventing her from moving down. At this point, I found water soothing, and I spent time in the shower, hanging off the shower walls (which my concerned husband supported from the other side!) with each contraction,

Chris called my doctor, Peter, who arrived around 2:00 P.M. and had to take off his shoes to examine me in the shower, much to Emma's amusement. Peter offered to break my waters, which I agreed to. Once out of the shower, I let him hold the lip of my cervix back while I pushed my baby's head through.

Through this intense time, sound was a strong ally, helping me to express my body's feelings and to find my surrender into the unknown. I was grateful to be at home, where I had loud, uninhibited freedom, and to be with caregivers who were familiar with my predicament and were not offended, even when I swore at them! Emma and her helper Ginny were a little reserved, especially at the noisy height of my contractions, but it felt good to have them nearby. Nicholas was my rock, and I clung to his neck as I half-squatted to birth this baby, just as I had depicted in drawings earlier.

Once Zoe was past my worried cervical lip, the pain eased and she was born, face up (persistent occipito-posterior, or POP) with relief and only a few pushes. My midwife Chris caught her and passed her through my legs, and I collapsed on the floor. I felt enormous surprise and pleasure, merging into ecstasy, as I held my warm, wet, soft, new baby. Her placenta soon followed with ease and no cutting, a perfect shape for the bag I had sewn. Her sex was a surprise for all of us (with the exception of Emma, who had predicted a sister). She went to my chest, skin, breast, and we bathed in her radiance and softness.

My face in those early photos has no lingering hint of pain, but Nicholas looks drawn and exhausted, reminding me that the role of birth supporter is also enormous, but without the ability to release the energy and fear through noise and movement.

Although Zoe's birth had been medically uncomplicated and had involved only minor intervention, the experience impacted me enormously. In the days, weeks, and months that followed, I went through layers of tears and sadness, and I felt much of my old self falling away.

Zoe's presence earthside soothed me enormously through this time: she had a beautiful, calming energy and she later told me that she had loved being a baby. Even through the stressful months in which I worked as a family physician and attended homebirths, she was balanced and happy in my arms or sling and on my breast.

Looking back, I can see the enormous changes that Zoe's birth brought to me. Before Zoe, I was a different creature—cocooned, perhaps—with a harder exterior woven with my thoughts and worries. Zoe's birth ripped me apart, but somehow with compassion and tenderness. Her birth and ongoing presence brought me the gifts of soft resilience; surrender rather than effort as a path; the ability to hold opposing perspectives; and, yes, a sense of freedom and flight.

Is it surprising that Zoe, on the verge of womanhood, tells me that her peak circus skill is Lyra (the aerial hoop) with which she can fly high with pleasure, skill, and daring?

chapter 4

YOUR BODY, YOUR BABY, YOUR CHOICE
A Guide to Making Wise Decisions

The number of decisions that women are now facing, even in an un-complicated pregnancy, is immense. This chapter gives some general principles and guidelines for making informed choices and also specific information to help with decision-making about screening for gestational diabetes, testing for group B strep in late pregnancy, and induction for "going overdue."

Women's experiences of pregnancy and birth have changed enormously in the past few decades. For example, our grandmothers and great-grandmothers may have accessed medical or midwifery care, but their pregnancies would have been overwhelmingly social rather than medical experiences, and neither their bodies nor their babies would have been subjected to the intense scrutiny and complex decision-making that twenty-first-century pregnancy, labor, and birth bring.

The medicalization of pregnancy begins in the earliest days and weeks, with a series of choices and tests offered at regular intervals over the next nine months. Today's parents need to make important and unprecedented decisions; for example:

- Which care provider will we choose?
- What tests will we have for mother and baby?
- What will we do if our baby is discovered to have a major abnormality during pregnancy?
- Where will our baby be born?
- Will we agree to a scheduled induction or cesarean?

Even today the complexity of these choices is increasing, as research-ers seek more ways to prevent common (and not-so-common) problems for mothers and babies. This is a worthy aim; however, like many tech-nological advances, the new drugs and treatments associated with these preventative measures can also have side effects for mother and baby. And because of the delicate balance of the pregnant woman's body, and the extreme vulnerability of her unborn baby, obstetric drugs and procedures are particularly liable to cause long-lasting side effects, many of which have been discovered only in retrospect.

These include the use of X-ray on pregnant women from the 1930s, which was discovered to increase the risk of cancer in exposed children only in 1956;[1] the use of diethylstilbestrol (DES), prescribed for threat-ened miscarriage from 1938 to 1971, which has been found to increase the risks of reproductive problems including infertility, miscarriage, prema-ture labor, and clear-cell cancers in exposed daughters, with effects even into the third generation;[2] and the recent use of misoprostol (Cytotec) for induction in women with a prior cesarean, which was discovered to dramatically increase the risks of uterine rupture only after it had been in use for several years. Moreover, many—in fact, most—obstetric drugs and interventions have not been tested for long-term effects, apart from birth defects, on exposed offspring.

It is now more important than ever for modern parents to be closely involved in decision-making and to carefully consider the choices that their care providers offer. This means making sense of complicated infor-mation not only intellectually but also with hearts and instincts. Today's parents also need ready access to obstetric technology when necessary, to get the most benefits with the least harm for mother and baby.

Accessing the best care and least harm may involve parents' assert-ing their wishes and desires over conventional care or "expert opinion." This can be very challenging, especially when it is the first encounter with the medical system. However, it is important to remember that it will be the parents, not the health-care professionals, who will live with consequences of these choices, so it is extremely important for parents to speak up for themselves and their babies.

This chapter offers a simple model that can be used in any decision-making situation, along with information about three common choices and interventions that are offered to expectant parents: testing for gestational diabetes; screening and treatment for group B strep; and induction for going overdue. Information on procedures such as ultrasound, epidurals, cesareans, cord clamping and cord blood banking, and homebirth are covered in separate chapters.

Making Decisions:
The BRAN Model for Parents-to-Be

This model uses an easily remembered formula to help make decisions. When you are offered a test or intervention, BRAN reminds you to ask about and consider the Benefits, Risks, and Alternatives and to also consider the effects of doing Nothing in this situation.

The benefits are usually easy to identify: in fact, this is what most health-care providers will mention first. Benefits will obviously depend on your situation, and you may even find that procedures that you had planned to avoid will be beneficial in some circumstances. For example, as described in chapter 9, sometimes unexpected complications will mean that there is a very good reason to accept a scheduled cesarean.

Health-care providers also will generally inform you of the major known risks, but you may need to do some of your own research to uncover all the risks of various procedures: this book provides information that may be helpful as well. There may also be major risks that are as yet unknown, because medical knowledge relies on researchers' formulating the right questions and having the funding and ability to conduct high-quality research to uncover all the implications of particular treatments. This can take many years.

It is also important to realize that care providers have their own beliefs and experiences, consistent with their personal and professional backgrounds. This may lead care providers to exaggerate some risks and underplay others. For example, obstetricians may emphasize the safety of cesarean surgery over vaginal birth, whereas midwives may emphasize the risks; the opposite is likely to be true for homebirth, with obstetricians emphasizing risks and midwives the benefits. Read on for more about risks.

Alternative courses of action may be difficult to find, as obstetrics has generally not explored or researched many alternatives to high-technology care, perhaps because of the belief that technology is always best for mothers and babies. Formal research into alternatives may also suffer from lack of funding. You may need to dig deep to find alternatives.

However, you can draw on the expertise and experience of other parents, and you may find that Internet support groups and parents' chat sites have a lot to offer. Be aware that this information is subjective and likely not tested scientifically. You may also wish to access the huge body of midwifery knowledge, either online (see www.sarahjbuckley.com for suggested sites) or by contacting a midwife in your area.

Midwives are the experts in normal birth, and they usually have excellent skills in exploring alternatives and facilitating decision-making. Other professionals who may have expertise in these areas include naturopaths, homeopaths, osteopaths, chiropractors, and traditional Chinese medicine (TCM) practitioners.

The *N* element of BRAN reminds you to ask: what if we do nothing? This is a valid alternative most of the time—although, because medicine is usually focused on "doing something," this course of action may be uncomfortable and even unknown for your care providers. Again, you may want to access midwifery knowledge, other practitioners, and/or other parents who have made this choice.

Choosing to do nothing can also be helpful in giving you more space to consider your options. You may want to check if it will be possible to later change your decision. Choosing to not accept a medical test for you or your baby may help you to avoid the "nocebo effect" (more on this later). Professional groups generally uphold the right of their patients/ clients to make an "informed refusal" of treatment, as I discuss in the following section.

Informed Choice

Using the BRAN model is an excellent way to make sure you have all the information that you need to make an informed choice. It is the duty of your health-care practitioner to provide this information in an understandable way. As the American College of Obstetricians and Gynecologists (ACOG) comments, "Patients are entitled to participate with their physician in a process of shared decision-making."[3]

Please remember that informed choice, including informed refusal, is your right in every situation in most countries of the world, even when you choose a path that could be considered life-threatening for your baby.

For example, the judicial system in most countries would not legally force a pregnant woman to undergo a cesarean for the welfare of her baby, just as they would not force a mother to undergo major surgery to donate an organ that would save the life of her child. The UK Royal College of Obstetricians and Gynecologists (RCOG) states, "If a competent woman refuses delivery by caesarean section, even after full consultation and explanation of the consequences for the fetus, her wishes must be respected."[4]

The American College of Obstetricians and Gynecologists (ACOG) Ethics committee further counsels members: "In the absence of extraordinary circumstances, circumstances that in fact, the Committee on Ethics cannot currently imagine, judicial authority should not be used to implement treatment regimens aimed at protecting the fetus."[5] However, there have been instances of court-ordered cesareans in some U.S. states.

ACOG offers this comment about informed refusal: "Once a patient has been informed of the material risks, benefits and alternatives, as well as the option to refuse, the patient has the right to exercise complete autonomy in deciding whether to undergo the recommended medical treatment, surgical procedure, or diagnostic test; to choose among a variety of treatments, procedures or tests; or to refuse to undergo these treatments, procedures or tests."[6]

Risks and "Soft Outcomes"

The concept of risk has come to dominate—one might say strangulate—discussions about choices in birth. Risk, which was originally a technical term used in merchant insurance,[7] is now used as sole justification for access to, or denial of, many options in maternity care, including vaginal breech birth and vaginal birth after cesarean (VBAC), even though the principles of informed consent and informed refusal are legally and ethically paramount.

It is important to realize that the obstetric concept of risk is based almost exclusively on measures of perinatal mortality (PNM): the chance of a baby dying around the time of birth. This is obviously an important outcome, but is also very narrow. It does not encompass, for example, possible risks to the physical or emotional well-being of mother or baby, nor include risks to the establishment of breastfeeding and attachment: processes that have been crucial for successful human survival for millennia and that are still vitally important today.

These factors—the physical and emotional well-being of mother and baby, and breastfeeding and attachment—are interrelated, and intrinsically connected with the processes of labor and birth. As described in chapter 6, the "ecstatic hormones" of labor and birth are designed to enhance safety, ease, and pleasure, and also optimize breastfeeding and attachment for mother and baby. For example, the late-labor surges of epinephrine and norepinephrine give energy and alertness to mother and baby at birth, priming both for an easy start to breastfeeding, and the peaks of oxytocin in the postpartum hour imprint love and connection for both partners and also enhance breastfeeding success.

It is therefore not surprising that, when we begin to interfere with the hormones and processes of labor and birth, we also risk losing ease, pleasure, and emotional well-being. In some situations, safety can also be compromised. Similarly, because breastfeeding and attachment are linked to the innate system of ecstatic birth, these longer-term processes can also be causalities of obstetric interference.

As described in chapters 11 and 12, breastfeeding and attachment are crucial for the ongoing physical and emotional well-being of our offspring, increasing the chances that they will survive and thrive to reproductive age and successfully produce more offspring who will survive and thrive. Because breastfeeding and attachment have been so critical to reproductive success and therefore to species survival, we could say that the evolutionary (and perhaps divine) purpose of labor and birth, in addition to producing a healthy mother and baby, is to ensure that mother and baby are optimally attached and will successfully breastfeed.

Breastfeeding and attachment will also benefit family well-being. Mother Nature intends that mother and baby will continue to share joy; reward; early, easy, and ongoing breastfeeding; and a continuing pleasurable mutual addiction, all reinforced by the ecstatic hormones—oxytocin, beta-endorphin, and prolactin—that are released with physical contact and breastfeeding. Mother Nature's recipe will ensure an ideal start to family life, creating ease and pleasure for the new father and other family members as well.

However, the importance of breastfeeding and attachment remains unrecognized under medicalized maternity care, with little attention toward or research into the impact of medical interventions on these "soft outcomes." There is even less research into the effects of medicalized births (including cesareans) on the emotional well-being of mother and baby, including serious outcomes such as postnatal depression (PND).

Note that, cross-culturally and historically, maternity care systems have always prioritized women's emotional well-being, from pregnancy through to postpartum, with special emphasis on loving care and support during labor and birth. Some traditional maternity systems have also considered the impact of birth care practices on the baby, who is an aware and extremely sensitive participant in these processes.[8]

More about Perinatal Mortality

It is also important to remember that measures of PNM only tell us how many babies will die (and how many will survive) during the few weeks that surround birth. PNM figures (usually expressed as "perinatal mortality rate," PNMR) do not tell us the risks of other serious medium- or long-term physical or behavioral problems for mother or baby that may be related to obstetric interventions at birth. Such possible outcomes are very poorly researched, although the published studies in this area give cause for concern: see chapter 6 and Michel Odent's important work.[9–11]

Parents must also understand that PNMR is actually an epidemiological measure based on population studies that assess this in relation to different conditions and treatments. These studies can give a general idea of risk and are usually used as the basis of obstetric advice, but they cannot predict the outcome in a specific situation. For example, although the PNMR increases somewhat after forty-two weeks, as described below, this does not mean that a woman who refuses induction at this time will endanger her baby's life, as she may be told.

Further, in high-income countries, PNM has reached very low levels, so that the capacity for obstetric interventions to further reduce this figure is fairly small. In western countries, the major causes of PNM are now stillbirth and prematurity, neither of which have been prevented (and in some places are actually increasing) under current obstetric care. Small gains in PNM may therefore require large numbers of interventions on healthy women, as we will discuss in detail.

These considerations do not negate the importance of PNM as an obstetric outcome. However, in modern times, we need wider consideration and measurement of the outcomes of maternity care. As a mother, I want my babies to do more than merely survive the birth; I want my children be as whole in brain and body as possible, without interfering with the development that is programmed into every human newborn, so that each can become the complete, happy, and loving person that it is our human birthright to be.

Because of this intense and extremely narrow focus on PNM—the bare bones of infant survival—and relative neglect of "soft" outcomes and long-term effects, all of which can enormously impact mother, baby, and family, we need to assess medical information on safety and risk using broader criteria, rather than accept standard medical definitions.

I suggest that, when making informed choices, mothers, fathers, and families gather the information that they need using BRAN, and also:

- Prioritize their feelings and instincts
- Take account of effects on emotional well-being, including that of their baby
- Think long-term
- Consider the possible impact on breastfeeding and attachment

The Nocebo Effect

"Nocebo effect" refers to the unintended negative effect of a medical diagnosis or treatment. It is particularly relevant to maternity care, because the mother's emotional well-being is so often neglected, as we have discussed. Michel Odent comments, "The nocebo effect is inherent in conventional prenatal care, which is constantly focusing on potential problems. Every visit is an opportunity to be reminded of all the risks associated with pregnancy and delivery."[12]

In addition to increasing worry for pregnant women, the nocebo effect may contribute to adverse outcomes by increasing the levels of stress hormones.[13] High levels of stress hormones in pregnancy increase the risks of prematurity and low birth weight, and they can cause damage to the developing brain that leads to conditions such as ADHD and learning difficulties, with possible lifelong effects on offspring.[14]

The nocebo effect reminds us how important it is to guard emotional well-being in pregnancy and to choose caregivers who will increase joy, rather than reinforce fear and worry, at this time. Odent, who emphasizes the importance of joy in pregnancy, recommends that practitioners "create such interactions that a pregnant woman feels even happier after a prenatal visit than before . . . or at least less anxious."[13] This is an excellent rule of thumb with which to evaluate maternity care and caregivers.

We can help to counteract the nocebo effect through activities that give joy and physical pleasure: for example, regular massage in pregnancy will reduce stress and may even reduce the risk of giving birth prematurely.[15, 16] Rest, relaxation, and regular exercise are also very useful, and tuning in to the baby will often give reassurance when worries arise.

Using the BRAN Model

This model can be used in any decision-making and is especially relevant to maternity care. The following information uses this model to help you to make an informed choice in relation to:

- Testing for gestational diabetes
- Screening for Group B strep
- Induction when pregnancy is "overdue"

Please note that I bring some of my own bias to this information: my trust in the natural process, for the vast majority of women; my skepticism about the benefits of exposing large numbers of mothers and babies to significant interventions to prevent very uncommon problems; my own experience of going three weeks past my original due date and electing to have no testing or induction; and my choice to use alternative treatment for a positive Group B strep swab in late pregnancy.

Testing for Gestational Diabetes

Gestational diabetes mellitus (GDM) is defined as an elevated blood glucose (the body's primary sugar) that is first diagnosed in pregnancy. You are likely to be offered screening for GDM in mid- to late pregnancy and will need to decide whether to accept this.

Background

A diagnosis of diabetes generally signals that the hormone insulin is not working efficiently in the body, where its role is to clear glucose from the bloodstream and take it into the cells for use as an energy source. When insulin is not fulfilling this role, because of insufficient levels or because its effects are counteracted in some way (insulin resistance), glucose builds up in the bloodstream. Outside of pregnancy, high blood glucose levels (hyperglycemia) can cause detrimental effects on the body, especially if levels are very high, or if mild to moderate elevations continue for years.

However, diabetes during pregnancy is usually a mild condition that develops only in the later months, involves glucose levels that are generally insufficient to cause major short-term effects for the pregnant woman, and in fact usually causes no symptoms. Also, GDM is self-limiting by definition, so that women with GDM are not susceptible to these long-term effects.

However, women who are diagnosed with GDM are more likely to develop diabetes in the following years, as we will describe. It is also possible that some women who are first diagnosed with diabetes during pregnancy have actually had mild, undiagnosed diabetes prior to the pregnancy, which becomes "unmasked" because of the insulin-resisting effects of pregnancy hormones. Note also that mild hyperglycemia is a normal and important adaptation in pregnancy, due to these hormonal effects. This increase in maternal glucose levels ensures that an adequate amount of this essential fuel can easily cross the placenta and supply energy to the growing baby.

What is most controversial in this area are the possible effects of GDM on the baby—including effects during pregnancy, in the newborn period, and also in later life—and also whether treating the pregnant woman for GDM will benefit her baby at any of these times. Any possible benefits also need to be weighed against the expense (medical, financial, and personal) of the tests and treatment.

This is a rather difficult area for decision-making, as experts have very different opinions on the importance of diagnosing and treating GDM, and the medical evidence is still reasonably inconclusive about the possible benefits. These issues are compounded by different tests and definitions for GDM and by a lack of large high-quality studies in this area.

Screening for GDM

In medicine, "screening" means testing people without signs or symptoms of a particular condition in order to find those who are at high risk. Those with positive screening results, indicting higher risk of the condition, will then be offered a diagnostic test, which can definitely diagnose the condition but which is generally more expensive and sometimes more risky than the screening test.

Screening for GDM usually involves drinking a high-glucose drink containing 50 to 100 grams of glucose, the equivalent of ten to twenty teaspoons of sugar. Blood glucose levels are tested in the following hour or so. There are several different systems using different glucose loads, different timing, and different cutoff values.

If results are high (a positive screen), a full oral glucose tolerance test (OGTT) is usually required to definitively diagnose GDM. This involves an eight-hour fast and a standard glucose drink, with blood sampling before and two to three hours afterwards. Many women have a positive glucose screen, but fewer than one in five will actually have GDM, as diagnosed on OGTT.[17] Under some systems the OGTT is used for both screening and diagnosis, although mainly in the cases of high-risk women.

Controversies in Screening and Diagnosis

Note that the glucose load (50 grams, 75 grams, 100 grams) used in the OGTT and the cutoff values for diagnosing GDM are not standardized internationally, creating major difficulties with diagnostic criteria and research comparisons. For example, in 1998, the World Health Organization (WHO) recommended that even mild glucose elevations (previously called impaired glucose tolerance or IGT) be defined as GDM.[18] The WHO criteria are less strict than other criteria, leading to twice as many women getting the GDM label, without good evidence of benefit to mother or baby, according to some experts.[19]

One study found that, among women screened for GDM, timing since the last meal had a significant effect on results, with lower blood glucose readings recorded when the woman's last meal was two to three hours before the test.[20]

According to midwife and author Anne Frye, the woman's usual diet can also influence her glucose response to this large sugar load. She recommends that women who do not usually consume large amounts of simple sugars (such as sweet foods and junk foods) should eat an extra amount of good-quality carbohydrates (natural, high-fiber, low GI; more on this later in the chapter) in the preceding days, to increase their insulin response.[21]

Frye also suggests another logical alternative to glucose-load screening: testing the glucose response to food that is closer to the woman's normal diet. For example, a two-hour postprandial (after-meal) test could be performed following a breakfast with at least 75 to 80 grams complex carbohydrates and 600 calories (values on food labels can be used to calculate this), with moderate exercise encouraged between the meal and the test.[21]

There is no agreement at present on whether to offer a screening test to all women or only those who have risk factors such as the following that make them more likely to have GDM:

- Overweight: body mass index [BMI—weight (kg)/height (m^2)] greater than 25, and especially greater than 30 (obese)
- Age older than twenty-five, and especially older than forty
- Family members with diabetes, especially parents or siblings
- GDM or a large baby (over 4 kilograms/8 pounds 13 ounces and especially over 4.5 kilograms/9 pounds 15 ounces) in a previous pregnancy
- Member of a high-risk ethnic group, including Native American, Asian, Hispanic, and Pacific Islander. UK studies show that black Caribbean and Middle Eastern women are also at higher risk.

However, such risk-scoring is not very useful, as around 90 percent of pregnant women will have one of more of these factors.[17] UK guidelines have suggested that age alone should not be used as a criterion for GDM risk,[22] which would reduce this number.

Currently the U.S. Preventive Services Task Force does not recommend routine screening.[17] ACOG recommends that every woman be screened, either by assessing for risk factors or by testing her blood sugar. The American Diabetes Association recommends blood screening only for women at high risk. The Society of Obstetricians and Gynaecologists of Canada (SOGC) recommendations make screening, either by risk factors or glucose tests, optional,[19] and in the UK, screening by OGTT is recommended only for women with risk factors apart from age.[22]

Screening is usually done at twenty-four to twenty-eight weeks or later, when growing levels of pregnancy hormones begin to create insulin resistance. Diabetes diagnosed before this is likely due to preexisting diabetes. Note that testing the urine for glucose by "dipstick" in pregnancy is not an accurate or useful way of detecting GDM.

Benefits for Mother and Baby

If you are diagnosed with GDM, the main outcome, which may be a benefit, is the knowledge that you have an increased risk of developing diabetes in the following years. This is probably because you have some degree of insulin resistance that becomes unmasked with the metabolic stresses and hormonal effects of pregnancy.[23]

This risk varies in different studies, and according to other factors such as initial glucose levels (reflecting severity of GDM), weight, and ethnicity. Overall, the United States National Diabetes Education Program estimates that women who have had GDM have a 20 to 50 percent chance of developing diabetes in the next five to ten years.[24]

Studies show that you can reduce this risk after pregnancy by reducing your weight, ideally to below BMI 25 (online charts based on kilograms or pounds are available)[25] and increasing your physical activity, ideally to thirty minutes five times weekly.[24, 26]

If you have had GDM, your glucose levels should be checked at six to twelve weeks postpartum and then every one to two years.[24]

It also seems to be reasonably certain that diagnosing and treating women for GDM will reduce the chance of having a large baby (macrosomia, large for gestational age—LGA—or larger than 4 kilograms or 8 pounds 13 ounces). In some studies this has also reduced the small risk of trauma to the baby due to shoulder dystocia, in which the shoulders become stuck during birth.[22] (GDM babies tend to be large overall, with extra-wide shoulders, which increases the risk of shoulder dystocia even compared with nondiabetic babies of the same weight.[27])

Uncertain Benefits

Some studies have suggested that women with GDM may be more likely to develop toxemia (preeclampsia)[27] and high blood pressure,[28] but it is not yet certain whether treating GDM will reduce this risk. There is also an increased risk of jaundice and low calcium levels for newborn GDM babies, related to high glucose levels in the womb,[27] which may not be improved with diagnosis and treatment.[29]

Some experts have suggested that the well-known risks of preexisting diabetes, especially Type I (insulin dependent diabetes or IDDM), may extend to GDM. These include an increased risk of stillbirth, but this has not been shown in, for example, the large hyperglycemia and adverse pregnancy outcomes (HAPO) study, which included more than twenty-five thousand women.[30]

In regard to possible long-term effects on offspring, one study found that children born from a pregnancy with GDM who were also large babies for their gestational age (LGA) were more likely to have markers of the metabolic syndrome (obesity, high blood glucose, high blood pressure, and high cholesterol) at age eleven.[31] Studies have indicated that obesity in pregnancy can also cause these changes,[31, 32] and both effects are likely due to higher insulin levels in the womb. It is not yet certain how diagnosis and treatment of GDM (or obesity) will affect these risks.

The medical evidence cannot yet tell us whether the mild hyperglycemia typical of GDM is significantly harmful to mother or baby[17] or whether the diagnosis and treatment of GDM actually benefits mother and baby in the short, medium, or long term, and whether such benefits might outweigh the risks of diagnosis and treatment.[33]

Risks for Mother and Baby

Possible risks of diagnosing and treating GDM include:

- Inconvenience and discomfort of monitoring blood glucose
- Possible hazards of drugs used for treatment
- Cost and other resources used in diagnosis and treatment
- Maternal worry and the nocebo effect

The diagnosis of GDM can also lead to higher cesarean[34] and induction rates,[22] which may also reflect the caregiver's extra precautions, once this diagnosis is made.[35, 36]

Although it may seem beneficial to induce (or deliver by cesarean) before the baby gets too big, and studies have shown that this does prevent macrosomia and reduce the chances of shoulder dystocia,[37] GDM babies can have a delay in lung maturity, especially if glucose levels have been very high in pregnancy, so it may be risky to deliver before the baby is ready to be born.[38] It has been estimated that over four hundred cesareans would need to be done on women with GDM to prevent one baby over 4.5 kilograms (9 pounds 15 ounces) from developing permanent nerve (brachial plexus) injury from a traumatic birth.[39]

One recent study found that newborns of women diagnosed with GDM (most of whom had mild GDM) were more likely to be admitted to NICU care than babies of mothers with untreated GDM, which may reflect increased induction of GDM babies in this study.[29]

Note that current evidence does not show overall benefit from inducing overdue GDM women who have had good glucose control before at least forty-one weeks.[27, 37, 38, 40] Similarly, a cesarean is not recommended routinely for women with GDM, although it may be considered if the baby is estimated to weigh over 5 kilograms (11 pounds).[27] Note, however, that ultrasound estimation of weight is not reliably accurate.[41]

Newborns of mothers with GDM have an increased risk of hypoglycemia (low blood sugar) in the early hours after birth. Hypoglycemia, which may affect around one in fifty GDM babies,[30] can be a serious condition, and at-risk newborns need to be checked with a finger-prick test and treated with breastfeeding or, if necessary, an oral or IV glucose solution. However, diagnosing and treating GDM may not lessen this risk overall, and it may actually increase risk for babies whose GDM mothers receive insulin.[29]

Note that cesarean babies are also more likely to be hypoglycemic (because they miss the CA surge; see chapter 6), but this has not been tested in relation to GDM. It is also likely that the chance of newborn hypoglycemia will be lessened when the baby has uninterrupted access to the mother's body and breastmilk.

Treatment of GDM requires the pregnant woman to monitor her blood glucose levels with a finger-prick test up to four times daily. Women who are unable to lower their glucose level with diet will be offered insulin, which involves daily injections.

There is a growing trend towards GDM treatment with oral hypoglycemic (glucose-lowering) drugs. Although insulin is thought to be safe for the fetus, as it does not cross the placenta, these drugs have not been subjected to rigorous testing and may have as-yet-unknown side effects for mother and/or baby that must be weighed against any potential benefits of treatment. For these reasons, the use of oral hypoglycemic drugs is currently considered experimental.[27, 42]

In regard to the nocebo effect, the U.S. Preventive Services Task Force reports: "In the first few weeks after screening, women who screened positive for gestational diabetes may report higher anxiety, more psychological distress, and poorer perceptions of their general health than women who screened negative."[43]

One study did find better health status and less depression at three months postpartum for women who were diagnosed and treated for GDM,[29] although this was studied in only a subset of study participants and may reflect the increased quality and quantity of care received (a placebo effect) rather than the medical treatment.

Alternatives

Reducing weight to normal levels before pregnancy[44] and limiting weight gain in pregnancy, especially if a woman is already overweight before pregnancy, will help to keep glucose levels low during pregnancy.[45, 46] Guidelines from the U.S. Institute of Medicine recommend weight gain between 15 and 25 pounds (6.8 to 11.4 kilograms) for overweight women (BMI of 19.9 to 25) and 15 pounds if obese (BMI of 30 or more).

However, as Frye notes, an excessive weight gain may only be worrying (or even possible) if the mother has consumed large amounts of high-sugar and/or high-fat junk food. Weight gain may therefore be less critical for women consuming a healthy diet.[21]

Exercise is also important, as it promotes insulin sensitivity as well as helping to burn calories. Diet and exercise during pregnancy have been shown to reduce the chances of developing GDM and also of having an overly large baby. Even fifteen to thirty minutes of light exercise such as walking three times weekly may be beneficial.[44–46]

Dietary changes that may benefit GDM, or even prevent its development, include: replacing foods with a high glycemic index (GI—a marker of how quickly the food raises glucose levels[47]) with low-GI carbohydrates; decreasing fat and increasing carbohydrates in the diet;[48] and increasing essential fatty acids in the diet.[49]

It is also sensible to ensure adequate levels of chromium, magnesium, vitamin E, selenium, vitamin B6, and zinc in the diet, which may help with glucose metabolism. Other food and herbs that may be helpful include onions and garlic, aloe vera, ginseng, fenugreek,[50] and liver in small quantities, fresh or dried in capsules.[21]

It is wise to ensure a good intake of antioxidants during pregnancy, which may help to prevent toxemia (preeclampsia) as well as optimize nutrition for you and your baby. You will get a good supply of antioxidants by ensuring a generous intake of fruits and vegetables.

Doing Nothing

Some experts believe that GDM is a serious condition and that every woman should be screened.[29] Others believe that GDM is a "diagnosis looking for a disease"[51–53] and that high glucose levels in pregnancy simply reflect the normal influence of placental hormones, which keep the mother's blood glucose high so that plenty of this essential fuel is available to her baby, as previously described.[53]

Michel Odent questions the usefulness of diagnosing GDM because this label can have a strong nocebo effect.[19] If a diagnosis of GDM causes high levels of stress and worry for the mother, her stress hormone levels can rise and be transmitted to her baby, increasing the risk of poor growth and premature birth, as already mentioned.

The U.S. Preventive Services Task Force recently reviewed all the studies in this area and concluded, "Although screening and early treatment of gestational diabetes reduce macrosomia, and although one trial suggests the possibility of other health benefits, the overall evidence is poor to determine whether maternal or fetal complications are reduced by screening."[54] This group also notes the inconvenience of this diagnosis and added health care costs for screening and OGTT.

Odent and others also rightly argue that the practical advice for women carrying the label of "gestational diabetes" is the same advice that all pregnant women can benefit from: eat well, following a diet with few simple sugars such as sucrose and glucose and plenty of complex carbohydrates with a low glycemic index; and exercise regularly, which helps the body burn up glucose and increases the effects of insulin.[53]

According to a major UK report, these measures are effective in controlling blood glucose levels for 80 to 90 percent of women with GDM.[22]

In Summary

You will need to consider all the consequences of accepting a test for GDM, especially the nocebo effect and possible increased risks of unnecessary interventions. Benefits to mother and baby from testing, diagnosis, and treatment of GDM are not yet proven, although it is likely that the chance of a very large baby is lessened.

There are many changes that you can make to your diet and exercise patterns that will reduce the chances of GDM, and its impact, should you be diagnosed with this condition. These changes will also generally benefit your own health and well-being and that of your unborn baby.

Screening and Treatment
for Group B Strep (GBS)

Group B streptococcus (GBS, beta-strep) is a type of bacteria that lives in the bowel and/or vagina as part of the normal flora during or outside of pregnancy. Between one in three and one in ten pregnant women are carriers of GBS, although GBS will come and go in the vagina and bowel for most women.

During labor and birth, the baby can be exposed to GBS in the womb (usually after the membranes have ruptured) or through contact with the mother's vaginal and bowel flora during birth. For some exposed babies, GBS will colonize (grow on) the skin and crevices. Much less commonly, GBS can enter the baby's body and cause serious infection, including infections in the lung (pneumonia), blood (septicemia), and brain (meningitis).

Although GBS is one of the leading causes of serious infection among newborns (early-onset or EOGBS, affecting babies under one week) and older babies (late-onset or LOGBS, affecting babies one week to three months), the actual number of affected babies is small. Currently fewer than one baby per two thousand in the United States contracts EOGBS (and an equal number with LOGBS), and one in twenty-five affected babies dies from GBS, totaling about eighty newborn deaths per year from EOGBS. Early-onset cases were around three times more common (1.5 per thousand) before the 1990s, when preventative measures began, and around half of affected babies died.[55]

Rates of GBS infection among newborns are similar in the UK, even without a preventative program: one baby per two thousand, per year, of whom around one in ten will die of GBS. UK rates of GBS carriage in pregnancy are also similar to those of U.S. women.[56] Lower rates of GBS carriage have been found among pregnant woman in countries such as Thailand, Myanmar, the Philippines, and Zimbabwe.[57]

Screening and Antibiotics to Prevent EOGBS

In recent years it has become common, and in some places almost mandatory, to test for GBS during pregnancy or at least to inform women of this option. Testing for GBS involves taking a swab from the pregnant mother's vagina and rectum; swabs are usually taken between thirty-five and thirty-seven weeks. Earlier swabs are not reliable for predicting whether the mother will be carrying GBS when she goes into labor, because, again, GBS carriage can be transient.

Technique is very important for accurate results. This includes using the right equipment and placing swabs in the correct transport media; however, swabs can be collected accurately by the woman herself. Swabs detect at least 85 percent of women with GBS colonization.[58]

If the swab is GBS positive, it is usually recommended that the woman be administered an antibiotic in labor to eliminate GBS from herself and her baby. Generally, this requires intravenous (IV) administration of penicillin every four hours until birth. Other broad-spectrum antibiotics such as ampicillin, erythromycin, and clindamycin can also be used, but these are not recommended routinely against GBS because they eradicate a wider range of bacteria, including more of the friendly bacteria in the gut and vagina, leading to possible overgrowth of potentially harmful microorganisms such as candida. Broad-spectrum alternatives may be needed for women who are allergic to penicillin.[55]

There has been international debate about whether all women should be swabbed and treated for GBS if positive (universal approach), or whether to adopt a risk-based approach and treat only women whose babies are at higher risk of EOGBS disease.

These risk factors include:

- Gestation of less than thirty-seven weeks
- Membrane rupture of more than eighteen hours

- Temperature over 100.4°F (38°C) in labor
- Having a previous GBS-affected baby
- Having GBS diagnosed on urine culture in pregnancy

In the United States, the Centers for Disease Control (CDC) have recommended universal screening, estimating that this approach will prevent twice as many EOGBS infections as risk-based approaches because around half of all babies who contract GBS do not have these risk factors.[58] Universal screening is judged to be cost-effective based on money saved in treating GBS babies.[55] Under the universal approach, around 30 percent of pregnant women would receive antibiotics in labor.

Canadian guidelines also recommend universal screening and treatment,[59] but this is not recommended at present in New Zealand[60] or in the UK,[56, 61] where the National Institute of Health and Clinical Excellence (NICE) judge that GBS screening is not justified because the clinical efficacy and cost-effectiveness are not certain.[61]

Under CDC recommendations, women who are planning a cesarean should still be screened, in case labor begins before surgery, but antibiotics are not necessary for a nonlabor cesarean delivery. If labor begins preterm, before swabs have been done, antibiotics are recommended.[55] Note that it takes forty-eight hours or so to get laboratory results from swabs.

Benefits of GBS Screening and Treatment

Overall, universal screening (when compared with risk-based treatment in labor) has been estimated to prevent EOGBS disease for 80 to 90 percent of susceptible newborns, preventing eight hundred infections and saving the lives of forty U.S. babies per year.[55] However, because lab tests may not be perfect and because clinical practice may not conform to guidelines, actual rates of effectiveness may be closer to 60 to 70 percent.[56]

For women without risk factors, the CDC estimates that screening and antibiotic use in labor will reduce the risk of GBS infection from one in two hundred to one in four thousand:[55] see below "doing nothing" for more GBS risks without antibiotics.

In the UK, the Royal College of Obstetricians and Gynecologists (RCOG) estimates that around twenty-four thousand women would need to be screened and seven thousand women would need to be treated with antibiotics to prevent one baby from dying from early-onset GBS. RCOG suggest that the benefits of universal screening (and treating more than two hundred thousand GBS carriers) may not be justified by the risks, at least in the UK.[56]

Note also that screening and treatment does not prevent late-onset GBS. Rates of LOGBS in the United States have remained stable at around one case per two thousand babies per year, despite widespread screening and use of antibiotics in recent years.[55]

Risks of GBS Screening and Treatment

The incidence of newborn GBS has certainly decreased in the United States since universal screening was adopted, but this benefit needs to be weighed against actual and possible risks for mothers and babies. These include the cost and inconvenience of screening, nocebo effects of positive results, risks to women with severe antibiotic allergies, possible increased risks of other late-onset infections, increased rates of antibiotic resistance, and impact on newborn gut flora. There may be other risks that are as yet unknown.

Universal screening, as recommended by the CDC, adds the time, expense, and perhaps discomfort of routine swabs to more than four million pregnant women in the United States every year. Those who test positive may experience several weeks of worry for themselves and/or their baby, especially if they have not been given good information about the relatively low risks involved. These factors can have a significant nocebo effect.

Women who wish to give birth in out-of-hospital settings (and their caregivers) may have difficulty accessing intravenous antibiotics, with little guidance from the CDC for this and other variations in care.

It has been estimated that between four in ten thousand and four in one hundred thousand women have a life-threatening (anaphylactic) allergy to penicillin. The CDC state that this is generally not a concern, because antibiotics are administered in a hospital setting where immediate response is possible.[55] However, RCOG estimates that two women could die every year from fatal anaphylactic reactions to penicillin if universal screening and prevention were undertaken in the UK.[56]

Around 10 percent of penicillin-allergic women may also have cross-reactions to other antibiotics in the cephalosporin family that may be used as alternatives, making it important to be very clear, preferably before labor, about the exact nature and history of any known antibiotic allergy.

The widespread administration of penicillin and other antibiotics to large numbers of women may lead to GBS bacteria developing resistance to these first-line drugs. So far this has not happened for penicillin, but GBS resistance to other antibiotics has developed. These effects are greater where clinicians are not following guidelines that recommend penicillin, and they are likely to increase with time.[55]

Resistance develops in this situation because broad-spectrum antibiotics kill off the sensitive (nonresistant) bacteria in the mother's gut and vagina and allow the overgrowth of bacteria that are resistant to antibiotics, which can then spread to the baby at birth. The increasing use of antibiotics in labor for GBS prevention has increased the proportion of newborn infections (GBS and non-GBS) that are resistant to antibiotics,[62] with a growing proportion of resistant infections among vulnerable premature babies.[63]

Using routine antibiotics around the time of birth may also predispose babies to later infections with non-GBS organisms. One U.S. study found that when term babies were exposed in labor to broad-spectrum antibiotics to prevent EOGBS, their risk of later serious bacterial infection (SBI) was five times higher than that of babies not exposed to antibiotics. The bacteria infecting these babies were more likely to be resistant to ampicillin—the usual antibiotic given to prevent GBS in labor in this setting. The U.S. rate of late-onset SBI in term babies is 1.6 cases per thousand.[64]

Concern also has been expressed about the effects of antibiotics in labor on the bacteria that first colonize the newborn baby's gastrointestinal tract. These bacteria come from the mother's bowel and vagina during birth, and the types of bacteria that are first established in the baby's gut (which is sterile until birth) will persist and significantly influence gut health and also immune function, including susceptibility to allergy, in the longer-term.

Antibiotics administered to the mother in labor could eradicate some of her good bacteria, allowing less-optimal bacteria (including bacteria that are resistant to antibiotics) to transfer to her baby, which could predispose the baby to short- and long-term problems, including immune dysfunctions and allergy.[65]

This effect is most likely with broad-spectrum antibiotics, which will kill more gut bacteria. For example, ampicillin has a moderate effect on bowel flora, and clindamycin and erythromycin have more significant effects, eradicating many helpful gut species (lactobacillus and bifidobacterium) and encouraging the overgrowth of harmful bacteria such as clostridium. Although narrow-spectrum antibiotics have much less impact, even penicillin can cause an overgrowth of candida (thrush) in the vagina in susceptible women.[66]

So far only one small study has looked at newborn bowel flora following exposure to antibiotics (in this case intravenous amoxicillin) in labor, and found more delay in gut colonization at day three among antibiotic-exposed babies, although numbers were too small for this finding to be statistically significant. Worryingly, babies in both exposed and unexposed groups had antibiotic-resistant bacteria in their gut flora, which may reflect colonization by resistant bacteria from the hospital environment.[67]

These studies have also shown that birth in the hospital, which is a foreign bacterial environment for mother and baby, is associated with a delay in gut colonization (even for babies unexposed to antibiotics)[67] and with colonization by less ideal bacteria.[68] These effects are probably due to sterile procedures and antibacterial washes and to colonization with bacteria transmitted from hospital staff to the baby. As UK neonatal pediatrician Bedford Russell notes, "[M]any infants are now becoming colonized by bacterial patterns probably unique in evolutionary history."[69]

Effects on the immune system are very possible. Bedford Russell comments further: "There is rapidly increasing evidence from experimental studies that the initial colonisation of the intestine is a moment of pivotal importance in long-term health, playing a profound role in imprinting of immune and systemic homeostasis."[70] According to animal studies, patterns of allergy and autoimmunity (where the body reacts against itself) are set by gut flora in the early weeks, although allergic and autoimmune disease may not be obvious until many years later.

Although poorly studied, altered gut flora colonization is likely to impact humans in a similar way. For example, one large study found that children exposed to antibiotics at delivery were 20 percent more likely to wheeze in the first two years and 40 percent more likely to have a wheeze persisting to age six or seven, compared with unexposed children.[71]

Similarly, a detailed long-term UK study found that offspring who had been cared for, as healthy newborns, in a communal nursery on the first night were more likely to report hay fever at age twenty-six compared with those who were not separated from their mothers. This study shows that even minor interventions that increase exposure to abnormal bacteria may influence the immune system and increase susceptibility to allergy.[72]

Anecdotally, some women have reported that their antibiotic-exposed babies have had gut dysfunctions in the early weeks and months that may be attributed to less-than-optimal gut flora, with possible longer-term effects as above.

Animal studies show that healthy gut flora may also be important for detoxifying. In one study the excretion of mercury in adult mice was significantly reduced by changes in gut flora following antibiotic administration.[73] One small human study showed higher mercury levels in the baby teeth of children with autism, who also had higher exposure to antibiotics in the first year of life.[74]

Changes in gut flora have also been linked to diabetes,[75–77] cancer, inflammatory bowel disease (Crohn's disease, ulcerative colitis),[78] and obesity,[79] which are all increasing in westernized societies.

In summary, medicine has focused on the short-term effect of eradicating GBS and neglected longer-term perspectives, especially in regard to the possible impact on gut flora. As one expert comments, "[The] common scenario of antibiotic administration to mother or newborn infant remains almost completely unstudied in anything but the short term."[70]

Alternatives

Alternatives to universal screening include the risk-based approach, as discussed in detail below. If GBS is found on screening, there are also some alternatives that may eradicate it, although these have not been scientifically tested.

Note that it is not recommended to treat GBS found on screening with antibiotics (unless it is associated with a urine infection) because it is likely that GBS will recur after treatment.[55] Similarly, if alternative treatments are used to eradicate GBS in pregnancy, it is important to swab again close to term to ensure that GBS has not recurred. Swabs should ideally be done within five weeks of birth.[55]

Alternative remedies that are aimed at eradicating GBS from the bowel as well as the vagina are likely to give longer-term benefits (and may prevent GBS recurrence before birth). This approach involves focusing on improving bowel flora overall.

Eradicating GBS in early pregnancy, if possible, may be beneficial as some studies have suggested that women who carry GBS may be more susceptible to premature labor. Other studies have found no extra risk, giving uncertainty in this area at present.

Treatments suggested by Anne Frye[21] include:

- Increasing fermented food in the diet—yogurt, kefir, miso, kombucha, sauerkraut
- Probiotic supplements orally and/or in the vagina
- A garlic clove scored and inserted into the vagina overnight; repeat with a fresh clove for at least four nights
- Grapefruit seed extract taken orally or by douche (such as Fem-Cleanse)
- General immune support using vitamin C, propolis, garlic, and echinacea

Note that most natural supplements have not been scientifically tested for safety in pregnancy (which is difficult and expensive), although it is likely that use of the suggested treatments in the last weeks for GBS is not harmful. More information is available online.[80]

Studies have also shown that washing the laboring woman's vagina with chlorhexidine can reduce GBS colonization in her baby, although studies have not so far shown an overall protection from neonatal GBS infection, possibly because of small study size.[81] Anne Frye suggests adding 1 tablespoon (12.5 milliliters) of Hibiclense to water to make 1 cup (200 milliliters) of water and using this solution (0.25 percent) as a douche or to wipe the inside of the laboring woman's vagina with cotton gauze every six hours until birth. If the mother is heavily colonized, this solution could also be used to wipe the baby.[21]

Finally, if antibiotics are given for GBS, it is preferable to use penicillin, except for women with significant allergy, because this will be less disruptive to the gut flora of mother and newborn.

Doing Nothing

Pregnant women could choose to avoid screening and opt to treat themselves (or their babies) only if there are risk factors. See the earlier list of risk factors accepted in the UK as justifying the use of antibiotics to prevent GBS.

According to Schrag and colleagues, whose 2002 study underpins CDC recommendations, administering antibiotics only to mothers with risk factors (but ensuring that all at-risk mothers are treated) would give newborns an overall risk of EOGBS of 0.44 per thousand (around one in 2,250) which is slightly higher than the one in 3,125 (0.32 per thousand) GBS risk for babies of mothers who are universally screened for GBS and given antibiotics if positive.[58]

For women who have screened GBS-positive, the UK RCOG estimates that the risk of GBS disease for the newborn, if the mother does not take antibiotics, is one in five hundred. Risks are lower if the swab was taken before thirty-five to thirty-seven weeks (in which case the GBS may have spontaneously cleared) and if there were no other risk factors. RCOG does not advise routine use of antibiotics, including for women who have tested positive for GBS in pregnancy but have no other risk factors—unless GBS was found in the urine, indicating a heavy colonization, which carries higher risks.[56]

In the United States the CDC estimate that newborns of GBS-positive mothers, with no other risk factors, have around a one in two hundred chance of being affected by GBS, based on figures from a 1985 study.[55] Note however that Schrag's 2002 study, just quoted, found an EOGBS risk of around one in seven hundred fifty for the newborns of low-risk GBS-positive mothers who did not receive antibiotics in labor.[58] A Canadian study estimated the chance of a newborn infection from a GBS-colonized mother at a little less than one in five hundred.[82]

GBS most commonly presents soon after birth, with 90 percent of affected babies showing signs of illness such as lethargy and poor feeding within twelve hours. These babies have almost certainly been infected in the womb by GBS that has ascended from the mother's vagina during labor. It is also possible for babies to become infected with GBS before labor, and in some cases even without the waters breaking.

It would therefore be sensible for women who wish to avoid antibiotics to also avoid, as far as possible, medical procedures that sweep bacteria from the lower vagina up to the cervix and uterus. Practices that have been shown to increase infection risks (although not specifically GBS) include: vaginal exams (especially if frequent and/or multiple); examinations or procedures in which the cervix is entered or transgressed, including artificial rupture of membranes; and use of a fetal scalp electrode,[55] which is screwed into the baby's head and provides a potential bridge for bacteria to cross from the mother's vagina to her uterus and baby. Membrane sweeping ("sweep and stretch" may also encourage ascending infection, although current studies have not shown extra GBS risks for mothers or babies.[55] It is also possible that upright positions in labor might discourage ascending infections.

Note also that, whether or not antibiotics have been used in labor, unwell newborns will always be admitted to a newborn intensive care unit (NICU) and treated promptly with antibiotics that will cover GBS as well as other causes of serious infection. Treatment in NICU involves early separation and broad-spectrum antibiotics; risks that must be taken into account by parents who choose to avoid antibiotics in labor. Modern treatment prevents death for 90 percent[56] to 96 percent[55] of newborns with GBS, although babies who survive a serious infection with GBS can be left with significant disabilities.

GBS Summary

Although universal screening and preventative treatment is the standard of care in many countries, it remains important to make an informed choice, weighing the risks of GBS affecting your baby against the possible effects of antibiotics on yourself and your baby. Although we know that administering antibiotics in labor will reduce the (reasonably small) chance of GBS infection, the full and long-term impact of antibiotic exposure on newborns is not yet known.

Induction for "Going Overdue"

Pregnant women today face an extraordinary amount of pressure to give birth according to the calendar, with the threat of induction should their labor not begin before a certain date.

Rates of induction have been increasing in recent years, with official U.S. figures showing that 22.8 percent of women were induced in 2005, compared with 9.6 percent in 1990.[83] However, even the current, highest-ever U.S. figures are likely to be an underestimate: 50 percent of respondents to the 2006 Listening to Mothers (LTM) survey reported that they or their caregiver had attempted to cause labor to begin, and 34 percent reported that their labor had been medically induced.[84]

Although official U.S. figures do not record the reason for induction, LTM respondents listed "caregiver concern that the mother was overdue" as the leading reason for medical induction, accounting for one-quarter of reported inductions.[84]

This "caregiver concern" has also increased in recent years, fueled by medical studies that report small decreases in perinatal mortality for post-term babies that are induced compared with "expectant management."[85] Although the post-term period has traditionally begun at forty-two weeks, recent reviews have recommended induction from forty-one weeks.[85–87]

As a consequence of these studies, which will be discussed, you are very likely to be offered an induction if your pregnancy continues past forty-one to forty-two weeks, usually with significant pressure to accept.

For many women, this pressure begins even earlier, based on the schedule of their caregiver, their own schedule, concerns about the baby's size, timing of ruptured membranes, or other previous or current health concerns.

When a woman does not accept induction, especially past forty-two weeks, her caregiver will almost certainly wish to have the pregnancy monitored at regular intervals until she goes into labor. In some locales she may not be able to continue with her preferred caregiver after a certain time because of local regulations and guidelines. All of these factors can create significant stress in what might otherwise be the blissful last days of pregnancy.

Estimated Dates

When induction is being considered because a pregnant woman has gone a certain time past her due date, it is obviously important to be sure that her due date is calculated accurately. In obstetric terms, the expected due date (EDD, expected date of delivery) is usually calculated at forty weeks from the first day of a woman's last normal menstrual period (LMP or LNMP). This is based on the assumption that she has a twenty-eight-day cycle and conceived fourteen days after the first day of her LMP.

"Menstrual dates" will be most accurate for women who know the actual date of conception and count thirty-eight weeks ahead. Alternatively, especially for those with a longer cycle, the probable day of ovulation (and therefore conception) can be calculated as fourteen days before the next expected period, according to usual cycle length: again, add thirty-eight weeks to get the obstetric EDD. Note that this is probably not the day you will naturally go into labor, which is likely to be a little later than your EDD, as we will address.

Some studies have shown that obstetric calculations based on women's LMP are likely to underestimate the due date compared with dating by ultrasound scan, leading to many inductions among women who are not actually overdue.[88] This discrepancy may occur because conventional obstetric calculations do not take account of variations in menstrual cycle length, as already noted. Note that some obstetric systems count forty weeks from the end, rather then the beginning, of the last menstrual period.[89]

Researchers who compared the LMP and obstetric dates of fourteen thousand healthy Danish women with spontaneous labor suggested that, where menstrual dates are used, another two days should be added, making the EDD 282 days—forty weeks and two days from LMP. This reduces the number of women who are judged to go beyond forty-two weeks from around 8 percent to close to 5 percent. Using dates from an ultrasound at between twelve and twenty-two weeks, and adding 282 days, would lead to only 2 percent of women being judged as post-term.[90]

Note that age, ethnicity, and previous births influence the average length of gestation. One U.S. study showed that healthy first-time white mothers had an average pregnancy length of 274 days from presumed ovulation, equating to forty-one weeks and one day from LMP.[89]

A very large study from Norway found an average gestation of 282 days overall, with slightly shorter gestations in December (midwinter).[91] Black women, women younger than nineteen or older than thirty-four, women with previous births, and women pregnant with male babies have tended, in these studies, to have shorter gestations.[91, 92]

Induction When Post-Term: The Benefits

The major justification for inducing pregnant women after forty-one to forty-two weeks is a small increase in perinatal mortality for babies who are still in the womb after this time. Perinatal mortality (PNM) includes those babies who die before labor (intrauterine fetal death or IUFD, stillbirth) and those who die during labor or after birth (intrapartum stillbirth and neonatal death). In post-term pregnancies, prelabor stillbirth makes the major contribution to increased PNM death rates, with post-term effects on intrapartum and neonatal deaths less clear.[93]

Stillbirth is also the largest cause of perinatal death overall[94] and is certainly a tragedy that we want to avoid. Stillbirth can occur at any stage of pregnancy, and the risk of stillbirth increases as pregnancy advances. According to one analysis, the chances of stillbirth in the subsequent week rise from one in 3,332 at thirty-seven completed weeks to one in 1,148 at forty weeks, one in 644 at forty-two weeks, and one in 486 after forty-three weeks, when the number of women who are still pregnant becomes too low for a statistically accurate assessment.[95, 96]

Note that different statistical methods can be used to derive post-term stillbirth figures. Some use the number of births during that week as the denominator and more recent analyses use the number of ongoing pregnancies, with the latter giving more dramatic figures for the risks for post-term babies.[93, 95, 97, 98]

Elective delivery at a particular time will prevent subsequent stillbirths, but this benefit needs to be weighed against the risks of induction or cesarean to mother and baby, including risks of prematurity—a leading cause of perinatal death. In some situations these risks may be justified, but parental informed choice should be paramount.

Complications during labor and birth are also somewhat more common among overdue babies. Although a review of relevant studies by the Cochrane Collaboration found a small increase in the risk of perinatal death in non-induced babies after forty-one weeks, including an extra risk of newborn death,[85] other large observational studies have not found increased risks of death in labor or the newborn period for babies from thirty-seven up to forty-two weeks gestation.[93, 99] However, there may be a small additional risk of intrapartum and neonatal deaths (around two per thousand) after forty-two weeks.[100]

Overdue babies who are smaller than expected (small for gestational age or SGA) may have lower reserves for withstanding labor and therefore a higher risk of death.[97] In post-term babies, this has been called post-maturity syndrome, although in fact these complications can occur at any time in pregnancy when the condition is called dysmaturity or intrauterine growth retardation (IUGR). This condition is thought to be caused by problems with the initial establishment of the placenta, leading to limitations in its capacity to supply the increasing needs of the growing baby.

It is obviously ideal for caregivers to recognize whether small overdue babies are constitutionally small and healthy or post-mature and at risk. Standard testing—including stress and nonstress heart rate tests, ultrasound, and biophysical profile (which includes an ultrasound and non-stress test), are aimed at detecting those babies who are at higher risk of stillbirth and perinatal death and who may require elective delivery.

Note that using ultrasound to detect low amniotic fluid (AF) levels (oligohydramnios) does not, by itself, give an accurate assessment of fetal well-being[97] and has been shown to lead to overdiagnosis of problems, resulting in high rates of induction for healthy babies.[101, 102] Although low AF levels can cause complications in labor, studies suggest that low levels in late pregnancy may reflect maternal dehydration, at least in some situations,[103–107] and may be corrected by drinking more water.

Overdue babies can also be larger than expected (large for gestational age, or LGA, usually greater than 4 kilograms or 8 pounds 13 ounces), and this may cause birth complications including shoulder dystocia and cesareans. However, according to some studies, large babies may have less, or even no, increased perinatal mortality when overdue, compared with term babies,[101] although larger babies may contribute to maternal complications, including cesarean.

Note also that induction is not generally recommended for predicted LGA babies for the following reasons: ultrasound weight prediction may not be accurate, induction will lead to increased intervention without evidence of better outcomes, cesarean rate is higher, and cesarean delivery does not necessarily prevent complications.[100, 108–110] However, there may be more pressure for induction if a post-term baby is estimated to be LGA.

If the baby is truly large, it is likely that the mother's body will have maximum pelvic softness and flexibility (due to peak levels of hormones such as progesterone) on the day she spontaneously goes into labor, giving her the best chance to accommodate and birth her large baby. Consistent with this, studies show that induction may actually increase the risk of difficulties in birth, such as shoulder dystocia,[111] perhaps reflecting the mother's less-than-ready pelvis.

Other complications that may be more common among overdue babies, according to some studies, include infection, fetal distress in labor, shoulder dystocia and birth trauma, birth asphyxia and low APGAR score (a measurment of condition at birth), meconium aspiration, cesarean birth, and postpartum hemorrhage (PPH),[100, 112, 113] although, as previously discussed, these findings are not consistent and may reflect post-maturity or macrosomia rather than complications due only to being post-term.

Assessing the Actual Risk for Overdue Babies

Even considering all of these risks, including possible (but not definite) increases in intrapartum and neonatal deaths, the actual number of babies who die post-term is still very low. One large Danish study that compared uninduced post-term pregnancies (including over six hundred pregnancies at forty-four weeks and fifty-five at forty-five weeks) to term pregnancies (between thirty-seven and forty-two weeks) found an overall PNM rate of four per thousand (289 babies out of 77,956) for post-term babies compared with three per thousand (92 babies out of 34,140) for term babies.[113]

One recent study has suggested that higher post-term stillbirth risks may not apply to parous women (those who have given birth previously). Researchers found stable PNM risks of around one per thousand ongoing pregnancies for parous women whose pregnancies continued up to and perhaps past forty-two completed weeks (numbers were too small for specific calculations past forty-two weeks), compared with risks of 1.4 and 3 per thousand at forty-one and forty-two weeks, respectively, for first-time mothers. The authors question the need for routine induction at forty-one weeks for parous women.[114]

It is also important to note that, with modern obstetric care and surveillance, many babies who would fare badly post-term (especially SGA babies) are likely detected and offered induction even before term. This means that babies who reach post-term may be even less at risk today that in the past.[101]

Intervention Studies

While the cited studies suggest small increased risks for babies who go overdue, it is still necessary for researchers to show that hastening labor and birth will lead to overall benefits. These are called intervention studies, of which there have been a number.

One major problem for post-term intervention studies is that the PNM risks are very low—on the order of one to two per thousand—which means that studies would need to include around sixteen thousand women to prove a benefit.[87]

Because no single study has included this many women (which would be a major undertaking) several smaller studies have been combined as a meta-analysis, with combined numbers that are statistically high enough to find a benefit. According to the authoritative Cochrane Collaboration systematic review, which included studies totaling almost eight thousand women, induction does reduce risks post-term, but five hundred inductions would be needed to prevent the death of one baby after forty-one weeks. The authors summarize, "the absolute risk is extremely small."[113]

Another recent systematic review, with studies that included sixty-five hundred women, found no statistically significant benefits for babies induced at forty-one weeks in terms of perinatal mortality rate, NICU admission, meconium aspiration (the baby inhaling its own feces during birth), meconium below the vocal cords, or abnormal APGAR scores. In this analysis, there was a small decrease in cesarean risk for induced women: 22 percent compared with 20 percent for expectantly managed women. This reduction was just barely statistically significant, and the authors listed this as the sole justification for this policy.[87]

In the UK, a recent report commissioned by the National Institute for Health and Clinical Excellence (NICE) also noted that, although there are small extra risks for post-term babies, induction has not been shown to improve the outcomes for overdue babies.[100] Similarly, population studies show that the shift to induction for post-term pregnancies, which consumes enormous maternity-care resources, has produced only small benefits for post-term babies. For example, a Canadian analysis showed that stillbirths at forty-one or more weeks' gestation decreased from 2.8 per thousand total births in 1980 to 0.9 per thousand total births in 1995, when routine induction past forty-one weeks became standard care. Parallel decreases in term stillbirths over this time suggest that around 40 percent of this benefit may be due to improvements in perinatal care, leaving a possible net prevention of around one stillbirth per nine hundred total births due to this policy.[116]

Balanced against this must also be the huge resource implications of inducing the 15 to 20 percent of women who are still pregnant at forty-one weeks. One Canadian review reports the death of a very ill pregnant woman because of limited access to labor facilities, filled to capacity with women judged to be post-term and therefore being induced.[117]

These authors also emphasize the extremely small risks of perinatal death at forty-one weeks—around one per thousand pregnancies, even without monitoring—and the large difference that shifting post-term induction policies from forty-one to forty-two weeks would make, with only 3 to 4 percent of women undelivered by this time.[117]

Similarly, a recent European analysis suggests that 527 women would need to be induced at forty-one completed weeks to avoid one baby's death, decreasing to 195 at forty-three weeks and one day. The authors comment, "[T]he risk was low, and numbers needed to induce to avoid one fetal or perinatal death were quite high."[118]

Post-Term Induction: The Risks

Much of the research previously quoted is based on the assumption that induction has no risks to mother or baby. As discussed at the start of this chapter, and detailed in chapter 6, this has not been adequately researched, especially in terms of breastfeeding, attachment, maternal emotional well-being, and long-term effects on induced offspring. Other possible risks, detailed here, include: precipitate labor; lack of blood and oxygen for the baby; increased maternal pain and need for pain relief; increased maternal risks of uterine rupture, postpartum hemorrhage, and cesarean; risks associated with breaking of the waters including infection, stress on the baby's skull bones, and possible bleeding in the brain; and uncommon but catastrophic effects including cord prolapse and amniotic fluid embolism.

Obvious adverse outcomes for babies, short of death, may also be inadequately recorded in some of the post-term studies, most of which have focused on mortality. For example, in the largest post-term trial, one induced baby apparently suffered a spinal cord injury and quadriplegia following severe fetal distress and a forceps delivery, after the mother experienced an overly fast (precipitate) labor induced by prostaglandin. This outcome has apparently not been disclosed in any trial report.[117]

It also highlights a major side effect of induction with any drug, which is the tendency to produce longer, stronger, and closer-spaced contractions for the laboring woman than she would experience with natural labor. In this situation, blood and oxygen supplies from the placenta will be more compromised than usual during contractions, and her baby will also have less time to "refuel" in between. Most healthy babies are well primed for a moderate lack of blood and oxygen during labor, even with induction drugs, but babies exposed to a precipitate induced labor, and/ or babies who have some vulnerability, may develop severe fetal distress that necessitates immediate delivery. Note that, in one post-term study, precipitate labor was almost three times more common among women who were induced post-term compared with women with expectantly managed pregnancies.[119]

An ongoing lack of blood and oxygen caused by induction drugs (including synthetic oxytocin/Pitocin/Syntocinon used for augmentation, or speeding labor) can also compromise the baby's health at birth, with low APGAR scores and acidosis more likely among babies who are exposed to induction drugs in labor.[120–123] A large European study of induction at term also found that more induced than non-induced babies of first-time mothers required NICU care.[124]

The longer, stronger, and more closely spaced contractions that follow induction will also be more painful for the laboring woman and will occur before she has the chance to produce her own pain-relieving hormones: beta-endorphin and oxytocin (see chapter 6). Therefore most women who are induced will require some form of pain relief, with more induced women using epidurals, which, as described in chapter 7, further increase the risks of labor complications for mother and baby.[125]

Links between induction and other obstetric interventions have not been well researched. One study of parous women—between thirty-seven and forty-two weeks—showed that those who were induced were more than one-third more likely to finish with a cesarean delivery.[125]

Other studies have found an approximately doubled chance of a cesarean among healthy nulliparous women—those in their first pregnancy—following induction at or beyond term.[126–130] In one observational study, only 43 percent of first-time mothers induced for post-term experienced a normal vaginal birth.[131]

Although the largest post-term intervention study supposedly showed lower cesarean rates among women induced for post-term (21.2 versus 24.5 percent for expectantly managed women[132]), this small difference may relate partly to different methods of induction between groups and to high rates of "cross-over": women randomized to induction who went into labor beforehand and women who were randomized to expectant management but who were actually induced.

According to a reanalysis of this trial based on the actual treatment received, women who were induced were twice as likely to deliver by cesarean,[117] which is consistent with other data, as discussed earlier. Note that most post-term trials have not looked at cesarean rates according to parity.

Note, too, that as mentioned earlier the average gestation for first-time mothers is forty-one weeks and one day, making them especially likely to be labeled and induced for post-term. In one large study, 40 percent of nulliparous women were induced, the majority for being "post-term," although few women were at or beyond forty-two weeks.[130] In this study, cesarean risk was doubled for nulliparous women, which may reflect their longer gestation and lack of readiness for labor.

Induction may also increase the chances of a longer second (pushing) stage and an instrumental delivery.[124, 131, 133] Studies also show an increase in the risk of postpartum hemorrhage following an induced labor,[134–136] which has been linked with a reduction (down regulation) in uterine oxytocin receptors in response to constant oxytocin exposure: see chapters 6 and 8.

Note that induction success is heavily influenced by the "ripeness" (softness, openness, length, and position) of the pregnant woman's cervix.

Although induction is more likely to be successful when her cervix is ripe, this also means that she is close to spontaneous labor. For example, one study found that 95 percent of women past forty-one weeks and three days with a ripe cervix gave birth within a week without induction.[110]

Induction with prostaglandins, or the use of these drugs to soften the mother's "unripe" cervix before induction with Pitocin, has become more common. For some women, this gives a more gentle labor compared with induction with Pitocin. However, prostaglandin drugs can unpredictably cause intense uterine contractions and fetal distress, with higher risks of rupture of the laboring woman's uterus, especially for women with a previous cesarean. Misoprostol (Cytotec, a drug designed to treat stomach problems) is especially dangerous in this situation (see chapter 9).

Induction by any means usually involves breaking the membranes (artificial rupture of membranes, or ARM) that protect the baby in pregnancy and labor. This is sometimes used as the first step in induction, especially if the woman's cervix is soft and already a little open in preparation for labor, and it may trigger labor without the need for drugs.

However, removing this protective bubble exposes the baby to increased risks of infection, especially if the laboring woman is given frequent vaginal examinations.[137, 138] For this reason, once membranes are ruptured a time limit for birth is usually given, commonly twelve to eighteen hours.

As well as "starting the clock," breaking the baby's waters also destroys the soft cushioning that the membranes and enclosed fluid provide, which usually persists until the last stages of labor.[139] Babies who experience ARM are more likely to show signs of distress on heart-rate monitoring, including both early decelerations and the more worrying late decelerations.[140–143]

Other evidence suggests that, by removing the cushioning "forewaters" in front of the baby's head, ARM may expose the baby's head to greater and more uneven mechanical stress in labor. Early researchers Schwatz, Caldeyro-Barcia, and colleagues suggested that pressure on the unprotected skull bones may cause tension on underlying brain structures, leading to tearing and bleeding inside the brain (intracranial hemorrhage, or ICH).[143]

This theory was supported by a recent ultrasound study of eighty-eight healthy, vaginally born newborns, of whom 26 percent were found to have a silent ICH. In this study, the membranes of all babies had been broken during labor, but babies with an ICH had a longer average time from ARM to birth. Almost all newborns with ICH had subdural hematomas[144] consistent with pressure on the skull bones. Potential long-term effects of ARM (and possible ICH) on the baby's brain have been little researched.[145–147] Rupture of the membranes can also increase the risk of cord prolapse, especially if the baby's head (or presenting part) is still high above the mother's cervix. This is an obstetric emergency.

Another rare but catastrophic complication of induction is rupture of the laboring mother's uterus. Rupture following induction is more likely in women who have had a previous cesarean[148] but can also occur in women without this history.[149, 150]

Other uncommon risks of induction include amniotic fluid embolism, which occurs when strong contractions force amniotic fluid into the mother's bloodstream. Although rare, fatal embolism is 3.5 times more likely following induction than in spontaneous labor.[151]

Induction After Forty-Two Weeks: The Alternatives

Many women who are recommended induction wish to avoid the medical hazards by inducing labor themselves.

Among Listening to Mothers II survey respondents, around one-fifth reported that they had attempted to self-induce, with one-third doing this to avoid a medical induction. The most common methods used were walking or exercise (82 percent); sexual intercourse (71 percent), which may be effective because prostaglandins from semen, deposited near the pregnant woman's cervix, can help to induce labor; and nipple stimulation (41 percent),[84] which can trigger labor by releasing oxytocin.

There are many other reported methods of "natural induction," but it is important to realize that the timing of labor and birth—the initiation of parturition—is regulated by complex and precise interactions between mother and baby that are still poorly understood. With the exception of premature birth and some other uncommon situations, labor will occur when mother and baby are optimally ready. This means the mother's body is primed for an efficient labor and the baby's body is ready to begin the changes necessary for life outside the womb. These processes may start days or weeks before labor.

We also do not yet understand the full implications of attempting to preempt this delicate process with any form of induction. We might also wonder about the imprint, in terms of prenatal and perinatal psychology, of hurrying the baby at this critical time and, conversely, the benefits that might come to us as parents when we trust our baby's own timing and process.

In summary, any method to induce labor before both mother and baby have signaled their readiness for birth (by actually going into labor) is not natural. As Michel Odent notes, "[T]here are no natural methods of induction. If a method is effective, it means that it is not natural, because it has preceded the signals given by the baby. We understand today that the fetus participates in the initiation of labor by sending messages that mean: 'I am ready.'"[152]

However, there are situations in which an ongoing pregnancy creates difficulties. For example, a midwife may be unable to continue care after a certain time (although it is preferable to avoid this by choosing a caregiver who is not under this duress, if possible), or there may be minor or even major concerns, and it may seem preferable to attempt to start labor.

Herbs have traditionally been used, and alternative treatments such as homeopathy, acupuncture, and kinesiology may also be helpful, although there has been little research into the risks and benefits. Evening primrose oil has also been used to ripen the pregnant woman's cervix, either taken orally or applied close to the cervix. This method takes many days, compared with herbal methods that can initiate labor within hours.[153]

If you wish to attempt to self-induce using nonmedical methods, please ensure that you have advice and preferably supervision from an experienced and knowledgeable practitioner. Castor oil and other herbs used to initiate labor can have significant side effects and risks, which include precipitate labor and fetal distress; they should be used with caution and monitoring.

Another common alternative to medical induction is a "sweep and stretch" of the membranes during late pregnancy. A routine sweep and stretch has been shown to reduce the chance of going post-term but may also have risks, including accidental rupture of the membranes, especially for women with cervical dilation of more than one centimeter.[154] It can also be a very uncomfortable procedure for women,[155] and it may not be wise for carriers of GBS, as previously discussed.

Sweep and stretch may sometimes induce an "overdue" pregnancy, avoiding the need for medical induction, but eight procedures would be needed to prevent one medical induction, according to Cochrane reviewers.[155] Sweep and stretch may be a useful procedure in conjunction with medical induction, when necessary, and can lead to a shorter labor.[156]

It is also possible that maternal anxiety may inhibit the onset of labor, an effect often noted by midwives. This could logically be a survival mechanism for mammals birthing in the wild, where the mother's instinctive assessment of safety would be necessary to ensure that labor and birth take place in the most advantageous surroundings. Sharing fears and concerns about labor and birth can maximize emotional readiness and may help to initiate labor, if the baby is truly ready. Here again gentle natural treatments such as homeopathy and kinesiology may be beneficial.

Doing Nothing

The evidence just presented suggests that extra risks probably exist for overdue babies, but they are very small, unless other risk factors are apparent. The risk of unexpected stillbirth is probably around one in one thousand after forty-one weeks, one in six hundred after forty-two weeks, and one in five hundred after forty-three weeks, as previously noted.

Extra risks during labor and birth are less clear, but may be confined to those babies who are truly post-mature rather than just post-term. It is also possible that risks are even lower for healthy mothers and babies who have been well cared for during pregnancy, so that preexisting complications have been excluded. It is likely that good maternal health and nutrition, before and during pregnancy, may be another protective factor.[157]

In the United States, ACOG advise that, for low-risk post-term women (after forty-two weeks) with a favorable cervix, there is insufficient evidence to determine whether induction or expectant management is preferable. For low-risk post-term women with an unfavorable cervix, ACOG notes that both expectant management and labor induction are associated with low complication rates and good perinatal outcomes.[158]

Doing nothing will help to avoid the risks of induction, including cesarean risks that are likely higher for women having their first baby. If you are in your first pregnancy, you may also consider adjusting your dates to allow for a longer gestation. Authors of the 2002 Agency for Healthcare Research and Quality report conclude: ". . . at least 500 inductions are necessary to prevent one perinatal death. Whether this is an acceptable trade-off at either the policy or individual level is unclear."

Doing nothing may therefore be a reasonable option, although it may be uncomfortable for your caregivers. Remember your right to "informed refusal," as discussed earlier. If you choose to do nothing, with or without formal monitoring, look for possible support from caregivers, family, and/or friends. And remember that every pregnant woman will go into labor eventually.

Induction for Post-Term: A Summary

Although induction for all women at around forty-one weeks has become the norm, it is important to consider your options in this situation. In particular, you will need to weigh the small extra risk of stillbirth against possible effects of induction.

Your Body, Your Baby, Your Choice

The theme of this chapter has been informed choice, which involves considering all the possible risks and benefits, looking also at alternatives and at the option of doing nothing.

The information is by no means comprehensive, and I would encourage you to seek more sources and resources (including emotional support) for whatever decision you are considering.

It is important to keep in mind that everything involves risk—"birth is as safe as life gets," as I quote in chapter 2—and that for most mothers and babies, pregnancy and birth will be relatively simple and uncomplicated.

Finally, please try to balance this complex information and decision-making with light and joyful activities, so that you can truly enjoy this amazing transition for yourself and your baby.

chapter 5

ULTRASOUND SCANS
Cause for Concern

Ultrasound is a very common procedure during pregnancy, and many parents enjoy seeing the first images of their unborn babies displayed on the screen. New ultrasound technologies, including 3-D and 4-D (moving) images, are especially compelling. However, it is important to realize that ultrasound technology is very new and relatively untested, in terms of safety, and its main purpose is to test for abnormalities, most of which cannot be treated before birth except by termination of the pregnancy. This chapter provides essential information for all parents-to-be, and details what we know—and don't know—about the safety and usefulness of ultrasound during pregnancy.

When I was pregnant with my first baby in 1990, I decided against having an ultrasound scan. This was a rather unexpected decision, as my partner and I are both physicians and had even performed pregnancy scans (sonograms) ourselves—rather ineptly, but sometimes usefully—while training in family practice obstetrics a few years earlier.

What influenced me the most was my feeling that I could lose something important as a mother if I allowed someone to test my baby. I knew that if a minor or uncertain problem showed up, which is not uncommon, I would be obliged to return again and again and that, after a while, I might feel as if my baby belonged to the system and not to me.

In the years since then I have had three more unscanned babies and have read many articles and research papers about ultrasound. Nothing I have read has made me reconsider my decision. Although a prenatal scan may sometimes be useful when specific problems are suspected, my conclusion is that it is at best ineffective, and at worst dangerous, when used as a screening tool for every pregnant woman and her baby.

History of Ultrasound

Ultrasound was developed during World War II to detect enemy submarines; it was later used in the steel industry. In July 1955 Glasgow surgeon Ian Donald borrowed an industrial machine and, using beefsteaks for comparison, began to experiment with the abdominal tumors that he had removed from his patients. He discovered that different tissues gave different patterns of sound wave "echo," leading him to realize that ultrasound offered a revolutionary way to look into the mysterious world of the growing baby.[1] Research into the potential of ultrasound for diagnosis and treatment began around the same time in Germany and the United States.[2]

This new technology spread rapidly into clinical obstetrics. Commercial machines became available in 1963[3] and by the late 1970s ultrasound had become a routine part of obstetric care.[4] Today ultrasound is seen as safe and effective, and scanning has become a rite of passage for pregnant women in most developed countries. In the United States it is estimated that around 65 to 70 percent of pregnant women have a formal scan in a diagnostic clinic,[5, 6] and many more woman may be scanned by their OB as part of their pregnancy visit.

However, there is growing concern as to its safety and usefulness. UK consumer activist Beverley Beech has called the routine use of ultrasound in pregnancy "the biggest uncontrolled experiment in history"[7] and the Cochrane Collaboration—considered the top authority in evidence-based medicine—concludes,

> . . . no clear benefit in terms of a substantive outcome measure like perinatal mortality [number of babies dying around the time of birth] can yet be discerned to result from the routine use of ultrasound . . . For those considering its introduction, the benefit of the demonstrated advantages would need to be considered against the theoretical possibility that the use of ultrasound during pregnancy could be hazardous, and the need for additional resources.[8]

The additional resources consumed by routine ultrasound are substantial. In the United States an estimated $1.2 billion would be spent yearly if every pregnant woman had a single routine scan.

In 1987, UK radiologist H. B. Meire, who had been performing pregnancy scans for twenty years, commented,

> The casual observer might be forgiven for wondering why the medical profession is now involved in the wholesale examination of pregnant patients with machines emanating vastly different powers of energy which is not proven to be harmless to obtain information which is not proven to be of any clinical value by operators who are not certified as competent to perform the operations.[9]

The situation today is unchanged on every count.

What Is Ultrasound?

The term ultrasound refers to the ultra-high-frequency sound waves used for diagnostic scanning: these waves travel at one to twenty million cycles per second, compared to one to twenty thousand cycles per second for audible sound.[3] Ultrasound waves are emitted by a transducer (the part of the machine that is put onto the body), and a picture of the underlying tissues is built up from the pattern of echo waves that return to the transducer. Hard surfaces such as bone will return a stronger echo than soft tissue or fluids, giving the bony skeleton an opaque or white appearance on the screen.

Ordinary scans use pulses of ultrasound that last only a fraction of a second; the machine uses the interval between pulses to interpret the echo that returns. In contrast, Doppler techniques—which are used in specialized scans, fetal monitors, and handheld fetal stethoscopes (sonicaids)—use continuous waves, giving much higher levels of exposure than pulsed ultrasound. Many women do not realize that the small machines used to hear their baby's heartbeat in pregnancy, and for monitoring during labor, are actually using Doppler ultrasound, although with fairly low exposure levels.

More recently, sonographers have begun using vaginal ultrasound, in which the transducer is placed high in the pregnant woman's vagina, much closer to her developing baby. This is used mostly in early pregnancy, when an abdominal scan can produce a poor picture. However, with vaginal ultrasound there is little intervening tissue to shield the baby, who is at a vulnerable stage of development, and heat may be transferred to the baby. Having a vaginal ultrasound is not a pleasant procedure for the woman; the term "diagnostic rape" was coined to describe how some women experience this procedure.

Another recent application for ultrasound is the nuchal translucency (NT) test, in which the thickness of the nuchal (neck) skin fold at the back of the baby's head is measured at around three months. A slight increase in the thickness of the fold makes a baby more likely, statistically, to have Down syndrome. When the baby's risk is estimated at more than one in 250 to 300, a definitive test is recommended. Around nineteen out of twenty babies diagnosed as high risk via the NT method of testing turn out not to be affected by Down syndrome, and their mothers will have experienced several weeks of unnecessary anxiety. An NT scan does not detect all babies affected by Down syndrome.

Nonmedical ultrasound, using 3-D and 4-D (moving) images, has also become popular as a way to "meet your baby before it is born." This "keepsake" use of ultrasound has been criticized as potentially harmful by the American Institute of Ultrasound in Medicine (AIUM),[10] the European Committee for Medical Ultrasound, Health Canada,[11] the Canadian Society of Diagnostic Medical Sonographers,[12] the American College of Obstetricians and Gynecologists,[13] and the U.S. Food and Drug Administration (FDA), which views it as an unapproved use of a medical device and suggests that consumers report organizations that offer nonmedical ultrasound.[14]

Information Gained from Ultrasound

Ultrasound is used for two main purposes in pregnancy—either to investigate a possible problem at any stage of pregnancy or as a routine scan at around eighteen to twenty weeks.

If there is bleeding in early pregnancy, for example, ultrasound may predict whether miscarriage is inevitable. Later in pregnancy, ultrasound can be used when a baby is not growing, or when a breech baby or twins are suspected. In these cases the information gained from ultrasound can be very useful in decision-making for the woman and her caregivers. However, the use of routine prenatal ultrasound (RPU), also known as a morphology or standard scan, is more controversial, as this involves scanning all pregnant women, whether they have complications or not, in the hope of improving the outcome for some mothers and their babies.

RPU is designed to check the size and integrity of the baby. The timing of RPU (at eighteen to twenty weeks) is chosen for practical reasons; it gives a reasonably accurate due date, along with a reasonable chance of finding most of the abnormalities that scanning can detect.

The assessment of the baby's due date, which is based on size, is most accurate at the early stages of pregnancy, when babies vary the least in size. For example, the estimated due date (EDD) calculated by a scan at seven to eight weeks will be accurate to plus or minus three or four days.[15] At eighteen to twenty weeks, the due date is accurate to around one week on either side of the given date, and some studies have suggested that an early examination, or calculations based on a woman's menstrual cycle, can be as accurate as RPU.[16, 17] Note that a later scan cannot give an accurate due date because of the large variation in size: after twenty-eight weeks, for example, a due date is only accurate to plus or minus three to four weeks.[15]

At eighteen to twenty weeks, the baby is also big enough to detect most of the abnormalities that can be diagnosed with ultrasound. However, this is also not infallible: RPU actually detects between 35 and 80 percent of the one in fifty babies that have significant abnormalities at birth.[18–21] Larger centers and sonographers with more experience tend to have higher detection rates, but even major centers will miss around 40 percent of abnormalities, with most of these abnormalities difficult or impossible to detect.[19, 20, 22] For example, heart and kidney defects are unlikely to be picked up on a routine scan; markers for Down syndrome are also hard to detect; and other major causes of intellectual disability, such as cerebral palsy and autism, are impossible to diagnose via pregnancy ultrasound.

When an abnormality is reported there is also a small chance that the finding is a false positive, where the ultrasound diagnosis is wrong and the baby is less affected or even unaffected. A UK survey showed that, for one in two hundred babies aborted for supposedly major abnormalities, the diagnosis on post-mortem was less severe than predicted by ultrasound, and the termination was probably unjustified. In this survey, 2.4 percent of the babies diagnosed with major malformations, but not aborted, had conditions that were significantly over- or underdiagnosed.[23] Two other studies have shown false positive results in around 10 percent of babies diagnosed with major structural abnormalities,[24, 25] making a repeat scan (preferably by another operator) important in this situation. There are also some conditions that have been seen to spontaneously resolve.[26]

As well as false positives, there are also uncertain cases, in which the ultrasound findings cannot be easily interpreted, and the outcome for the baby is not known. In one study involving women at high risk, almost 10 percent of scans were uncertain.[27] This can create immense anxiety for the woman and her family, and this worry may not be allayed by the birth of a normal baby; in the same study, mothers with uncertain diagnoses were still anxious three months after the birth of their baby.

These uncertainties include the so-called "soft markers": conditions that do not cause problems but are sometimes linked with more serious diagnoses such as Down syndrome. These include choroid plexus cysts in the brain; echogenic bowel and heart foci; short femur; short humerus; and pyelectasis of the kidney. Around 1 percent of babies, for example, have a choroid plexus cyst, but only 1 in 150 of these babies will have a chromosomal abnormality such as Down syndrome.[28] Because the diagnosis of soft markers can cause anxiety, and the overwhelming majority of babies with these markers are normal, some experts have suggested that soft markers should be disclosed to only those women at high risk of abnormality.[29]

In cases in which a chromosomal abnormality is suspected, the doubt can be resolved by further tests such as amniocentesis. In this situation, there may be up to two weeks of waiting for results, during which time a mother has to decide whether she would terminate the pregnancy if an abnormality is found. The process of amniocentesis also carries an additional risk of miscarriage. Some mothers who receive reassuring news have felt that this process has interfered with their relationship with their baby.[30]

In addition to estimating the due date and checking for major abnormalities, RPU can also identify placenta previa (a low-lying placenta) and can detect the presence of more than one baby at an early stage of pregnancy. However, almost all women who have placenta previa detected on an early scan will be needlessly worried; studies have shown that the placenta will effectively move up and not cause problems for 80 to 100 percent of women.[31–34] Some researchers have even suggested that a low-lying placenta seen on an early pregnancy scan does not require a follow-up scan.[33] Furthermore, detection of placenta previa by RPU has not been found safer than detection in labor.[26] No improvement in outcome has been shown for multiple pregnancies either; the vast majority of these will be detected before labor, even without RPU, with no difference in outcome found for mothers or babies.[8]

More recently, ultrasound has been used to assess specific markers such as the length of a pregnant woman's cervix (linked in some studies to premature labor) and the amount of amniotic fluid (AF) at the end of pregnancy, with low levels seen as a marker of risk. However, assessment of AF volume will overestimate the risk: for example, in one study three out of every four overdue babies (72 percent) with a low AF index had no major problems in labor and birth, and only 11 percent required special care after birth.[35] Note also that low AF (oligohydramnios) may reflect maternal dehydration and may be simply corrected by drinking more water, which is likely to also reduce the risks in labor and birth.[36]

A short cervix (less than 25 millimeters), as found on midpregnancy ultrasound, has been shown to be a useful predictor of premature birth only in women who are at high risk (for example, with a previous premature birth) and requires accurate assessment by experienced and well-trained sonographers.[37-39]

In its 2004 Practice Bulletin, the American College of Obstetricians and Gynecologists (ACOG) recommend scans only for specific reasons, including uncertain due dates and fetal assessment, and comments that routine scans are cost-effective only when done by ultrasound specialists working in high-level centers.[6] In a UK review, ultrasound was cost-effective for the health care system only when the majority of babies with ultrasound-diagnosed abnormalities were aborted.[40]

In Canada, guidelines recommend routinely offering a midpregnancy scan and emphasize that information on risks and benefits must be provided and informed consent obtained.[41]

Biological Effects of Ultrasound

Ultrasound waves (USW) are known to affect tissues in two main ways. First, the sonar beam can cause heating of the tissues being scanned. Elevations of temperature up to 1 to 1.5° Celsius (1.8 to 2.7° Fahrenheit) are presumed safe based on whole-body heating in pregnancy, which seems to be safe up to 2.5°C (4.5°F).[42] The degree of heating ultrasound causes will depend on the specific tissues; bone heats more than soft tissue, which heats more than fluid. Heating also depends on machine settings and output and will be greater with longer exposure, especially when the transducer is held stationary.[43]

Doppler scans, which use continuous waves, can cause even more significant heating especially in the baby's developing brain.[44] A recent tissue model suggests that heating in late-pregnancy human fetal tissues exposed to pulsed and Doppler ultrasound may be significantly higher than what is regarded as safe: up to 1.4°C and 5.8°C (2.5 to 10.4° Fahrenheit) respectively.[45]

The second recognized effect is cavitation, in which the small pockets of gas that exist within mammalian tissue vibrate and then collapse. In this situation

> . . . temperatures of many thousands of degrees Celsius in the gas create a wide range of chemical products, some of which are potentially toxic. These violent processes may be produced by micro-second pulses of the kind which are used in medical diagnosis . . . [42]

Cavitation is thought to occur mainly in tissues with significant pockets of gas, such as the lung and bowel after birth. A form of cavitation may be responsible for the bleeding in small blood vessels (capillary bleeding) seen in newborn mice exposed to ultrasound at usual diagnostic levels.[46] The significance of cavitation effects in human fetal tissue remains uncertain, although there is evidence that mammalian tissue may contain microbubbles that are subject to cavitation effects.[47]

As well as heating and cavitation, ultrasound waves may cause other mechanical effects such as acoustic streaming, in which a jet of fluid created by the ultrasound wave causes a mechanical shearing force at the cell surface. This force may change important cell membrane properties such as permeability (the degree to which substances flow into and out of the cell).[47] In a recent review, experts suggest that changes in membrane permeability may have adverse effects not only on embryogenesis (early development), but also on late prenatal and postnatal development. They comment: "protracted examinations using high intensities during periods of cell migration (second and third trimester) may pose some risk to the fetus."[47] Acoustic streaming may explain effects such as increased agglutination (stickiness) of red blood cells following exposure to ultrasound at usual diagnostic levels.[48]

A number of studies have suggested that these biological effects may be of real concern in living tissues. The first study suggesting problems was a study on cells grown in the laboratory. Cell abnormalities caused by exposure to pulsed ultrasound were seen to persist for several generations.[49] Another study involving newborn rats, who are at a similar stage of brain development to humans at four to five months in utero, suggested that pulsed ultrasound may damage the myelin that covers nerves,[50] indicating that the nervous system may be particularly susceptible to damage from this technology.

Another rodent study, published in 2001, showed that exposing adult mice to dosages typical of obstetric (pulsed) ultrasound caused a 22 percent reduction in the rate of cell division and a doubling of the rate of apoptosis (programmed cell death) in the cells of the small intestine.[51]

Other experts in this area have expressed concern in relation to heating of the developing central nervous system, whose tissues are sensitive to damage by physical agents including heat. Barnett, a biomedical physicist, notes that heating of the fetal brain is more likely after the first trimester (three months), as the skull bone is more developed and can reflect and concentrate the ultrasound waves.[44]

One study found brain hemorrhages in mouse pups exposed in the womb to pulsed ultrasound at doses similar to those used on human babies. Researchers comment that this damage, which occurred only at specific ultrasound frequencies, may be due to yet another mechanism, perhaps a mechanical force on tissue near the fetal skull (and other bones).[52] Other researchers found that a single ten-minute pulsed ultrasound exposure in pregnancy affected the locomotor and learning abilities of mouse offspring in adulthood, with a greater effect from longer exposure time.[53]

In another recent study, researchers examined the brains of ten-day-old mice exposed to standard (pulsed) prenatal ultrasound for varying lengths of time and found abnormalities in cell migration—the process by which brain cells move upward from the base of the brain into their appropriate place during development. (In humans this occurs from around eleven to twenty-four weeks). Effects on neuronal migration were greater with longer exposure. No mice exposed to 600 minutes of ultrasound survived to ten days, which may reflect the stress of the procedure in addition to direct ultrasound effects. Researchers suggest that the neuronal damage may be nonthermal and noncavitational, and comment, "There are also some reasons to think that the USW may have a similar or even greater impact on neuronal migration in the human fetal brain."[54] Neuronal migration abnormalities are recognized in human conditions including autism and dyslexia.

There is also evidence that ultrasound waves can produce actual sound within the womb. Researchers placed a microphone beside the amniotic sac during scanning and recorded sound corresponding to 84 decibels when the ultrasound probe was aimed at the microphone.[55] This noise level is as loud as an alarm clock, and recognized as potentially damaging. (Note that Doppler ultrasound does not produce such noise.) Other researchers have confirmed an increase in fetal activity during scanning,[56] which may reflect discomfort due to sound or other sensations.

Cavitation, which also creates tissue-damaging free radicals, may be significant in relation to amniotic fluid. Researchers have found an increase in free radical formation following Doppler application to samples of amniotic fluid, the authors suggest that this effect may also apply to pulsed ultrasound.[57]

One primate study exposed monkey fetuses to frequent (up to ten minutes five times weekly) but low-dose ultrasound and found lower birth weight and lower numbers of white cells in the blood up to five months of age.[58, 59] Researchers suggest that lower weights may be due to disruption of growth hormones. Low birth weight was also found in one human Doppler study, described later.

Research has found that ultrasound also induces bleeding in the lung among other mammals, including newborns and young animals. The American Institute of Ultrasound in Medicine (AIUM) recently concluded thusly:

> There exists abundant peer-reviewed published scientific research that clearly and convincingly documents that ultrasound at commercial diagnostic levels can produce lung damage and focal haemorrhage

> in a variety of mammalian species . . . The degree to which this is a clinically significant problem in humans is not known.[60]

This is likely due to cavitational effects and therefore unlikely to affect babies in the womb, whose lungs are not aerated. However, these solid research findings add extra concerns, for example, about ultrasounds performed on newborn babies.

Human Studies

Single or small studies on humans exposed to ultrasound have shown that possible adverse effects include premature ovulation,[61] preterm labor or miscarriage,[26, 62] low birth weight,[63, 64] poorer condition at birth,[65] perinatal death,[66] dyslexia,[67] delayed speech development,[68] and less right-handedness.[69–72] Nonright-handedness (left-handedness and ambidexterity) is a consistent finding in many ultrasound studies, including the more authoritative randomized controlled trials, and is, in some circumstances, a marker of damage or disruption to the developing brain.[73]

A large UK study found that healthy mothers and babies randomized to two or more Doppler scans to check the placenta, beginning in mid-pregnancy, had more than double the risk of perinatal death compared to babies unexposed to Doppler.[66] Similarly, an Australian randomized Doppler study involving high-risk mothers and babies found more fetal distress in labor and lower APGAR scores at birth among Doppler-scanned babies.[65]

Another Australian study showed that babies randomized to five or more Doppler ultrasounds during pregnancy were 30 percent more likely than babies randomized to routine (pulsed) ultrasound to develop intrauterine growth retardation (IUGR)—a condition that ultrasound is often used to detect.[64] This may be related to higher exposure levels with Doppler, as more IUGR has been found in high-exposure animal studies, but not in lower-exposure human studies using pulsed ultrasound.[74]

Two studies have followed up offspring involved in randomized controlled trials (RCT) in Sweden and Norway in the late 1970s and compared exposed and unexposed (or less exposed) children's development at eight to nine years old. Neither study found any measurable effect on hearing, vision, growth, or learning.[75–80] However, there was more nonright-handedness (left-handedness and ambidexterity) in the offspring in these[69, 71, 72] and several other nonrandomized studies.[70, 81]

Although RCTs are the "gold standard" in medical research, it is difficult to gain reassurance from these trials because, for example, in the Swedish study, 35 percent of the supposedly unexposed group actually had a scan,[69] and in the major branch of the Norwegian trial, scanning time was only three minutes.[77] Scanning intensities used today are also much higher than in 1979–1981; outputs have been estimated to have increased six times between 1991 and 1995 alone.[82]

A recently published follow-up to the Australian Doppler trial, comparing outcomes in offspring randomized to single (pulsed)- or multiple (Doppler) scans, produced some degree of reassurance, finding no differences in the learning and motor functions of offspring followed to eight years old.[83] This study did not, however, include a group of unexposed children, making it unclear whether these children's outcomes are actually normal. It is also noteworthy that almost 45 percent of the single scan group received two or more scans, and that exposures in this study date back to 1989–91. The researchers state, "our results do not lessen our need to undertake further studies of potential bio-effects of prenatal ultrasound scans."[8] Further, as veteran ultrasound researcher Kjell Salvesen notes, "there are no epidemiological [large population] prenatal ultrasound studies with commercially available ultrasound devices produced after 1990."[85]

Note that the preceding evidence does not prove that a single ultrasound examination at low to medium exposure will cause definite harm to a developing baby. However, it tells us, as parents and practitioners, to be cautious about applying this new technology—especially with high and/or repeated exposures—and to always balance the known benefits against possible risks in each individual situation.

In a 2002 review of the safety of ultrasound in human studies, published in the prestigious U.S. journal *Epidemiology*, the authors comment:

> Continued research is needed to evaluate the potential adverse effects of ultrasound exposure during pregnancy. These studies should measure the acoustic output, exposure time, number of exposures per subject, and the timing during the pregnancy when exposure(s) occurred.[86]

These reviewers concluded: "Until long-term effects can be evaluated across generations, caution should be exercised when using this modality during pregnancy."[87]

Ultrasound Exposure and Dose

As these authors imply, we need to know the exposure involved in all studies of ultrasound, but this is not easy to measure because there is a huge range of output, or dose, possible from a single machine. Ultrasound machines can give comparable pictures using a lower output or an output five thousand times higher—and because of the complexity of machines, it has been difficult to quantify the output for each examination.[89]

Furthermore, the incredibly fine details that we are now seeing on scans come at the cost of substantial increases in output. Changes to U.S. FDA regulations since 1993 allow operators to use ultrasound machines with very high outputs, exposing unborn babies to intensities up to eight times higher than what was previously allowed, provided the output is displayed (as thermal and mechanical indices) on the machine.[89]

This new regulation gives operators an incredibly high degree of self-regulation, and its success in protecting unborn babies from harm depends on an appreciation, by each operator, of complex biophysical interactions (which are not well understood) and of the risk-benefit ratio involved in every examination.[46] Such expectations may not be realistic; in the United States, Australia, the UK, and most other countries, ultrasonography training is voluntary, even for obstetricians, and the skill and experience of operators varies widely. It also seems that few operators are aware of research findings such as those just discussed, and sonographers in nonmedical settings may be even less aware of safety issues.

If you choose to have a scan, I recommend that you copy the form on page 91 and ask the doctor who orders your test, as well as the sonographer who performs the test, to fill in the details and to sign it. This will give you a record of your baby's exposure and will also raise the technician's awareness of the dosage that is used on your baby.

The American Institute of Ultrasound in Medicine noted in 2000:

> . . . the responsibility of an informed decision concerning possible adverse effects of ultrasound in comparison to desired information will probably become more important over the next few years.[90]

My Baby's Ultrasound Exposure Record

The following procedure requires the use of ultrasound _____

_____

_____

This is necessary to obtain the following information _____

_____

_____

To my knowledge, there is no current alternative method available to obtain this

information that carries less risk to _____ and her baby

(mother's name)

Signature _____ Date _____

(doctor or midwife)

The ultrasonographer is asked to specify:

Manufacturer and model of ultrasound equipment _____

_____

_____

Date of last calibration _____

Type or combination of types of ultrasound used _____

_____

Intensity of exposure (W/cm sq or mW/cm sq) _____

_____

Maximum thermal index _____

Maximum mechanical Index _____

Time commenced _____ Time completed _____

Duration of exposure _____

Name of hospital or clinic _____

Carried out by _____

Qualifications _____ Position _____

Signature _____ Date _____

Source: Adapted with permission from Beech BL, Robinson J. Ultrasound unsound? *AIMS Journal* Spring 1993;5:1.

Women's Experiences of Ultrasound

Women have not been consulted at any stage in the development of this technology, and their experiences and wishes are presumed to coincide with, or be less important than, the medical information that ultrasound provides.

For example, ultrasound has been presumed to increase bonding or attachment between mother and baby. Research suggests that ultrasound may seem to increase attachment before women experience quickening (feeling the baby move) but not after this.[91, 92]

Ultrasound is also said to provide reassurance: however, women's anxiety has been shown to increase before an ultrasound and then decrease back to previous levels.[91]

Some studies have shown that women have high expectations and enjoy having a scan (unless an abnormality is found),[93] which may reflect an increasing emphasis on a visual rather than felt experience of the baby.[94] As feminist Germaine Greer commented in relation to ultrasound, "We don't believe anything is real these days unless we see it on TV."[95] A visual representation, as in a ultrasound photo or video of the baby, may also be an increasingly important social marker of pregnancy,[94] which may explain the popularity of "keepsake" 3-D and 4-D scans.

Other studies have suggested that women are not fully informed about the risks and benefits of ultrasound,[93, 96] with a Canadian study finding that 46 percent of women did not realize that ultrasound is a screen for abnormalities, 18.6 percent were uncertain about safety, and 37.2 percent were uncertain about the limitations of testing.[96] Researchers comment, "it is beyond the purpose and capability of this routine ultrasound screening programme to meet the current expectations of the women and to provide the level of assurance about fetal well-being that they are seeking."[97]

Supporters of RPU also presume that early diagnosis and termination—the main purpose of ultrasound—is beneficial to the affected woman and her family. However, the discovery of a major abnormality on RPU can lead to very difficult decision-making.

Some women who agree to have an ultrasound are unaware that they may get information about their baby that they do not want, as they would not contemplate a termination.[41] Other women can feel pressured to have a termination, or at the least feel some emotional distancing, when their baby is diagnosed with a possible abnormality.[30]

Furthermore, there is no evidence that women who have chosen termination for a baby with a lethal abnormality are, in the long term, psychologically better off than women whose babies have died at birth; in fact, there are suggestions that the opposite may be true in some cases.[98, 99, 100] And when termination has been chosen, women are unlikely to share their story with others and can experience considerable guilt and pain from the knowledge that they themselves chose the loss.[101]

When a minor abnormality is found—which may or may not be present at birth, as discussed earlier—a woman can feel that the pleasure has been taken away from her pregnancy, and significant stress added.[98] And the process of prenatal diagnosis can cause harm if it generates a high degree of anxiety—and high levels of stress hormones—in the mother, especially early in pregnancy.[102] Women's experiences with ultrasound, and other tests used for prenatal diagnosis are thoughtfully presented in the books *Defiant Birth: Women Who Resist Medical Eugenics* by Melinda Tankard Reist[98] and *The Tentative Pregnancy* by Barbara Katz Rothman.[103] These authors document the heartache that women can go through when a difficult diagnosis is made; for some women, this pain can take years to resolve.

To my mind, ultrasound also represents yet another way in which the deep internal knowledge that a mother has of her body and her baby is made secondary to technological information that comes from an expert using a machine; thus the cult of the expert is imprinted from the earliest weeks of life.

Furthermore, by treating the baby as a separate being, ultrasound artificially splits mother from baby well before this is a physiological or psychic reality. This further emphasizes our culture's favoring of individualism over mutuality and sets the scene for possible—but to my mind artificial—conflicts of interest between mother and baby in pregnancy, birth, and parenting.

Conclusions and Recommendations

I would urge all pregnant women to think deeply before they choose to have a routine ultrasound. It is not compulsory, despite what some may say, and each mother must consider the risks, benefits, and implications of scanning for herself and her baby, according to their specific situation.

If you choose to have a scan, be clear about the information that you do and do not want to be told. Have your scan done by an operator with a high level of skill and experience (usually this means performing at least 750 scans per year), and ask for the shortest scan possible. Ask them to fill out the form on page 91, or to give you the information so you can fill it out, and to sign it.

If an abnormality is found, ask for counseling and a second opinion as soon as practical. And remember that it's your baby, your body, and your choice.

chapter 6

UNDISTURBED BIRTH
Mother Nature's Blueprint for
Safety, Ease, and Ecstasy

With the huge increases in obstetric intervention in recent decades, and the decline in low-technology choices of care such as homebirth and birth centers, many are asking: can natural birth survive, and is it worth saving? This chapter presents the affirmative argument and describes in scientific terms the exquisite hormonal orchestration of "undisturbed" birth and its multiple in-built safety factors for mothers and babies. The impact of common interventions on the laboring mother's hormonal processes is also detailed; a model that provides a scientific base for the "cascade of intervention" in which one intervention leads to another, with the final outcome being a high-technology and possibly frightening birth experience for the mother, her partner, and likely the baby as well. Finally, this chapter has recommendations for enhancing ease, pleasure, and safety in birth that will be useful for mothers, fathers, families, birth supporters, and maternity care providers.

The term undisturbed birth came to have great meaning for me when I gave birth to my fourth baby in darkness, in private, and with only my family present. It describes well this beautiful experience, which awakened me anew to the ecstasy of birth, and I realized that the process of birth can be very simple if we can avoid disturbing it. Comparing this birth with my three previous home births, and with home and hospital births that I had attended, I saw also how ingrained is our habit of disturbance and that our need, as care providers, to "do something" so often becomes self-fulfilling in the birth room.

I realized that birth is also very complex, and that the process is exquisitely sensitive to outside influences. The parallels between making love and giving birth became very clear to me, not only in terms of passion and love, but also because we need essentially the same conditions for both experiences: to feel private, safe, and unobserved. Yet the conditions that we provide for birthing women are almost diametrically opposed to these; no wonder giving birth is so difficult for most women today.

What Disturbs Birth?

As I imply, anything that disturbs a laboring woman's sense of safety and privacy will disrupt the birth process. This definition covers most of modern obstetrics, which has created an entire industry around the observation and monitoring of pregnant and birthing women. Some of the techniques used are painful or uncomfortable, most involve some transgression of bodily or social boundaries, and almost all techniques are performed by people who are essentially strangers to the woman herself. All of these factors are as disruptive to pregnant and birthing women as they would be to any other laboring mammal—with whom we share the majority of our hormonal orchestration in labor and birth.

Underlying these procedures is an ingrained distrust of women's bodies and of the natural processes of gestation and birth. This attitude in itself has a strong nocebo, or noxious, effect.

On top of this is another obstetric layer devoted to correcting the "dysfunctional labor" that such disruption is likely to produce. The resulting distortion of the process of birth—what we might call "disturbed birth"—has come to be what women expect when they have a baby, and perhaps, in a strange circularity, it works. Under this model women are almost certain to need the interventions that the medical model provides, and to come away grateful to be saved no matter how difficult or traumatic their experience.

These disturbances are counterproductive for nurses and midwives also. When a midwife's time and focus is taken up with monitoring and recording, she is less able to be "with woman"—the original meaning of the word midwife—as the guardian of normal birth.

When a midwife's intuitive skills and ways of knowing are increasingly sacrificed to technology, she'll need more and more invasive procedures to get information that, in other times, her heart and hands would have illuminated. And when a woman misses out on the ecstasy of birth, so does her midwife, which will influence her job satisfaction as well as her future expectations of birth.

Undisturbed Birth

However, our women's bodies have their own wisdom, and our innate system of birth, refined over one hundred thousand generations, is not so easily overpowered. This system, which I am calling undisturbed birth, has the evolutionary stamp of approval not only because it is safe and efficient for the vast majority of mothers and babies, but also because it incorporates our hormonal blueprint for ecstasy in birth. When birth is undisturbed, our birthing hormones can take us into ecstasy—outside (*ec*) our usual state (*stasis*)—so that we enter motherhood awakened and transformed. This is not just a good feeling; the post-birth hormones that suffuse the brains of a new mother and her baby also catalyze profound neurological changes. These changes give the new mother personal empowerment, physical strength, and an intuitive sense of her baby's needs,[1] and they prepare both partners for the pleasurable mutual dependency that will ensure a mother's care and protection and her baby's survival.

Undisturbed birth represents the smoothest hormonal orchestration of the birth process, and therefore the easiest transition possible; physiologically, hormonally, psychologically, and emotionally, from pregnancy and birth to new motherhood and lactation, for each woman. When a mother's hormonal orchestration is undisturbed, her baby's safety is also enhanced, not only during labor and delivery, but also in the critical postnatal transition from womb to world. Furthermore, the optimal expression of a woman's motherhood hormones, including the fierce protectiveness of her young, will ensure that her growing child is protected and well nurtured, adding another layer of evolutionary fitness to the process of undisturbed birth.

Undisturbed birth does not necessarily mean unsupported or solitary birth. Some anthropologists believe that human females have sought assistance in birth since we began to walk on two legs, because the change in our pelvic shape that accompanied this upright stance added uniquely complex twists and turns to our babies' journeys during labor and birth. According to Rosenberg and Trevathan, human babies' unique occipito-anterior (OA, back of head to mother's front) position at birth makes an unassisted birth more difficult than for other mammals.[2] It does mean having supporters whom we have specifically chosen as our familiar and loving companions, who are confident in our abilities, and who will intervene as little and as gently as possible.

Undisturbed birth does not imply that birth will be pain-free. The stress hormones released in birth are equivalent to those of an endurance athlete,[3] which reflects the magnitude of this event, and explains some of the sensations of birth. And like a marathon runner, a woman's task in birth is not so much to avoid the pain—which usually makes it worse—but to realize that birth is a peak bodily performance, for which our bodies are superbly designed. Undisturbed birth gives us the space to follow our instincts and to find our own rhythm in an atmosphere of support and trust, which will also help to optimize our birth hormones, aiding us further in transmuting pain.

Undisturbed birth does not guarantee an easy birth. There are many layers, both individual and cultural, that can impede us at birth, and we can also consider that birth has been significantly disturbed in our culture for many generations.

However, when we provide physiological conditions during labor and birth—that is, conditions in which the laboring woman feels private, safe, and unobserved—we are optimizing the functioning of birth hormones for both mother and baby. This, coupled with our unparalleled levels of hygiene and nutrition, gives us a better chance of an easy and safe birth than was the case for almost any of our foremothers, from whom we have also inherited, through evolution and natural selection, the female anatomy and physiology that gives birth most easily and efficiently.

Note also that the processes of human birth are built on the evolutionary foundation of mammalian birth, which stretches back 175 million years. Like our mammalian cousins, human females are designed to give birth safely and efficiently in the wild, and the system of human birth includes inbuilt mammalian mechanisms to ensure that, as far as possible, mother and baby will birth successfully even in the absence of companions. It is even possible that, for some women, birth will proceed most smoothly in the absence of "supporters," who may unwittingly interfere with her mammalian needs for privacy and safety.

The Hormones of Birth

The hormonal orchestration of birth to which I refer is exceedingly complex. Despite a great amount of research over the last fifty years, involving both humans and other mammals, many fundamental processes are still not understood.

For example, we still do not understand what causes the onset of human parturition (childbirth). Many factors are likely to be involved, including hormones and other information passing between mother and baby to ensure readiness of both partners.

The hormones estrogen,[4] progesterone,[5] cortisol,[6] and corticotrophin-releasing hormone (CRH)[7] are all implicated, as is SP-A, a protein made by the maturing fetal lung that enters the amniotic fluid and may directly stimulate the mother's uterus.[8]

In this chapter, I will be primarily discussing the hormones oxytocin; beta-endorphin; the catecholamines, epinephrine and norepinephrine (adrenaline and noradrenaline); and prolactin. As the hormones of love, pleasure and transcendence, excitement, and tender mothering, respectively, these form the major components of an ecstatic cocktail of hormones that nature prescribes to aid birthing mothers of all mammalian species.

Levels of these hormones generally build during an undisturbed labor, peaking around the time of birth or soon after for both mother and baby, and subsiding or reorganizing over the subsequent hours or days. An optimal hormonal orchestration provides ease, pleasure, and safety during this time for mother and baby. Conversely, interference with this process will also disrupt this delicate hormonal orchestration, making birth more difficult and painful, and potentially less safe.

All of these hormones are produced primarily in the middle or mammalian brain, also called the limbic system or emotional brain. For birth to proceed optimally, this more primitive part of the brain needs to take precedence over our neocortex—our "new" or higher brain—which is the seat of our rational mind. This shift in consciousness, which some have called "going to another planet," is aided by (and also aids) the release of birthing hormones such as beta-endorphin, and is inhibited by circumstances that increase alertness, such as bright lighting, conversation, and expectations of rationality.

If we were to consider giving birth as the deepest meditation possible, and give birthing women the appropriate respect, support, and lack of disturbance, we would provide the best physiological conditions for birth. Alternatively, we can consider the parallels between birth and sexual activity, which involves an almost identical pattern of hormone release.[9] In birth, as in lovemaking, we need to feel safe and private so that we can let down our guard, let our hormones flow, and reap the rewards of the processes—which include, in both situations, an ultimate dose of hormonal ecstasy.

Mother Nature's pragmatic and efficient principles dictate that these hormones should also help the baby at birth, and this is being increasingly confirmed by scientific research. This hormonal interdependence contradicts the common medical response to natural birth as the mother's prizing of her own experience over her baby's safety, and underlines the mutual dependency of mother and baby, even as they begin their physical separation.

Estrogen and Progesterone

In our current understanding, the prime movers—the hormones that are involved in setting the scene, which includes activating, inhibiting, and reorganizing other hormone systems—are the sex steroids progesterone and estrogen (of which there are three distinct types). In pregnancy, the placenta's progesterone production increases ten to eighteen times higher than nonpregnant levels, while placental production of estriol, the dominant type of pregnancy estrogen, rises by more than one thousand times[10] with an estrogen surge close to the onset of labor.

These hormones are thought to play a critical and complex role in the initiation of labor, possibly through changes in their levels and/or ratios, or perhaps through local (paracrine) effects within the expectant mother's uterus.[4]

Estrogen also increases the number of uterine oxytocin receptors[11] and gap junctions (connections between muscle cells)[12] in late pregnancy, effectively "wiring up" the uterus for coordinated contractions in labor. Estrogen and progesterone together activate opiate painkilling pathways in the brain and spinal cord in preparation for birth.[10]

Oxytocin

Oxytocin has been called the hormone of love[13] because of its connection with sexual activity, orgasm, birth, and breastfeeding. In addition, oxytocin is produced in social situations such as sharing a meal,[14] making it a hormone of altruism or, as Michel Odent suggests, of "forgetting oneself."[15]

Oxytocin is also the most powerful uterotonic (contraction-causing) hormone, and its release is associated with the contractions of labor and birth in all mammalian species.[16]

Oxytocin is made in the hypothalamus, deep in the middle brain, and is stored in the posterior pituitary, from which it is released in pulses into the bloodstream. Pulses occur every three to five minutes during early labor, becoming more frequent as labor progresses. Levels are difficult to measure in the human because of oxytocin's pulsatile pattern of release and because, in pregnancy, the placenta makes a specific enzyme, oxytocinase, to metabolize oxytocin. Oxytocinase activity increases even more in labor,[17] which may be important in ensuring that oxytocin levels drop substantially between pulses, so that the laboring woman's uterus is exposed to oxytocin only episodically and remains sensitive to its effects. The half-life of oxytocin (the time taken to reduce blood level by half) has been variously estimated as three and a half minutes,[18] ten to twelve minutes,[19] and fifteen minutes.[20]

The number of oxytocin receptors in a pregnant woman's uterus increases substantially late in pregnancy, increasing her sensitivity to oxytocin. Circulating levels do not actually rise until late in labor, as we will discuss.[21] Receptors are most dense in the woman's fundus (the top of her uterus),[19] which helps to coordinate efficient contractions in labor.

Oxytocin is thought to be the prime initiator of the rhythmic uterine contractions of labor, although it is not the only hormonal system involved—mice who have had their oxytocin gene inactivated are still able to deliver, but not to breastfeed, their young.[22] It has been hypothesized that prostaglandins, which are produced locally in the uterus, take over this uterotonic role later in labor.[18] Oxytocin has also been shown to have a painkilling effect in rats and mice.[23]

The baby also releases large amounts of oxytocin from the pituitary during labor, and there is some evidence that this oxytocin may be transported back through the placenta into the mother's circulation.[18, 24] Oxytocin is also produced by the placenta and fetal membranes, as well as being present in amniotic fluid.[18] Some researchers have therefore suggested that fetal oxytocin may directly stimulate the mother's uterine muscle, and that this may be important in the process of labor.[25]

Oxytocin catalyzes the final powerful uterine contractions that help the mother to birth her baby quickly and easily. At this time, the baby's descending head stimulates stretch receptors in a woman's lower vagina, which trigger oxytocin release from her pituitary. This oxytocin release causes more contractions that promote more fetal descent, inducing more stretch-receptor stimulation and therefore even more release of pituitary oxytocin.[26] This "positive feedback loop" is also known as the Ferguson reflex. When labor has been largely undisturbed, this effect may be amplified by epinephrine/norepinephrine, as will be described later, producing an even more powerful mechanism called the fetus ejection reflex (FER).[27]

After the birth, ongoing high levels of oxytocin, augmented by more pulses released as the baby touches, licks, and nuzzles the mother's breast,[28] help to keep her uterus contracted and so protect her against postpartum hemorrhage. Skin-to-skin and eye-to-eye contact between mother and baby also help to optimize oxytocin release.[29] Blood oxytocin levels peak at around thirty minutes postpartum and subside towards the end of the first hour.[30] Oxytocin levels in the brain, which switch on instinctive maternal behavior, may be elevated for substantially longer.[31]

Newborn oxytocin levels also peak at around thirty minutes after birth[32] so that during the first hour after birth, both mother and baby are saturated with high levels of oxytocin, the hormone of love. Newborn babies have elevated levels of oxytocin for at least four days after birth,[32] and oxytocin is also present in breastmilk.[33]

Oxytocin is also involved with the olfactory system, which is known to play an important role in mammalian birth. In labor, stimulation of the olfactory sense augments oxytocin release, and after the birth, smell is thought to be important in the establishment of mothering behavior.[10, 34] For example, one study found that monkeys delivered by cesarean rejected their offspring unless the babies were swabbed with secretions from the mother's vagina.[35] Newborn babies are attracted to the smell of amniotic fluid (which is soothing[36]) and of their mother's nipple,[37] which may help them with locating and attaching to the mother's breast after birth. (Norepinephrine is also involved in postpartum olfaction; see the discussion that follows.) The large number of human genes that are involved with smell—1 to 2 percent of the total[38]—suggests that smell is of evolutionary importance in mother-infant bonding in our species.

As well as reaching peak levels after birth, oxytocin is secreted in large amounts in pregnancy, when it acts to enhance nutrient absorption and conserve energy by making pregnant women more sleepy.[39] The well-documented suppression of the hypothalamic-pituitary-adrenal (HPA) stress pathway during pregnancy and lactation—which keeps pregnant and breastfeeding mothers more relaxed, more resistant to stress, and experiencing more positive mood states—may be due, at least in part, to oxytocin.[10]

Animal studies have shown that the effects of oxytocin, administered to a caged animal, also extend to its untreated cagemates.[40, 41] It seems likely that there is an olfactory or pheromonal transmission (via substances secreted outside the body) involving oxytocin. This transmission may also explain the positive emotions that birth helpers can feel when attending a woman who is birthing with peak levels of oxytocin.

During breastfeeding, oxytocin mediates the milk ejection, or let down, reflex and is released in pulses as the baby suckles. During the months and years of lactation, oxytocin continues to act to keep the mother relaxed and well nourished, by enhancing the efficiency of her digestion. Swedish oxytocin expert Kerstin Uvnas Moberg calls it "a very efficient anti-stress situation, which prevents a lot of disease later on." According to her research, mothers who breastfed for more than seven weeks were calmer, when their babies were six months old, than mothers who did not breastfeed at all.[39]

The oxytocin system has also been implicated in aggressive-defensive behavior in lactating females,[42] although opiate mechanisms are also known to be involved.[43]

Other studies indicate that oxytocin is also involved in cognition, tolerance, and adaptation, and researchers have recently found that oxytocin also acts as a cardiovascular hormone, with effects such as slowing the heart rate and reducing blood pressure.[44]

Uvnas-Moberg describes a "relaxation and growth response" to oxytocin release, which reflects its ability to turn on the parasympathetic nervous system, which is involved with digestion and growth, and to reduce activity in the sympathetic "fight-or-flight" system.[45] Other research suggests that the female response to stress is marked by a "tend and befriend" pattern, which may be mediated by oxytocin.[46] Malfunctions of the oxytocin system have been implicated in conditions such as schizophrenia,[47] autism,[48] cardiovascular disease,[49] and drug dependency,[50] and it has been suggested that oxytocin may mediate the antidepressant effect of drugs such as Prozac.[51]

Beta-Endorphin

Beta-endorphin is one of a group of naturally occurring opiates (drugs derived from the opium poppy), with properties similar to meperidine (Demerol, pethidine), morphine, fentanyl (Sublimaze), and opiate-like drugs such as Nubain and Stadol, and it has been shown to work on the same receptors of the brain. It is secreted from the pituitary gland under conditions of pain and stress, when it acts to restore homeostasis (physiological balance); for example, by acting as a natural painkiller. Beta-endorphin also activates the powerful mesocorticolimbic dopamine reward system, producing reward and pleasure in association with important reproductive activities including mating, birth, and breastfeeding. Beta-endorphin is also released during episodes of social and physical contact, reinforcing pro-social behaviors among all mammals. In pregnant rats, beta-endorphin causes an increased tolerance to pain.[52] Beta-endorphin also suppresses the immune system, which may be important in preventing a pregnant mother's immune system from acting against her baby, whose genetic material is foreign to hers.

Like the addictive opiates, beta-endorphin reduces the effects of stress and induces feelings of pleasure, euphoria, and dependency. Beta-endorphin levels increase throughout labor;[53] with levels of beta-endorphin and CRH (the executive stress hormone) reaching those found in male endurance athletes during maximal exercise on a treadmill.[3] Maternal blood levels peak at the time of birth, subsiding significantly in the first one to three hours and reaching normal levels one to three days after birth.[54] Levels in the new mother's limbic system are likely to be elevated for much longer, as beta-endorphin takes more than twenty-one hours to break down within the brain and cerebrospinal fluid (CSF).[55]

In labor, such high levels help the laboring woman to transcend pain, as she enters the altered state of consciousness that characterizes an undisturbed birth. In the hours after birth, elevated beta-endorphin levels reward and reinforce mother-baby interactions, including physical contact and breastfeeding, as well as contributing to intensely pleasurable, even ecstatic, feelings for both.

The baby also secretes beta-endorphin during labor from the fetal pituitary[56] as well as directly from placental tissue and membranes,[57] and levels in the placenta at birth are even higher than those in maternal blood.[58] Kimball speculates that early cord cutting may "deprive mothers and infants of placental opioid molecules designed to induce interdependency of mothers and infants."[59]

Beta-endorphin has complex and incompletely understood relationships with other hormonal systems.[52] For example, high levels of beta-endorphin inhibit oxytocin release. It makes sense that when pain or stress levels are very high, contractions will slow, thus "rationing labor according to both physiological and psychological stress."[60]

Beta-endorphin may also be involved in preventing premature birth by inhibiting the action of oxytocin before labor begins,[61] and may be one of the "brakes" that lifts with the onset of normal labor.[10] Beta-endorphin facilitates the release of prolactin during labor,[62, 63] which prepares the mother's breasts for lactation and also aids in lung maturation for the baby.[64]

Beta-endorphin is also important in breastfeeding. Levels peak in the mother twenty minutes after commencement,[65] and beta-endorphin is also present in breastmilk.[66] Researchers have found higher levels, at four days postpartum, in the breastmilk of mothers who have had a normal birth, compared with cesarean mothers; they speculate that this extra dose of beta-endorphin is designed to help the newborn with the stressful transition to life outside the womb.[67]

Beta-endorphin, as a component of ongoing mother-baby interactions, induces a pleasurable mutual dependency for both partners, reinforcing and rewarding behaviors such a breastfeeding and physical contact that are associated with long-term well-being and survival.

Catecholamines

The fight-or-flight hormones epinephrine and norepinephrine (adrenaline and noradrenaline) are part of the group of hormones known as catecholamines (CAs) and are produced by the body in response to stresses such as hunger, fear, and cold, as well as excitement. Together they stimulate the sympathetic nervous system for fight or flight.

During labor, maternal CA levels slowly and gradually rise, peaking around transition.[68] However, high epinephrine levels in early labor, which reflect activation of the woman's fight-or-flight system in response to fear or a perception of danger, have been shown to inhibit uterine contractions,[69] therefore slowing or even stopping labor. Norepinephrine also acts to reduce blood flow to the uterus and placenta and therefore to the baby.[70] This reflex makes sense for mammals birthing in the wild, where the presence of danger would activate the fight-or-flight response, inhibiting labor and diverting blood to the major muscle groups so the mother can fight or, more likely, flee to safety. In humans, high levels of epinephrine have been associated with longer labor and adverse fetal heart rate (FHR) patterns, which indicate that the baby is low in oxygen (hypoxic),[71] consistent with CA-mediated reductions in uterine blood flow.

Research has also shown that very high CA levels can paradoxically stimulate uterine contractions,[69] which may contribute to the fetus ejection reflex (FER), as described by Michel Odent.[27] According to Odent, this reflex occurs at transition, or perhaps even earlier in labor, and almost always follows an undisturbed birth, perhaps because low CA levels in early labor are necessary for its full expression. The mother experiences a sudden and enormous increase in CA levels, giving her a rush of energy and strength; she will be upright and alert, with a dry mouth and shallow breathing and perhaps the urge to grasp something. She may express fear, anger, or excitement, and the CA surge will produce, in concert with high oxytocin levels (associated with the Ferguson reflex), several very strong and irresistible contractions that will birth her baby quickly and easily.[27, 71]

Some birth attendants have made good use of this reflex when a woman is having difficulties in the second (pushing) stage of labor. For example, as reported by Odent,[27] one anthropologist working with an indigenous Canadian tribe recorded that when a woman was having difficulty in birth, the young people of the village would gather together to help. They would suddenly and unexpectedly shout out close to her, with the shock increasing her catecholamines and triggering her fetus ejection reflex, giving a quick birth.

After the birth, the new mother's CA levels drop steeply. If she is not helped to warm up, the cold stress will keep her CA levels high, which will inhibit her uterine contractions and therefore increase her risk of postpartum hemorrhage[72] (see chapter 8).

Norepinephrine, as part of the ecstatic cocktail, is also implicated in instinctive mothering behavior. Mice bred to be deficient in norepinephrine will not care for their young after birth unless this hormone is injected back into their system.[73]

For the baby also, labor is an exciting and stressful event, reflected in increasing CA levels. In labor these hormones have a very beneficial effect, protecting the baby from the effects of hypoxia (lack of oxygen) and subsequent acidosis by redistributing cardiac output (blood supply)[74] and by increasing the capacity for anaerobic glycolysis (metabolism of glucose at low oxygen levels).[75]

The baby experiences a marked surge in CA hormones, especially norepinephrine, close to the time of birth, probably triggered by pressure on the head.[76] This surge plays a very important role in the baby's adaptation to extrauterine life. It aids newborn metabolism by increasing levels of glucose and free fatty acids,[77] which protect the newborn's brain from the low blood sugar that can occur in the early newborn period when the baby loses the placental supplies of glucose.[78]

In addition, catecholamines enhance respiratory adaptation to life outside the womb by increasing the absorption of amniotic fluid from the lungs and stimulating surfactant release.[76] (Surfactant is essential for smooth inflation of the newborn lungs). CAs also assist with the necessary newborn shift to nonshivering thermogenesis (heat production),[79] increase cardiac contractility, stimulate breathing, and enhance responsiveness and tone in the newborn.[75]

High CA levels at birth also ensure that the baby is wide-eyed and alert at first contact with the mother. The baby's CA levels also drop steeply after an undisturbed birth, being soothed by contact with the mother, but norepinephrine levels remain elevated above normal for the first twelve hours.[80] High newborn norepinephrine levels, triggered by a normal birth, have been shown to enhance olfactory learning during this period,[81] helping the newborn to learn the mother's smell.

Prolactin

Prolactin, known as the mothering (or nesting) hormone, is released from the pituitary gland during pregnancy and lactation. Prolactin is named for its well-known prolactation effects, preparing a pregnant woman's breasts for lactation and acting postnatally as the major hormone of breastmilk synthesis.

Prolactin's lactogenic (milk-producing) effect is blocked during pregnancy by high levels of progesterone, produced by the baby's placenta. When progesterone levels drop with the birth of the placenta, prolactin can begin stimulating milk production. All mammalian species also produce a placental hormone with lactogenic effects—in the human this is human placental lactogen (hPL). Human placental lactogen, like prolactin, increases throughout pregnancy and also helps to organize the expectant mother's brain for maternity.[82]

Prolactin is an important hormone in reproduction; mice bred with abnormalities in prolactin are unsuccessful in reproduction and lacking in maternal behavior.[83] In all mammalian species, prolactin is thought to play a major role in postpartum maternal behavior through its actions on the nursing mother's brain.[82]

The mother's prolactin levels rise progressively during pregnancy but decline during labor, reaching the lowest point when her cervix is fully dilated. Prolactin then rises again steeply in the moments after birth[84] (perhaps due to stimulation of the mother's cervix during delivery[85]), reaching peak levels in the following two to three hours. After this, levels decline again slowly and reach another nadir from nine to twenty-four hours postpartum.[84, 86–88]

This postpartum maternal surge in prolactin provides maximum levels, available to brain and body, in the hour or so after birth. This elevation may be important in optimizing maternal behaviors at this time, as well as ensuring successful lactation.

During lactation, prolactin levels are directly related to suckling intensity, duration, and frequency,[82] although prolactin levels actually peak at night.[89] After a nursing episode, breastfeeding mothers are calmer, with an elevation in mood and increased resistance to stress: these effects are likely to be due to the lactational peaks of oxytocin and prolactin, both stress-reducing hormones.[00]

There are more than three hundred known bodily effects of prolactin,[83] including induction of maternal behavior, increase in appetite and food intake, suppression of fertility, stimulation of motor and grooming activity, reduction of the stress response, stimulation of oxytocin secretion and opioid activity, alteration of the sleep-wake cycle and increase in REM sleep, reduction in body temperature, and stimulation of natural analgesia.[82] Prolactin, along with growth hormone (GH), is one of the hormones of growth and lactation (HGL) and as such has a crucial influence in the development and function of the immune system.[91]

This spectrum of prolactin effects has been called the maternal subroutine (MS) and is associated psychologically with the perceived need to take care of a child. For example, elevations of prolactin can be triggered by surrogate maternity.[92, 93]

Prolactin is also a hormone of submission or surrender. In some studies of primate troupes, the dominant male has the lowest prolactin level,[94] while other troupe members have higher prolactin levels and are more subordinate and obedient.[15] In the breastfeeding relationship, these prolactin effects may help the mother to put her baby's needs first.

Animal studies show that prolactin release is also increased by carrying infants,[95, 96] and its association with paternal nurturing[97] (including in humans[98]) has earned it the added title "the hormone of paternity."[99] Human studies have shown that just before the birth, fathers-to-be have elevated prolactin levels, which parallel the rise of prolactin in their partners.[90] New fathers with higher prolactin levels are more responsive to newborn cries.[100]

The baby produces prolactin in utero, and prolactin is also present in breastmilk, with a significant amount being transferred intact into the newborn circulation, at least in the rat.[101] According to one researcher, "there is evidence that prolactin plays an important role in the development and maturation of the neonatal [newborn] neuroendocrine [brain-hormone] system."[102] This may partly explain the enhanced IQ and brain development of breastfed babies.[103, 104]

Impact of Obstetric Procedures

Induction and Augmentation with Synthetic Oxytocin

Induction can be a useful and even life-saving intervention in complicated pregnancies. However, our current rates of induction, and the use of oxytocic ("fast labor") drugs to speed up labor (known as augmentation, stimulation, or acceleration), are extreme.

The most commonly used drug for induction and augmentation is synthetic oxytocin, known as Pitocin or Syntocinon. In the 2006 U.S. Listening to Mother's II survey, 34 percent of women reported that their labor had been medically induced, with Pitocin used for 80 percent of these inductions. Pitocin was also reportedly administered to 55 percent of vaginally birthing women to augment their labor.[105]

Official U.S. figures give a 22.3 percent induction rate in 2005; more than double the 1990 rate (9.5 percent).[106] Elsewhere, induction rates were 25.6 percent in Australia (2005)[107] and around 20 percent in England (2005 to 2006)[108] and Canada (2001 to 2002).[109]

As with all medical interventions, the balance between benefit and risk becomes weighted toward risk when powerful drugs and procedures are used on essentially healthy individuals. Drugs used for induction and augmentation can cause harm to mothers and babies because they produce an abnormal labor. These drugs can also interfere with the orchestration of the mother's ecstatic hormones and possibly with the brain-hormone system of her baby as well.

Synthetic oxytocin is administered intravenously (IV) in labor and acts very differently from a laboring woman's intrinsic oxytocin, which is largely released from her limbic system and so permeates her brain, as the hormone of love, as well as her body.

First, the uterine contractions produced by IV Pitocin are different from natural contractions—possibly because it is administered continuously rather than in a pulsatile manner[110]—and this can cause detrimental effects to the baby in the womb. Pitocin-induced contractions will be longer, stronger, and closer together than a woman's natural contractions, especially early in labor. This can cause stress to the baby because there is insufficient time to recover from the reduced blood flow that occurs when the placenta is compressed with each contraction. Pitocin also causes the resting tone of the uterus to increase, further restricting refueling.[111] Such overstimulation (hyperstimulation) can deprive the baby of the necessary supplies of blood and oxygen, and so produce abnormal FHR patterns, fetal distress (leading to cesarean section), and even, by overstimulating the mother's uterus, lead to uterine rupture.[111]

Birth activist Doris Haire describes the effects of Pitocin on the baby:

> The situation is analogous to holding an infant under the surface of the water, allowing the infant to come to the surface to gasp for air, but not to breathe.[112]

This assessment is supported by a recent study that used an intrauterine catheter to directly measure the uterine pressure (IUP) among laboring women, most of whom had Pitocin infusions. Those women who had longer contractions, higher maximum pressure, and shorter intervals between contractions were more likely to have newborns with acidosis, as measured in cord blood at birth. Acidosis at birth implies some degree of oxygen deprivation during labor and is associated with a low APGAR score, signifying poor condition at birth, and increased need for NICU (neonatal intensive care unit) care and assisted ventilation (breathing) in the newborn period.[113]

Although the direct effects of induction on acidosis and newborn well-being have not been well researched, one Swedish study found a doubled risk of acidosis in babies born following induced compared to spontaneous labor,[114] and a large Belgian study, including over 7,000 mothers and babies, found an increased need for transfer to neonatal care for the newborns of low-risk first-time mothers who had been electively induced (induced for nonmedical reasons), compared to babies born following spontaneous labor.[115]

The U.S. Pitocin package insert warns that Pitocin can cause fetal heart abnormalities (bradycardia, premature ventricular contractions and other arrhythmias—all signs of fetal distress); low five-minute APGAR scores; neonatal jaundice; neonatal retinal hemorrhage; permanent central nervous system or brain damage; and fetal death.[116]

A U.S. hospital study using low or high-dose protocols for induction with Pitocin found that 42 and 55 percent of induced women respectively experienced hyperstimulation (usually remedied by turning down the infusion rate), and 3 and 6 percent respectively required a cesarean for fetal distress.[117] A Swedish study showed an almost three times higher risk of asphyxia for babies born after augmentation with Pitocin,[118] and in a study in Nepal, where monitoring is not optimal, induced babies were five times more likely to have signs of brain damage at birth.[119]

Note that the ability of the baby to tolerate low levels of oxygen is naturally increased in late labor (when maternal contractions are at their most powerful) through the catecholamine surge that occurs close to the time of birth, triggered by pressure on the fetal head, as discussed earlier. It is likely that this protective mechanism is less active for babies in earlier stages of labor, when the head is higher in the mother's pelvis. This may explain the increased vulnerability of babies who are exposed to powerful Pitocin-induced contractions early in labor (and the need for monitoring), compared with babies in spontaneous and nonaugmented labor.

Stronger contractions are also more painful for the laboring woman, who is very likely to require painkilling drugs or an epidural. And because synthetic oxytocin, administered IV, cannot cross through the adult blood-brain barrier into the limbic system, women receiving this drug do not receive the psycho-emotional benefits of oxytocin during labor (including analgesia) nor do they benefit from enhanced feelings of calm and connection during labor or after birth.

Although Pitocin stimulates uterine contractions, this has minimal effects on the dilation of a laboring woman's cervix, compared with a normal labor.[120] This creates the possibility of a "failed induction"— in which, despite the presence of regular, and sometimes very painful, contractions, labor does not progress, the woman's cervix fails to dilate, and a cesarean becomes necessary.

Pitocin can cause other negative effects for the laboring woman. For example, there is ample evidence that women who are administered a Pitocin infusion for induction or augmentation are at increased risk of postpartum hemorrhage.[121–123] Research indicates that this is because prolonged exposure to nonpulsatile synthetic oxytocin in labor leads to a dramatic reduction in the numbers of oxytocin receptors in the laboring woman's uterus.[124] This makes her uterus insensitive to oxytocin and her own postpartum oxytocin release ineffective in preventing hemorrhage in the crucial minutes after birth. In these circumstances, extra doses of Pitocin are likely to be necessary.

Although we are gaining in understanding of the physical effects of synthetic oxytocin, administered in labor, we do not yet understand the full psychological, or psychoneuroendocrine (mind-brain-hormone) effects of interference with the oxytocin system at the time of birth.

In one study, women whose labors were augmented with Pitocin did not experience an increase in beta-endorphin levels in labor,[125] indicating the complexities that may result from interference with any of the hormonal systems of birth. Hormonal disruption may also explain the findings, in some studies, of a reduced rate of breastfeeding following induced labor.[126–128] (This has occurred even among women who intended to breastfeed[128] and when controlling for other variables associated with low breastfeeding rates.[126]) Another contributing factor could be the extra stress of an induced or augmented labor: stress in labor has been linked with a reduction in breastmilk production.[129]

Other research has suggested that, in humans, oxytocin may pass through the placenta to the baby,[24, 130] and a recent rat study looking at the fetal brain during labor has provided evidence that maternal oxytocin can not only cross to the offspring but also enter the fetal brain at this time, because of an immature fetal blood-brain barrier.[131] These findings suggest that the fetal oxytocin system may also be affected by administration of synthetic oxytocin in labor.

However, there have been few direct studies, animal or human, of the effects of induction and augmentation on the offspring. Observational studies have shown differences in newborn resting brain activity[132] and in neurological development at age two months[133] compared with babies born after spontaneous delivery, but other researchers have found no difference in psychomotor development at thirty months (for induction using prostaglandins)[134] and in motor, IQ, auditory, and visual development at five years of age.[135] A recent dissertation study using a pilot survey of mothers has linked the use of Pitocin in labor with subtle shifts in psychosocial functioning among three-year-olds.[136] More research is obviously needed.

Another recent study assessed changes in temperature during skin-to-skin nursing among newborns exposed to different drugs in labor. Babies exposed to synthetic oxytocin in labor showed an exaggerated temperature response to skin-to-skin contact and breastfeeding. Researchers suggest that the autonomic nervous system, which regulates basic body functions including temperature, may be altered by this intervention.[137]

Animal models using exogenous oxytocin (from external sources) in the perinatal period raise more concerns about the possible longer-term effects of such exposure. In one study, prairie voles that were exposed to a single dose of synthetic oxytocin a few hours after birth showed abnormalities in sexual and parenting behaviors in adulthood.[138]

The hypothesis that induction may predispose to neurobehavioral abnormalities such as autism has been proposed[48, 139, 140] because interference with the oxytocin system has been implicated in autism in animal[141–143] and human studies.[144–146] There is some evidence, from epidemiological (population-based) studies, that induction may be a risk factor,[147] but studies thus far have not supported a direct causal effect.[148, 149] It is likely that conditions such as autism have many causative factors,[150] although this may include, especially for vulnerable individuals, exposure to Pitocin around the time of birth.

Note also that, under western obstetric care, synthetic oxytocin is routinely administered to the mother as her baby is being born, as part of the active management of third stage. If oxytocin can cross the placenta and the fetal blood-brain barrier, the majority of newborn babies could be exposed to this substance. (See chapter 8 for more detail about management of the third stage, and chapter 4 for more about induction risks.)

Opiate Painkillers

In the United States, opiates such as nalbuphine (Nubain), butorphanol (Stadol), alphaprodine (Nisentil), hydromorphone (Dilaudid), and fentanyl (Sublimaze) have been traditional mainstays of labor analgesia. Meperidine (Demerol, pethidine), which is the usual opiate administered in Australia and the UK, has also been frequently used, but the popularity of these drugs has decreased due to the rise in epidural availability and use. In the 2006 U.S. Listening to Mothers II survey, 22 percent of women reported using opiates during labor.

Opiates are simple to administer, and in many places the midwife or labor and delivery nurse can prescribe and inject these drugs during labor. However, research has questioned their efficacy, with some research showing that opiates produce excessive sedation and little pain relief,[151] with an overall reduction in pain of only about 20 percent with these drugs.[151–153]

All opiates used in labor can cause side effects such as nausea, vomiting, sedation, pruritus (itching), hypotension (low blood pressure), and respiratory depression. For the baby, these drugs can cause FHR abnormalities (usually related to drowsiness), respiratory depression, impaired early breastfeeding, and altered neonatal neurobehavior (behavior reflecting brain function),[154] largely due to their sedating effects and ready passage through the placenta.

Use of these drugs may also reduce a laboring woman's own opioid hormone release,[155] which may be helpful if excessive levels are inhibiting labor. However, the use of pethidine has been shown to slow labor in a dose-response way.[156] In one randomized trial, morphine administered in labor directly reduced oxytocin release,[157] which is consistent with research showing that, within the mammalian brain and limbic system, opiates reduce the release of oxytocin.[158]

Given that the release of opiates within the brain is connected with maternal behavior, it is not surprising that animal research has found that these substances (given, in these studies, after the establishment of lactation) can disrupt various aspects of early mothering.[159–162]

Again, we must ask, "What may be the effects for mother and baby of laboring and birthing without peak levels of this hormone of pleasure and transcendence?" Some researchers have described our endogenous opiates as the reward system for reproductive acts; that is, our endorphins keep us making babies, having babies, and breastfeeding.[15, 163] Anecdotally, I notice that women who have pleasurable experiences of birth and breastfeeding tend to have larger families and, on a global scale, countries that have embraced the obstetric model of care, which prizes drugs and interventions above birthing pleasure and empowerment, have experienced steeply declining birth rates in recent years.

More serious are the implications of Swedish research into the use of opiates at birth,[164] recently repeated in a U.S. population.[165] In the first study, researchers looked at the birth records of two hundred opiate addicts born between 1945 and 1966, and compared them to their nonaddicted siblings. Offspring whose mothers used analgesia in labor (opiates, barbiturates, and nitrous oxide gas) were more likely to become addicted to drugs (opiates, amphetamines) as adults, especially when multiple doses were administered. For example, when a mother had received three doses of any of these drugs in her labor, her child was 4.7 times more likely to become addicted to opiate drugs in adulthood compared with unexposed offspring. This figure was replicated almost exactly in the U.S. study.

Animal studies suggest a mechanism for such an effect. It seems that, as with the research on oxytocin and prairie voles cited earlier,[138] drugs and hormones administered in the perinatal (late pregnancy and early newborn) period can cause effects in brain structure and function in offspring that may not be obvious until adulthood.[166–173]

For example, Csaba and colleagues have found that, among rats, adult behavior (and especially reproductive behavior) can become abnormal after a single perinatal administration of substances including beta-endorphin[174] and serotonin[175, 176] (another natural brain chemical).

In one of their studies, changes in brain chemistry after one dose of beta-endorphin administered in late pregnancy persisted through three generations,[177] and these researchers summarize:

> Perinatally, the first encounter between the maturing receptor and its target hormone results in hormonal imprinting, which adjusts the binding capacity of the receptor for life. In the presence of an excess of the target hormone or foreign molecules than can be bound by the receptor, faulty imprinting carries life-long consequences.[172]

Note also that, in these studies, administration of a single dose of Vitamin K soon after birth caused changes in sexual behavior in adulthood[178] and increased the number of uterine estrogen receptors among female offspring.[179]

Along with the possibility of hormonal imprinting, there may be direct, toxic effects from any drugs that the baby is exposed to during labor and birth. Researchers warn, "During this prenatal period of neuronal [brain cell] multiplication, migration, and interconnection, the brain is most vulnerable to irreversible damage."[180]

Epidural and Spinal Drugs

Epidural pain relief has major effects on all of the hormones of labor we have discussed here. Epidurals inhibit beta-endorphin production[53, 181–183] as do spinals.[184] Both will therefore also inhibit the alteration in consciousness that is part of a normal labor, and their popularity may partly reflect our lack of understanding of the hormonal processes and of the need for laboring women to shift their state of consciousness. Most modern birth settings are also lacking in the experience, training, and environmental facilities to accommodate this most basic requirement for birth.

Epidurals reduce oxytocin production[185, 186] or stop its rise[181, 182] during labor. When an epidural is in place, the oxytocin peak that occurs at the time of birth is also inhibited because the stretch receptors of a birthing woman's lower vagina, which trigger this peak, are numbed. This effect probably persists even when the epidural has worn off and sensation has returned, because the nerve fibers involved are smaller than the sensory nerves and therefore more sensitive to drug effects.[187] A woman laboring with an epidural therefore misses out on the final powerful contractions of labor and must use her own effort, often against gravity, to compensate for this loss. This explains the increased length of the second stage of labor and the increased need for forceps when an epidural is used.[188]

The use of epidurals also inhibits catecholamine release for the laboring woman.[189, 190] This may be advantageous for the mother in the first stage of labor; however, close to the time of birth a reduction in CA levels will likely inhibit the fetus ejection reflex and prolong the second stage. Some studies have shown excessively high CA levels among epidural babies,[191] suggesting high levels of stress: this may contribute to alterations in newborn blood glucose and lipid (fat) levels, both important energy sources, in the hours after birth.[192, 193]

Release of the uterine-stimulating prostaglandin F2 alpha is also adversely affected by epidurals. Levels of this hormone naturally rise during an undisturbed labor, consistent with its presumed role as the major mediator of uterine contractions later in labor. However, in one study, women with epidurals experienced a decrease in PGF2 alpha, and a prolongation of labor.[186] In this study, average labor times increased from 4.7 to 7.8 hours.

All of these hormonal disruptions explain some of the most recognized consequences of epidurals on the processes of labor, as described in chapter 7. Effects include a lengthening of labor (by an average of twenty-six minutes in first stage and fifteen minutes in second stage[194]), doubled chance of oxytocin augmentation,[194, 195] doubled need for instrumental delivery,[195] doubled risk of a severe perineal tear (third or fourth degree),[194] and a 1.5 times increased risk of cesarean.[188] In six of nine studies reviewed in one paper, less than half of women who received an epidural had a spontaneous vaginal delivery.[188]

Note that most of the comparison groups used in these studies involve women using opiate drugs, which also disrupt the hormonal processes of labor, although to a lesser extent. It is likely that a comparison with women using no drugs in labor would have found even more significant effects.

Drugs administered by epidural enter the mother's bloodstream within minutes and go straight to the baby at equal (and sometimes effectively greater) levels as in the mother.[196, 197] A baby's immature system takes longer to eliminate epidural drugs: for example, the half-life for the commonly used local anesthetic Bupivicaine is 2.7 hours in an adult but around eight hours in a newborn baby.[198]

Studies using the comprehensive Brazelton Neonatal Behavioral Assessment Scale (NBAS) have found deficits in newborn abilities consistent with toxicity from these drugs.[188]

Epidural anesthesia used for cesareans has also been associated with more acidosis in healthy newborn babies compared with general anesthetic, an indication that epidurals can compromise fetal blood and oxygen supply.[199, 200] This effect is probably due to the well-recognized drop in maternal blood pressure that epidurals cause.[188]

Another indication that epidurals may have unintended hormonal effects for mothers and babies comes from French researchers who gave epidurals to laboring sheep.[201] The ewes failed to display their normal mothering behavior especially those in their first lambing that were given epidurals early in labor. Seven out of eight of these mothers showed no interest in their offspring for at least thirty minutes.

Some studies indicate that this disturbance may also apply to humans. Mothers given epidurals in one study spent less time with their babies in hospital, in inverse proportion to the dose of drugs they received and the length of the second stage of labor.[202] In another study, mothers who had epidurals described their babies as more difficult to care for one month later.[203] Such subtle shifts in relationship and reciprocity may reflect any or all of these factors: hormonal dysfunctions, drug toxicity, and the less-than-optimal circumstances that often accompany epidural births: long labors, forceps, and cesareans.

For more about labor epidurals, including effects on breastfeeding, see chapter 7.

Cesarean Surgery

In the Western world we are experiencing an epidemic of cesareans, and we have somehow come to believe that this is a safe—and perhaps even safer—way of delivering our babies. Medical evidence does not support this assertion. As described in chapter 9, cesarean surgery involves major abdominal surgery and increases the risk of maternal death overall by about four times,[204–206] and, for elective surgery on a healthy mother and baby, by around three times.[207] Increasing evidence suggests that cesarean babies may also be more at risk—even healthy, low-risk babies[208, 209]—and that elevated risks continue in every subsequent pregnancy for both mother and baby, as discussed in chapter 9.

With a cesarean, there will be an absent or curtailed labor and the maternal hormonal peaks of oxytocin, endorphins, and catecholamines are absent or reduced. The multiphasic pattern of prolactin secretion is eliminated in elective cesarean.[88]

Studies of babies delivered by elective cesarean also show significantly lower levels of oxytocin,[210] endorphins,[57] catecholamines,[211] and prolactin.[88, 212] Some of the well-documented risks of cesareans may be due to these hormonal deficits—particularly, for the baby, to the absence of the catecholamine surge. This means that babies born after cesareans are at increased risk of respiratory compromise[213–216] for up to a week after birth,[217] as well as low blood sugar[77] and poor temperature regulation.[218]

Brain oxygenation is lower immediately after cesarean versus vaginal birth,[219] possibly because of the lack of blood redistribution from the catecholamine surge and/or the loss of the placental transfusion with cesarean delivery.[220] (See chapter 8 for more about the placental transfusion.)

Recent research in rats,[131] mentioned earlier, suggest that the laboring mother's natural oxytocin crosses to her baby's brain and reverses the function of the brain chemical gamma-aminobutyric acid (GABA), leading to reduced brain activity and therefore less need for blood and oxygen. This neuroprotective effect likely applies to human babies and, again, babies born via elective cesarean will miss it.

These changes may explain the slower neurological adaptation after birth in cesarean babies,[221–223] which may in turn explain the cesarean baby's delay in adapting to a diurnal pattern of sleep.[224]

Recent research has found many more differences in the physiology of cesarean newborns. These include differences in levels of the hormones of calcium metabolism,[225] renin-angiotensin (fluid and blood pressure regulating) hormones,[226–228] human atrial natriuretic peptide (a hormone produced by the heart),[229] progesterone,[230] the muscle enzyme creatinine kinase,[231] brain dopamine pathways,[232] nitric oxide synthesis[233] (which helps with lung maturation),[234] the insulin-like hormone IGFBP1,[235] melatonin,[236] thyroid hormones (which normally decrease during labor and surge in the hours after birth),[237] and liver enzymes.[238]

In the immune and blood systems, cesarean babies have depressed neutrophil function[239] and survival;[240] fewer neutrophils, lymphocytes, and natural killer cells (all white cells that fight infection);[241] less IgG (a type of immunoglobulin or antibody);[242] different phagocyte function (a white cell that ingests bacteria—this difference persists for six months);[243] lower hematocrit, reflecting fewer red cells;[244] less erythropoietin (a substance that signals red cell production);[245] decreased transfer of antibodies against Herpes simplex through the placenta;[246] less activation of monocytes (white cells that make antibodies);[247] decreased ability of monocytes to make cytokines (which kill foreign cells);[248] down-regulated lymphocyte adenoreceptors;[249] changes in coagulation factors;[250] and lower levels of leukotrienes (which mediate inflammation and healing).[251]

Gut function also differs for cesarean babies, whose stomachs are less acid than vaginally born babies' after birth,[252] and who secrete less of the gut hormones gastrin[253] and somatostatin.[210] Cesarean babies have an altered bowel flora compared with vaginally born babies, which persists for at least six months, and possibly lifelong.[254] This bowel flora abnormality (which occurs because the cesarean baby is not exposed to the mother's bowel flora at birth) may explain the increased susceptibility of premature cesarean babies to newborn gut infections,[255] and possibly the increased risk of asthma[256, 257] and allergies[258] (including food allergies[258]) for cesarean offspring in later life. (See chapters 4 and 9 for more about newborn gut flora.)

The processes of labor and birth are known to produce oxidative stress for the baby,[259] which is heightened when the newborn is suddenly exposed to the oxygen-rich environment after birth. Term labor triggers an increase in antioxidants in the baby's blood that may act to protect against this sudden hyperoxia (high levels of oxygen).[260] (See also chapter 8 for information about the antioxidant properties of bilirubin.)

Another protective system is the transfer of the amino acid tryptophan from mother to baby during labor, which is used by the baby to make kynurenine. This substance protects the newborn's vulnerable brain against, for example, seizures and brain damage due to low oxygen levels. This transfer is reduced for cesarean babies.[261]

Many of these differences may be due to a reduced activation of the baby's stress hormones with cesarean delivery, especially elective cesarean: in a normal labor, the baby's stress hormones are thought to activate many of the hormonal and metabolic systems just described. In more simple terms, we could say that the processes of labor and birth are designed to fully awaken the baby to prepare for life outside the womb.

These stress hormones—which include cortisol, adrenocorticotropic hormone (ACTH, which releases cortisol from the adrenal), and arginine vasopressin (AVP, also known as antidiuretic hormone, ADH), as well as beta-endorphin and the catecholamines[262]—follow the hormonal pattern described earlier for vaginally born babies; they are elevated in labor, peak at birth, then slowly decline. Levels in cesarean babies are reduced overall and the pattern may also be different; for example, beta endorphin levels are elevated at birth but are maintained or continue to rise in the following hours,[263] perhaps reflecting the fact that the cesarean baby lacks the normal preparation for birth and so is maximally stressed in the hours afterward.

After a cesarean mothers and babies are usually separated for some hours (which may be another reason for stress in a cesarean newborn), so the first breastfeeding is usually delayed. Both will also be affected to some extent by the drugs used in the procedure (epidural, spinal, or general anesthetic) and for postoperative pain relief.

The maternal consequences of such radical departures from our genetic blueprint are suggested in the work of Australian researchers who interviewed 242 women in late pregnancy and again after birth. The 50 percent of women who had given spontaneous vaginal birth experienced, in general, a marked improvement in mood and an elevation of self-esteem after delivery. In comparison, the 17 percent of women who had cesarean surgery were more likely to experience a decline in mood and self-esteem. The remaining women had a forceps or vacuum delivery, and their mood and self-esteem were, on average, unaltered.[264]

Another study looked at the breastfeeding hormones prolactin and oxytocin on day two, comparing women who had given birth vaginally with women who had undergone emergency cesarean surgery. In the cesarean group, prolactin levels did not rise as expected with breastfeeding, and oxytocin pulses were reduced or absent. In this study, first suckling had been at 240 minutes average for cesarean babies and 75 minutes average for babies vaginally born. The authors of this study believe that these differences may be partly explained by the delay in the first breastfeed, and conclude,

> These data indicate that early breastfeeding and physical closeness may be associated not only with more interaction between mother and child, but also with endocrine [hormonal] changes in the mother.[265]

The possible consequences of these hormonal changes are explored in a recent study of 185 breastfeeding new mothers and babies. The study found that healthy, breastfeeding cesarean babies had a significantly lower breast milk intake for the first six days, compared with babies born after a normal birth, even when controlling for the mothers' previous birth and breastfeeding experience and for delay in first feeding. These researchers found that only 20 percent of cesarean babies had regained their birth weight by day six, compared with 40 percent of babies in the normal birth group.[266] The authors conclude that there is a lag in breast milk transfer (BMT) after a cesarean.

Other research has shown that early and frequent suckling positively influences milk production and the duration of breastfeeding.[267, 268]

Many other studies and reviews have shown significantly reduced breastfeeding rates after cesarean surgery,[269–271] which may reflect all of the effects just detailed. These findings also highlight the extra assistance that cesarean mothers and babies may need with early breastfeeding.

These cesarean studies not only indicate important links between birth, hormones, and breastfeeding, but also show how an optimal birth experience is designed to enhance the long-term health of mother and baby. For example, successful and long-term breastfeeding confers advantages such as reduced risk of breast cancer and osteoporosis for the mother, and reduced risk of diabetes and obesity, along with increased intelligence, long-term, for the child. (See chapter 12 for more details.)

The connections between events at birth and long-term health certainly deserve more study.[272] But we cannot afford to wait many years for researchers to prove the benefits of an undisturbed birth. Perhaps the best we can do is to trust our instincts and vote with our birthing bodies, choosing (and supporting) models of care that increase the chances of undisturbed—and therefore safer, easier, and more ecstatic—birthing.

Early Separation

There are many animal studies that show that removing newborns from their mothers has negative effects on maternal-infant care and on the growing offspring. For some species there is an inviolable need to lick and smell the offspring; without this, attachment will not occur. There seems also to be a critical period for mammals—the first hour or so after birth—when this process is most easily disrupted.

Human studies also support the importance of not disturbing this early contact. Swedish researchers noted that if an infant's lips touched the mother's nipple in the first hour of life, the mother kept her infant with her for an extra fifty-five minutes every day, compared with mothers who did not experience suckling until later.[273]

Early breastfeeding also confers a lifelong benefit to the baby's gut system. Klaus, quoting research by Uvnas-Moberg,[274] comments:

> . . . when the infant suckles from the breast, there is an outpouring of 19 different gastrointestinal hormones in both the mother and the infant, including insulin, cholecystokinin, and gastrin. Five of these hormones stimulate the growth of intestinal villi in the mother and the infant. As a result, with each feeding, there is an increased intestinal surface area for nutrient absorption. The hormonal release is

stimulated by the touch of the mother's nipple by her infant's lips. This increases oxytocin in both the mother's brain and the infant's brain, which stimulates the vagus nerve, then causes the increase in the output of gastrointestinal hormones. Before the development of modern agriculture and grain storage 10,000 years ago, these responses in the infant and mother were essential for survival when famine was common.[275]

Undisturbed early contact, especially skin-to-skin, fulfills the newborn's physical needs, giving efficient temperature regulation, easy access to the mother's breast, and less crying than among babies who are wrapped and placed in cribs.[276] One study showed that newborns who experienced "kangaroo care"—that is, uninterrupted skin-to-skin contact with the mother—in the first hour after birth were less stressed and more organized in their behavior, cried less, and slept longer, compared with babies who were routinely separated.[277] In another study, elevated skin temperatures, indicating lower levels of stress and CA hormones, were found to persist for twenty-three hours in babies who had been skin to skin with their mothers after birth.[278]

Researchers have also identified a separation distress call in the human neonate, equivalent to that in other mammalian species. This cry, which is almost certainly genetically encoded, signals the newborn's need for close body contact with the mother after birth and ceases at reunion. The authors note, "These findings are compatible with the opinion that the most appropriate position of the healthy full-term newborn baby after birth is in close body contact with the mother."[279]

There are also good reasons for continued contact between mother and baby, if the baby is distressed at birth. For example, the baby can be resuscitated with the cord intact, which gives the advantage of an ongoing supply of blood and oxygen to support this transition. (For more about this, see chapter 8.)

Beyond the early hours after birth, there is a vulnerable period when attachment is still developing; separation at this time also has negative long-term consequences for all mammalian species. For example, researchers found that infant rats removed for five hours a day in the first week of life had increased responsiveness to stress in adulthood, associated with alterations in HPA (stress) hormone regulation.[280] In humans the duration of this vulnerable period is not known, but some experts believe that it could last for weeks to months.[281]

In humans, extra contact "allowed" in hospitals decreases the risks of abandonment, abuse, neglect, and failure to thrive in childhood. These benefits have been noted in many hospitals that have adopted the WHO Baby-Friendly Hospital Initiative (BFHI), which includes early contact and routine rooming in for mother and baby (rather than putting the baby in a nursery). [282]

For example, in one hospital in Thailand abandonment was reduced from thirty-six per ten thousand to one per ten thousand after becoming "baby-friendly."[283] In an earlier study, U.S. researchers found substantially less "parental inadequacy" as well as improved child development for those high-risk mothers randomly allocated to rooming in with their babies.[284]

In another study, mothers who had experienced extra early contact with their babies spoke differently to their children at two years of age, using more questions, adjectives, and words per proposition, along with fewer commands and content words.[285]

The wisdom of undisturbed mother-baby contact after birth is well described by Joseph Chilton Pearce in his book *Evolution's End: Claiming the Potential of Our Intelligence.* According to Pearce, when the newborn baby is in skin-to-skin contact, at the mother's left breast, which is where new mothers in all cultures instinctively cradle their babies, and in contact with her heart rhythm, "a cascade of supportive confirmative information activates every sense, instinct and intelligence needed for the radical change of environment . . . Thus intelligent learning begins at birth."[286]

For the mother also, "A major block of dormant intelligences is activated . . . the mother then knows exactly what to do and can communicate with her baby on an intuitive level."[287] Such intuitive capacities are sorely needed in our human culture, in which we are heavily reliant on outside advice from books and experts to tell us how to care for our babies.

More scientifically, Lin and colleagues state, "Parturition [birth] plays a critical role in the full expression of maternal behavior in postpartum females, yet the precise mechanism remains unclear."[288] Animal research is consistent with the hypothesis that the processes of birth activate areas of the brain involved with mothering behaviors via the peaks of hormones such as oxytocin, catecholamines, and prolactin.[288–290]

Breastfeeding: A Second Chance

It is also noteworthy that breastfeeding involves three of the four ecstatic hormones of labor and birth: oxytocin, beta-endorphin, and prolactin. When birth has been difficult or disturbed, when mother and baby have been separated, or when the mother has missed her ecstatic hormonal cocktail, she can use breastfeeding and skin-to-skin contact with her baby to stimulate these hormones, helping her to fall in love with her baby, and vice versa.

Constant or near-constant contact between mother and baby (ideally using a sling or baby carrier in the day and cosleeping at night, with as much skin contact as possible) will also help to optimize these pleasurable hormones, which also reduce stress for both mother and baby, as noted earlier.

When the baby's breastfeeding behavior and/or nipple attachment is suboptimal, which may be due to perinatal drugs and procedures, or to separation in the hours after birth, some have suggested using skin-to-skin contact in a bath to reenact the time after birth,[291] allowing the baby to use the amazing primitive reflexes, which are only present for the early weeks, to crawl up the mother's body, find the nipple, and self-attach.[292]

Undisturbing Birth

How can we avoid disturbing the process of birth and align our practices with our evolutionary blueprint? This can seem difficult in a culture in which birth has been disturbed, one way or another, for many generations. Yet it is really very simple. If we were to provide conditions of privacy, and a sense of safety for birth—which, as the late Jeannine Parvati Baker reminds us, "is orgasmic in its essence"[293]—most women would experience a spontaneous, ecstatic, and relatively easy birth.

Dutch professor of obstetrics, G. Kloosterman, offers a succinct summary, which would be well placed on the door of every birth room:

> Spontaneous labor in a normal woman is an event marked by a number
> of processes so complicated and so perfectly attuned to each other that

any interference will only detract from the optimal character. The only thing required from the bystanders is that they show respect for this awe-inspiring process by complying with the first rule of medicine—*nil nocere* [do no harm].[294]

Suggestions for Undisturbing Birth for Women and Their Caregivers

For women:
- Take responsibility for your health, healing, and wholeness before and during the childbearing years.
- Care for yourself well during pregnancy, focusing on lowering stress and having a good diet, adequate rest, and regular exercise.
- Consider using centering activities such as yoga and meditation.
- Choose a model of care that enhances the chance of a natural and undisturbed birth, especially homebirth, birth center, and/or one-on-one midwifery care.
- Arrange support according to your individual needs—trust, a loving relationship, and continuity of care with support people are important.
- Consider having an advocate at a hospital birth; ideally your own private midwife or doula, who can help protect your birthing space and also support your partner, if present. Also note the following caregiver recommendations.

For caregivers:
- Ensure an atmosphere in which the laboring woman feels private, safe, and unobserved, and free to follow her own instincts.
- Reduce neocortical (higher-brain) stimulation by keeping lighting and noises soft, and reducing words to a minimum.
- Cover the clock and any other technical equipment.
- Avoid procedures (including obvious observations) unless absolutely necessary.
- Avoid talking to the laboring woman unless absolutely necessary.
- Avoid drugs unless absolutely necessary.
- Avoid cesarean surgery unless absolutely necessary.

For the hour following birth:

- Don't separate mother and baby for any reason, including resuscitation, which will be more effective with the cord attached.
- Keep lighting low, and the room very warm, beginning just before birth.
- Maintain an atmosphere of quiet and calm for mother and baby.
- Facilitate immediate and uninterrupted skin-to-skin contact between mother and baby. Weighing, measuring, bathing, and washing are unnecessary at this time.
- Support breastfeeding soon after birth, ideally allowing the baby to find the nipple and self-attach without disturbance.

Maia's Birth—A Family Celebration

In our family, we call Maia's birth "a-Maia-zing" and it truly was. Through my pregnancy and leading up to her birth, I made some unconventional and very personal choices, based on my own beliefs and feelings at the time and drawing on a deep faith in my body and in the natural processes of labor and birth. I also trusted my preparation and knowledge, and my ability to know when help was (and wasn't) needed. Ultimately, we were all blessed, as you will read.

The night that Maia, my fourth baby, was born, I was cooking soup for dinner. I leaned over in the pantry for ingredients and—pop!—floods of clear fluid, and the smell of babies and birth.

Two photos of our family at dinner are the only pictures that we have from Maia's birth. Each of us wears the expression of that night's experiences. I look like I am in a state of total bliss. My beloved, Nicholas, looks proud. Nine-year-old Emma looks excited; four-year-old Jacob looks uncertain; and six-year-old Zoe radiates blessings.

Maia's birth was to be witnessed only by the family. It was my strong instinct, right from the start, that this was what my baby wanted. Nicholas had not been entirely comfortable with this option; like me, he was trained in family physician obstetrics, and he was very aware of the possible complications and of his responsibilities. However, toward the end of the pregnancy he accepted my wishes, and we stopped arguing about medical versus alternative responses. He simply prepared his medical kit—IV fluids and Syntocinon (Pitocin) in case of bleeding—and I prepared my box of homeopathics and herbs for my baby and myself.

Along with the decision to give birth without outside assistance, I committed myself to being optimally prepared on every level. My body was well nourished and I practiced yoga and meditation daily. I had regular massage, osteopathic and craniosacral treatments, and later in my pregnancy shiatsu, which revitalized and balanced my body wonderfully. In my daily yoga practice I worked with pain, stretching into tight and painful areas and finding the bliss at the center. I wondered how it would be in this labor—could I find the ecstasy at the heart of giving birth?

I opted against medical care or tests—even blood pressure tests—in this pregnancy. I trusted my body and my baby to tell me, through feelings, dreams, and impulses, what was needed. Through my meditation I developed a series of affirmations, one for each level of my body, which I used in the last months. In the final weeks, it was only the last affirmation that I needed: *I totally surrender and trust*.

That night, as my labor deepened, I moved into our bathroom where I had my trusty yoga mat on the floor to protect me from the cold tiles. My expansions (not contractions) were very close together. I couldn't even get back to our adjoining bedroom to read the birth blessings sent to me by my women's circle in Melbourne, or to gaze at the birthing mandalas that the children had colored so exquisitely during my pregnancy. No time either for music, dancing, essential oils, or water. As my friend Davini wished for me, this birth was to be "simple and present"

By this time I was standing, moaning, and circling my pelvis with each expansion. Then a new space opened up for me, and for the remainder of my labor I was looking into the eyes of my beloved, telling him: "I love you, I love you, I love you, I love you . . ." peaking and subsiding with each wave.

After an hour or so, I felt a familiar catch in my throat—a feeling that the urge to push was close. "This baby will be born soon," I said. Nicholas filled the tub and woke Emma and Zoe. As he left again to wake Jacob, I had a sudden desire for water. I jumped into the bathtub, finding a beautiful position in the triangle of the tub; upright and kneeling with my feet supported on the sides as I pushed.

I felt every inch of my baby descending, and I could hold the growing pressure in my vagina without contracting against it. In this way, progress was very quick; two or three pushes, and not even a strong stretching feeling. I said, "I'm crowning." One more push and, "Here's the head." Yet strangely I had no feeling of my push finishing easily at the baby's neck.

We were in candlelight, and I was tucked into the darkest corner of the bathtub. Nicholas had a flashlight ready, and he shone it into the water to check the baby. "It's a foot!" he said. I turned, baby still half in my body, and saw a left leg waving in the water. Nicholas leant down—I still don't know how he did it without getting wet—and freed the other leg, which was straight against her belly, held up only by the foot.

I asked Nicholas to feel the cord—she was born past her umbilicus by now. "It's not pulsating," he said. We both knew what this meant; our baby needed to be born quickly, as the cord was being compressed between her head and my pelvic bones, cutting off her blood supply. "I'll stand up," was my instinctive response.

Standing with ease, I leaned forward, my hands supporting her slippery little legs and bottom. Without waiting for the next wave, I pushed. Out came her chest, arms spilling out, cord tumbling and tangled, then finally, with one push, her head.

I scooped her up into my arms, to the warmth of my heart. She was like a little bundle of kelp: floppy, blue, and not breathing. "We love you, baby, we love you!" the children cried, calling her in. After twenty or thirty seconds—it seemed longer, but Nicholas was watching her closely—she opened one eye, squeaked, and took a breath, pinking up straight away.

From blue kelp to pink flesh, here was our little breech mermaid, born tail in the water and top out! Emma and Zoe both saw deep blue and pink—her colors—surrounding her at birth, and Jacob saw "Blue, pink, purple, yellow, and orange." Emma had the important job of recording the time of birth—10:48 P.M., July 26, 2000.

Nicholas helped me out of the tub and back to the bedroom, and I lay on the bed, skin to naked newborn skin, all of us in the purest bliss. The children were very keen to know her sex, but Nicholas and I needed a bit of time to recover, which we did with joyous laughter. After a few minutes, we pulled back the towel to see that our baby was, as we had guessed, our own girl—Maia Rose!

I put her to my breast—her eyes were open now—and she suckled straight away. Zoe went to get our friend Suzanne, who was sleeping over with her two children.

She had heard the whole process from the other end of the house, including our laughter, which told her that all was well. She helped with the children and with cleaning up, and prepared us a beautiful plate of fruit along with the juice that I hadn't had time to drink in labor. I sat up after half an hour or so—it was getting a bit uncomfortable—and squatted to deliver Maia's placenta.

We didn't cut Maia's cord, as we had chosen lotus birth (as we had for Zoe and Jacob), in which baby, cord, and placenta remain whole and attached until natural separation. My perineum was totally unscathed—I have been blessed this way with all of my births—and I bled barely at all. My body felt amazing.

"Perfect!" said Nicholas. "An evening birth, then a full night's sleep." Well, almost!

In the days that followed, I was respectful of the enormous opening that my body had been through, and I stayed in bed, in a quiet space, with my baby. Maia's cord came away, without any fuss, on her third evening. It was seven days before I even left the bedroom, and I didn't go past the mailbox or in a car for a full six weeks. Nicholas had arranged one month off work to care for our household, which he did beautifully. As well as this, friends and neighbors brought meals and flowers and gave practical help. We were fully nourished and our community shared in the magic of birth and baby.

Maia's birth blessed our household for this time and beyond. The love that I had felt pouring through my body as I birthed her continued to radiate and fill us all; we were truly "in love" for weeks afterward.

As Maia has grown, I have seen, as with my other children, the imprint of her character on her birth. At seven, she is a strong, present girl: passionate, energetic, and loving. Her birth, too, was strong and passionate, and she was born with the sun sign Leo: sign of drama, courage, and love.

Maia's birth continues to be a source of gratitude, inspiration, and nourishment for me in all facets of my life. Her birth was a major opening that has transformed me, making me the mother that Maia needs me to be, as well as deepening my understanding of, and commitment to, gentle, instinctive, and undisturbed birth.

chapter 7

EPIDURALS

Risks and Concerns for
Mothers and Babies

The use of epidural pain relief in labor has been increasing in recent years throughout the westernized world, with epidurals now accepted as an almost routine aspect of modern labor care in many countries, including the United States. However, epidurals carry significant and often unacknowledged risks and side effects for mothers and babies, and may have long-term impacts on breastfeeding and mother-baby relationships. This chapter presents current information from medical studies to help women make an informed choice about the use of epidurals for themselves and their baby.

The first recorded use of an epidural was in 1885, when New York neurologist J. Leonard Corning injected cocaine into the back of a patient suffering from "spinal weakness and seminal incontinence."[1] More than a century later, epidurals have become the most popular method of pain relief (analgesia) in U.S. birth rooms. In the Listening to Mothers II survey (published in 2006), more than three-quarters of women reported that they were administered an epidural, including 71 percent of women who had a vaginal birth.[2] In Canada in 2005–2006, 53.7 percent of women who birthed vaginally used an epidural, with wide variation among provinces and territories,[3] and in England, in 2005–2006, 22 percent of women overall had an epidural before or during delivery.[4]

Epidurals involve the injection of a local anesthetic drug (derived from cocaine) into the epidural space—the space around (*epi*) the tough coverings (*dura*) that protect the spinal cord. A conventional epidural will block nerve signals from both the sensory and the motor nerves as they exit from the spinal cord, giving very effective pain relief for labor (sensory block) but making the recipient unable to move the lower part of her body because of the motor block. In the last five to ten years, epidurals have been developed with lower concentrations of local anesthetic drugs and with combinations of local anesthetics and opiate pain killers (drugs similar to morphine and meperidine) to reduce the motor block and to produce a so-called "walking" epidural.

Spinal analgesia ("spinal" for short) has also been increasingly used for pain relief in labor to reduce the motor block and ideally allow women to move during labor. Spinals involve drugs injected right through the dura and into the spinal (intrathecal) space, and produce very fast and effective short term analgesia. To prolong the pain-relieving effect for labor, epidurals are now being co-administered with spinals, as a combined spinal epidural (CSE).

Epidurals and spinals, collectively known as regional or neuraxial analgesia, offer laboring women the most effective form of pain relief available, and women who have used these analgesics rate their satisfaction with pain relief very high. However, satisfaction with pain relief does not necessarily reflect overall satisfaction with birth,[5] and epidurals are associated with major disruptions to the processes of birth. These disruptions can interfere with a woman's ultimate enjoyment of, and satisfaction with, her labor experience, and may also compromise the safety of birth and the well-being of mother and baby.

Epidurals and Labor Hormones

Epidurals significantly interfere with some of the major hormones of labor and birth (described in detail in chapter 6), which may explain their negative effect on the processes of labor. As the World Health Organization (WHO) comments, "Epidural analgesia is one of the most striking examples of the medicalization of normal birth, transforming a physiological event into a medical procedure."[6]

For example, oxytocin, introduced in chapter 6 as the hormone of love, is also a natural uterotonic—a substance that causes a woman's uterus to contract in labor. Epidurals lower the mother's production of oxytocin, as measured in her bloodstream,[7] or stop its normal rise during labor.[8] The effect of spinals on oxytocin release is even more marked.[8] Epidurals also obliterate the maternal oxytocin peak that occurs at birth[7, 9]—possibly the highest oxytocin activity of a mother's lifetime—that catalyzes the final powerful contractions of labor, giving timely hormonal help to the mother as she pushes her baby out. Oxytocin is also released in the new mother's brain, helping her fall in love with her baby at first meeting; release of oxytocin within the brain is also inhibited when an epidural is used in labor, according to evidence from animal studies.[10] Another important uterotonic hormone, prostaglandin F2 alpha, is also reduced in women using an epidural.[11]

Beta-endorphin is the stress hormone that builds up in a natural labor to help the laboring woman to transcend pain; beta-endorphin is also associated with the altered state of consciousness that is a normal aspect of labor. Being "on another planet," as some describe it, helps the mother-to-be to work instinctively with her body and her baby, often using movement and sound. Epidurals dramatically reduce the laboring woman's release of beta-endorphin,[12, 13] and levels immediately after birth can be reduced to one-fifth of normal following epidural use in labor.[14] Perhaps the widespread use of epidurals reflects our ignorance of the importance of this hormonal shift, our difficulty with supporting women in this altered state, and our cultural preference that laboring women be quiet and compliant.

Epinephrine and norepinephrine (adrenaline and noradrenaline)—collectively known as the fight-or-flight hormones or catecholamines (CAs)—are released under stressful conditions, and levels also naturally increase during normal labor.[15] At the end of an undisturbed labor, a natural surge in these hormones gives the mother extra energy to push her baby out, and makes her excited and fully alert at first meeting with her baby.

However, early labor is inhibited by high CA levels,[16] which may be released when the laboring woman feels hungry, cold, fearful, or unsafe. This makes evolutionary sense: if the mother senses danger or does not have the energy for labor, her fight-or-flight hormones will slow or stop labor and give her the time to flee to find a safer place to birth or to replenish herself. (The roles of these hormones in birth are discussed in more detail in chapter 6.)

Epidurals reduce the laboring woman's release of epinephrine from placement through birth. This may be helpful if stress is inhibiting the early stages of labor; however, in late labor and birth, a reduction in the natural surge of CA hormones may be disadvantageous. In one study, women with epidurals had epinephrine levels at birth that were 75 percent lower than those of women using other forms of pain relief in labor.[17] This reduction in the late-labor CA surge may contribute to the difficulty that women laboring with an epidural can experience in pushing out their babies and to the increased risk of instrumental delivery (forceps and vacuum) that accompanies the use of an epidural, as noted in the following section.

Epidural effects on norepinephrine are much less,[18, 19] leading to a change in the epinephrine:norepinephrine ratio that may unbalance the CA hormones and cause hyperstimulation of the laboring mother's uterus, as will be discussed.

Effects on the Processes of Labor

Epidurals slow labor, possibly through the just-described effects on the laboring woman's oxytocin release, although there is also evidence from animal research that the local anesthetic drugs used in epidurals may inhibit contractions by a direct effect on the muscle of the uterus.[20] One study has suggested that large volumes of saline, used as an epidural preload, may also reduce the laboring woman's uterine activity in active labor.[21]

On average the first stage of labor is twenty-six minutes longer in women who use an epidural, and the second (pushing) stage is fifteen minutes longer.[22] Loss of the final oxytocin peak probably also contributes to the doubled risk of an instrumental delivery—vacuum or forceps—for women who use an epidural,[23] although other mechanisms may be involved.

For example, an epidural paralyzes not only the laboring woman's lower body, but also her pelvic floor muscles, which are important in guiding her baby's head into a good position for birth. Researchers have found that when an epidural is in place, the baby is up to four times more likely to be persistently posterior (POP; that is, face up) in the final stages of labor—13 percent compared with 3 percent for women without an epidural in one study.[23] A POP position decreases the chance of a spontaneous vaginal birth; in one study, only 26 percent of first-time mothers (and 57 percent of experienced mothers) with POP babies experienced spontaneous vaginal birth; the remaining mothers had an instrumental birth (forceps or vacuum) or a cesarean.[24] According to another study, the risk of anal sphincter injury is seven times greater for women who birth their babies POP than for those with normally positioned babies, which is related to the increased need for instrumental assistance.[25]

Anesthesiologists have hoped that low-dose epidural or CSE will increase the chances of a spontaneous vaginal birth, but the improvement seems to be modest. In a large randomized UK study (known as COMET—Conventional Obstetric Mobile Epidural Trial), 37 percent of women with a conventional epidural experienced instrumental births, compared with 29 percent of women using low-dose epidural infusion and 28 percent of women using CSE.[26] (In this study, more babies from the low-dose group needed resuscitation, likely because of exposure to the drug fentanyl, which will be discussed further.)

Other centers have attempted to increase the rate of spontaneous vaginal birth by allowing the epidural to wear off late in labor. A recent review concluded that this policy is associated with more pain (possibly because the laboring mother has not built up her beta-endorphin levels) and that there is not enough evidence to suggest that it is useful in avoiding instrumental delivery.[27]

The impact of an instrumental delivery is substantial for both mother and baby. For the mother, instrumental delivery increases her risks of episiotomy and tears to her vagina and perineum, and of major tears that can damage her anal sphincter and lead to bowel incontinence. Two studies have shown that severe perineal lacerations are around twice as common after epidurals.[28, 29] After an instrumental delivery, women report more sexual problems, perineal pain, and urinary incontinence, compared with women who have had a spontaneous birth.[30–32] For example, an Australian population survey of women six to seven months after birth found that, compared with women who had spontaneous vaginal birth, women who had instrumental deliveries were four times more likely to have perineal pain, twice as likely to have sexual problems, and almost twice as likely to experience urinary incontinence.[31]

For the baby, instrumental delivery can increase the short-term risks of bruising, facial injuries, displacement of the skull bones, and cephalohematoma (blood clot in the scalp).[33] The risk of intracranial hemorrhage (bleeding inside the brain) was increased in one study by more than four times for babies born by forceps compared with spontaneous birth,[34] although two studies showed no detectable developmental differences for forceps-born children at five years old.[35, 36]

Another study found that, when women with an epidural had a forceps delivery, the force used by the clinician to deliver the baby was almost doubled, compared with the force used when an epidural was not in place.[37]

As well as increasing all of these risks, epidurals also increase the need for Pitocin (Syntocinon) to augment labor, probably due to the slowing of labor just mentioned. Women laboring with an epidural in place are up to three times more likely to be administered Pitocin. [22] The combination of epidurals and Pitocin, both of which can cause fetal heart rate (FHR) abnormalities and fetal distress (reflecting a critical lack of blood and oxygen), markedly increases the risks of operative delivery (forceps, vacuum, or cesarean delivery). In an Australian survey, up to two-thirds of first-time mothers who were administered both an epidural and Pitocin had an operative delivery.[38]

Epidurals increase the risks of pelvic floor problems,[39] which may reflect the increased pelvic floor risks associated with epidural co-interventions and effects including the use of Pitocin, instrumental delivery and episiotomy,[40] longer second (pushing) stage of labor,[39–41] and coached pushing.[42]

The impact of epidurals on the risk of cesarean is controversial. One recent review suggests no increased risk;[22] another points to a 50 percent increased risk.[43] A critical look at the research suggests that epidurals combined with low-dose oxytocin augmentation regimes—most commonly used North America are likely to increase cesarean risks, whereas more aggressive, higher-dose regimes—common in research but not in practice—may prevent the progression from epidural to cesarean.[44] In practice, this means that women accepting an epidural in a setting that uses low-dose Pitocin regimes are likely to increase their cesarean risk. First-time mothers accepting an epidural in a setting using low-dose Pitocin may be up to three times more likely to have a cesarean.[45]

Note that many of the studies used to arrive at these conclusions are randomized controlled trials (RCTs), in which the women who agree to participate are randomly assigned to epidural or nonepidural pain relief. Nonepidural pain relief usually involves opiates such as meperidine (pethidine), which can itself significantly impact labor and birth for mother and baby. Many of these studies are also flawed from high rates of crossover—women who were assigned to nonepidural but who ultimately had an epidural, and vice versa. Also, note that most studies have no true controls—that is, women who are not using any form of pain relief—so we cannot know the impact of epidurals on mothers and babies compared with birth without analgesic drugs from these studies.

Epidural Techniques and Side Effects

The drugs used in labor epidurals are powerful enough to numb and usually paralyze the mother's lower body, so it is not surprising that they can produce significant side effects in mother and baby. Side effects range from minor to life threatening and depend, to some extent, on the specific drugs used. Local anesthetic drugs (usually lidocaine, bupivacaine, or ropivacaine) depress the electrical conduction of nerve impulses, leading to numbing at the site of injection; these drugs are also commonly used for dental procedures and minor surgery. When injected via epidural, these drugs target the sensory nerves as they exit the spinal cord through the epidural space, as mentioned previously. Opiate drugs (usually morphine, fentanyl/Sublimaze, or sufentanil) injected into the epidural space produce analgesia by acting on opiate receptors in the spinal cord, as does a laboring woman's natural beta-endorphin release.

However, any drug injected into the epidural space will enter the mother's bloodstream within minutes, generating possible whole-body (systemic) effects for the mother. Epidural drugs also cross the placenta, creating potential side effects for the baby. As Golub notes, "Probably the most widespread exposure of the developing brain to central nervous system active agents occurs at birth."[46]

Opiate drugs administered as a "spinal" also act on spinal cord receptors and have been shown to move rapidly upward in the cerebrospinal fluid to the brain stem (lower brain), where they can cause breathing problems by depressing the brain stem respiratory center.[47]

Many of the epidural side effects we will soon discuss are not improved with low-dose or walking epidurals, because women using these techniques may still receive a substantial total dose of local anesthetic, especially when using patient-controlled boluses (repeated large doses) or continuous infusions over many hours.[26] The addition of opiate drugs in epidurals or CSE can introduce further risks, such as pruritis (itching) and the respiratory depression already mentioned.

Further, the ability of women with a walking epidural to actually walk will be compromised by the presence of an IV and monitor, by the need for constant one-to-one caregiver support while walking, and likely by the fear of legal liabilities. Some studies show that women using a walking epidural or CSE may have impaired balance[48] and low blood pressure,[49] which can also affect the ability to walk.

Maternal Side Effects

The most common side effect of epidurals is a drop in maternal blood pressure. This effect is almost universal and usually preempted by administering IV fluids before placing an epidural. Even with this preloading, episodes of significant low blood pressure (hypotension) occur for up to half of all women laboring with an epidural,[30, 51] especially in the minutes following the administration of a drug bolus. Hypotension can cause complications ranging from feeling faint to cardiac arrest[52] and can also affect the baby's blood supply, as we will discuss. Hypotension can be treated with more IV fluids and, if severe, with injections of epinephrine (adrenaline).

Some researchers believe that the hypotensive effect of epidurals and spinals may be caused by the sudden relief of pain, which disrupts the laboring mother's balance of CA hormones (epinephrine and norepinephrine). These hormones help maintain and balance the mother's blood pressure and heart rate, as well as influence the strength of her contractions. A shift in CA hormones can also cause her uterus to contract too strongly (hyperstimulation), as previously mentioned, which reduces the baby's supplies of blood and oxygen and can lead to fetal distress.

Other common side effects of epidurals include inability to pass or hold urine (and thus the requirement for a urinary catheter), for up to two-thirds of women;[51] itching of the skin (pruritis), for up to two-thirds of women administered an opiate drug via epidural;[50, 51] shivering, for up to one in three women,[53] possibly due to abnormalities in temperature control, as will be discussed; sedation, for around one in five women;[51] and nausea and vomiting, for one in twenty women.[51]

Epidurals can also cause a rise in temperature in laboring women. Fever over 100.4°F (38°C) during labor is five times more likely overall for women using an epidural.[22] This rise in temperature is more common for women having their first babies and more marked with prolonged exposure to epidurals.[43, 54] For example, in one study, 7 percent of first-time mothers laboring with an epidural were feverish (febrile) after six hours; this increased to 36 percent after eighteen hours.[55] This effect appears to be predictable: in another study, the 22 percent of first-time mothers who later developed a fever displayed small temperature elevations in the hour after epidural placement.[54]

The cause of this fever is not known, although various explanations have been proposed. These include: a direct effect on the woman's heat-regulating system; inflammation or infection of the uterus and membranes (chorioamnionitis); and a false effect, because most trials compare women having epidurals with women administered (nonepidural) opiate drugs, which reduce temperature.[56] Maternal fever can have a significant effect on the baby, as will be discussed.

Opiate drugs, especially when administered via spinals and CSE, can cause unexpected breathing difficulties for the mother, which may come on hours after birth and may progress to respiratory arrest. DeBalli comments "Respiratory depression remains one of the most feared and least predictable complications of . . . intrathecal [spinal] opioids."[57] Drugs with low lipid solubility such as morphine have a slower action, and are more likely to cause delayed respiratory depression, than drugs such as fentanyl, which is now more commonly used.

Many observational studies have found an association between epidural use and bleeding after birth (postpartum hemorrhage, PPH).[58–63] For example, a large UK study found that women were twice as likely to experience PPH if they had used an epidural in labor.[58] This may be related to the increase in instrumental births and perineal trauma (causing bleeding) or may reflect hormonal disruptions that can prevent the new mother's uterus from contracting efficiently after birth. (See chapter 8 for more about PPH and hormones.)

An epidural gives inadequate pain relief, including one-sided effects, for around 10 to 15 percent of women,[50] and the epidural catheter requires reinsertion in about 5 percent.[64] For around 1 percent of women, the epidural needle punctures the dura (dural tap); this causes a severe headache, which requires absolute bed rest for several days, and usually is treated with an injection into the epidural space.[65, 66]

More serious side effects are rare. If the epidural drugs are inadvertently injected into the bloodstream, local anesthetics can cause toxic effects such as slurred speech, drowsiness, and, at high doses, convulsions. This occurs in around one in twenty-eight hundred epidural insertions.[64] Overall, life-threatening reactions occur for around one in four thousand women.[52, 64, 67, 68] Death associated with an obstetric epidural is very rare,[69] but may be caused by cardiac or respiratory arrest or by an epidural abscess that develops days or weeks afterward.

Later complications include weakness and numbness in four to eighteen women per ten thousand, most of which resolve within three months.[52, 67–70] Longer-term or permanent problems can arise from damage to a nerve during epidural placement; from abscess or hematoma (blood clot), which can compress the spinal cord; and from toxic reactions in the covering of the spinal cord, which can lead to paraplegia.[52]

A recent review found some evidence that women who had used an epidural were more likely to experience urinary retention in the hospital and stress urinary incontinence in the first year after birth. This may be related to the longer labors and higher rates of instrumental delivery associated with epidurals.[43]

Side Effects for the Baby

Some of the most significant and well-documented side effects for the unborn baby (fetus) and newborn derive from effects on the mother. These include, as noted already, effects on her hormonal orchestration, her blood pressure, and her temperature regulation. As well, epidural drugs can cause directly toxic effects to the fetus and newborn, whose drug levels may be even higher than the mother's drug levels.[71]

Fetal Heart Rate Changes

Epidurals can cause changes in the fetal heart rate (FHR), indicating that the unborn baby is lacking blood and oxygen (fetal distress). This effect is well recognized following the administration of an epidural, usually within the first thirty minutes; it can last for twenty minutes, and it is particularly likely following the use of opiate drugs administered via epidural and spinal. In these situations the fetal heart rate can drop to very low levels (fetal bradycardia).

This fetal bradycardia (and other FHR abnormalities) may relate to the sudden drop in maternal CA hormones, which can cause hypotension and uterine hyperstimulation, as noted earlier.[72] Co-administration of epidurals and uterine stimulating drugs, including Pitocin and prostaglandins, may further increase hyperstimulation risks.[72] The use of spinals, including in CSE, is even more likely to cause fetal bradycardia,[73, 74] most probably because spinal opiates cause more hyperstimulation than epidurals.[73]

Drug toxicity may also contribute to the FHR effects: Capogna notes that FHR abnormalities peak at the same time as maternal drug levels,[72] and Hill and others propose that high doses of local anesthetics may cause spasm in the uterine arteries, impairing the blood supply to the uterus and baby and causing fetal distress.[75]

Note that the use of meperidine (Demerol, pethidine) for labor analgesia can also cause FHR abnormalities. This makes the real effects of epidurals on FHR hard to assess, because in randomized trials epidurals are usually compared with meperidine and other opiate drugs.

Studies looking at FHR abnormalities after the administration of spinal opiates have found that 10 to 15 percent of babies develop FHR changes,[72] and one in twenty-eight develops a significant bradycardia (slow heart rate).[76] One RCT has suggested a dose response, with more FHR abnormalities with higher doses of spinal sufentanil.[74] FHR changes will usually resolve spontaneously with a change in position; more rarely, they may require drug treatment.[77] More severe changes, and the fetal distress that they reflect, may require an urgent cesarean.

Capogna notes that the supine position (lying on the back) may contribute significantly to hypotension and FHR abnormalities when an epidural is in place:[72] one researcher found that the supine position (plus epidural) was associated with a significant decrease in fetal cerebral oxygenation (oxygen supply to the baby's brain).[78] Side-lying may be safer.

Effects from Maternal Fever

An epidural-induced rise in the laboring mother's temperature can also affect the baby. In one large study of first-time mothers, babies born to febrile mothers, 97 percent of whom had received epidurals, were more likely to be in poor condition (low APGAR) at birth; to have poor tone; to require resuscitation (11.5 percent versus 3 percent); and to have seizures in the newborn period, compared with babies born to afebrile (not feverish) mothers.[79]

The authors of this study express concerns about these effects and note that in primate studies[80] maternal hyperthermia (high temperature), even without infection, can cause low oxygen and low blood pressure in both mother and fetus as well as newborn acidosis, a sign of lack of blood and oxygen in labor. They note further, "Other animal studies have demonstrated that an increase in brain temperature of even 1°C or 2°C [1.8°F or 3.6°F] increases the degree of brain damage resulting from an ischemic insult [injury due to lack of blood]."[79]

Another reviewer notes, "Maternal fever has been associated with adverse neonatal outcomes, including birth depression, neonatal encephalopathy, neonatal seizures, and neonatal mortality in preterm and term infants. Maternal fever has been associated with cerebral palsy."[81] Other studies have found a fourfold increased risk of newborn encephalopathy (a sign of possible brain damage)[82] and upward of 1.3 times mortality in babies born to febrile mothers.[83]

Maternal fever in labor can also directly cause problems for the newborn. Because fever can be a sign of infection involving the uterus, babies born to febrile mothers are almost always evaluated for sepsis (infection). Sepsis evaluation involves prolonged separation from the mother, admission to special care, invasive tests, and most likely administration of antibiotics until tests results are available. In one study of first-time mothers, 34 percent of epidural babies were given a sepsis evaluation compared with 9.8 percent of nonepidural babies.[79]

Drugs and Toxicity

These effects on the baby are likely to increase when other drugs and co-interventions are used, although, incredibly this has not been well studied. In older studies babies born to women who were induced (with Pitocin or by artificial rupture of membranes, or ARM) and also received an epidural were more likely to be mildly hypoxic (lacking in oxygen) at birth,[84] and mothers who were induced using intravenous prostaglandins along with an epidural had an extremely high incidence of hyperstimulation, and their babies had some severe, although temporary, FHR abnormalities. The authors comment, "the combined application of an intravenous prostaglandin and continuous epidural analgesia should not be introduced into obstetrical practice."[85] There are no similar studies, to my knowledge, using modern vaginally administered prostaglandins, which are commonly used with epidurals.

There are also few studies of the condition of epidural babies at birth, and almost all of these compare epidural babies with babies born after exposure to opiate drugs, which are known to cause drowsiness and difficulty with breathing. These studies show little difference between epidural and nonepidural (usually opiate-exposed) babies in terms of APGAR score and umbilical cord pH (which reflects the baby's condition in labor).[43] However, a large population survey from Sweden found that use of an epidural was significantly associated with a low APGAR score at birth.[86]

There are also reports of newborn toxicity from epidural drugs, especially opiates,[87] which are administered via epidural at doses similar to those given by injection into muscle or vein. These drugs will enter the mother's and then the baby's circulation within minutes. Opiate overdose can make the baby unresponsive and not breathing at birth. Newborn opiate toxicity seems more likely when higher dose regimes are used, including those that allow the mother to self-administer extra doses, although it also seems that there are wide differences in individual newborn sensitivity.[87]

It is also important to note that a newborn baby's ability to process and excrete drugs is much less than that of an adult. For example, the half-life (time to reduce drug blood levels by one-half) for the local anesthetic bupivacaine (Marcaine) is 8.1 hours in the newborn, compared with 2.7 hours in the mother.[88] One study found detectable amounts of bupivacaine metabolites in the urine of exposed newborns for thirty-six hours following spinal anesthesia for cesarean.[89]

As well, drug levels may not accurately reflect the baby's toxic load, because drugs may be taken up from the blood and either stored in newborn tissues such as brain and liver or bound to blood proteins,[71] from which they are more slowly released. This is especially likely for drugs such as fentanyl, which are very fat-soluble (lipophilic) and so can cross easily into the brain.[90] See a later discussion for the possible impact of epidural fentanyl on newborn breastfeeding ability.

A recent review also found higher rates of jaundice for epidural-exposed babies, which may be related to the increase in instrumental deliveries (which causes jaundice through bruising) or to the increased use of Pitocin.[43] Jaundice may cause drowsiness and problems with breastfeeding, and if treatment under ultraviolet lights is prescribed, may involve maternal-newborn separation.

There is also some evidence that local anesthetic drugs used in epidurals may have a negative effect on the newborn immune system. One study showed that lidocaine can directly cause a reduction in the activity of natural killer (NK) cells, possibly by activating the stress response. These authors also suggest that the increase in stress hormone levels among epidural babies, found in several studies, may be a direct effect of epidural local anesthetic drugs, which raise levels of the primary stress hormone corticotrophin releasing hormone (CRH).[9]

Neurobehavioral Effects

Although we are increasingly recognizing the importance of the baby's abilities in the hours after birth, the impact of labor drugs, including epidurals, on the newborn remains poorly researched.

Older studies comparing babies exposed to epidurals with unmedicated babies found significant neurobehavioral effects, whereas more recent studies have not found differences. However, these older studies used the more comprehensive (and more difficult to administer) Brazelton Neonatal Behavioral Assessment Scale (NBAS, devised by pediatricians), whereas more recent tests have used less complex tests, especially the Neurologic and Adaptive Capacity Score (NACS, which was devised by anesthesiologists). The NACS is easier to administer, aggregates all data into a single figure, and has been criticized by many as insensitive and unreliable.[56, 92-95] All three observational studies that compared epidural-exposed with unmedicated babies using the NBAS found significant differences between groups.[43]

Murray and colleagues compared fifteen unmedicated with forty epidural-exposed babies and found that the epidural babies had more abnormalities in NBAS score at twenty-four hours. There was some recovery at day five, but NBAS remained elevated (indicating worrisome neurobehavior), with particular difficulty in "control of state," which was consistent with diaries kept by the mothers showing that epidural babies cried more frequently. The twenty babies whose mothers who had received oxytocin as well as an epidural had even more abnormal NBAS scores at day five and were drowsy and unresponsive, which may be explained by these babies' higher rates of jaundice.

At one month NBAS was not different between groups, but epidural mothers reported that their babies were "less adaptable, more intense and more bothersome in their behaviour."[96] These differences remained after controlling for forceps use and length of labor. Furthermore, maternal testing at twenty-four hours after birth using the Cohler's Maternal Attitude Scale had suggested no early between-group differences in maternal interactive style, indicating that the findings were not likely to reflect differing maternal attitudes and mothering styles among the women who chose epidurals.[97]

Sepkoski et al. compared thirty-eight epidural babies with twenty-two unmedicated babies and found less alertness and ability to orient, and less mature motor abilities, for the first month of life. The epidural mothers spent less time with their babies in the hospital. These findings were in proportion to the dose of bupivacaine administered, suggesting a dose-related response to epidural drugs.[98]

Rosenblatt compared fifty-nine epidural babies with thirty-five undrugged babies using NBAS from birth to six weeks and found maximal epidural effects on the first day. Although there was some recovery, at three days epidural babies still cried more easily and more often compared with unmedicated babies, and aspects of this problem ("control of state") persisted for the full six weeks. Effects were dose-related, with more depression of visual skill and alertness from day one through six weeks among babies with higher cord blood bupivacaine levels. Epidural babies also had more response to stress, more tremulousness and startling, and cried more when handled up to the age of six weeks.[99]

Although these older studies concerned conventional epidurals, the total dose of bupivacaine administered to the mothers (mean doses 61.6 milligrams,[97] 112.7 milligrams,[98] and 119.8 milligrams[99] respectively) was reasonably comparable to more recent low-dose studies (for example, 67.5 milligrams,[71] 91.1 milligrams,[100] 101.1 milligrams[26]).

These neurobehavioral studies highlight the possible impact of epidurals on newborns and on the evolving mother-infant relationships. The researchers comment: "Although direct biochemical drug effects may wear off in the first days . . . the mother's early impressions may remain to influence how rewarding she finds her baby and the manner in which she responds to her baby's initiatives at 1 month of age."[101]

One study has suggested that newborn neurobehavior may be less affected when drug doses are lower. This study used ultra-low-dose bupivacaine/fentanyl epidurals, with newborn bupivacaine levels around one-half to one-third of other studies. Assessment with the NACS showed no significant overall differences between twenty-eight epidural babies compared with twenty-eight babies unexposed to labor analgesics; however, babies with higher bupivacaine levels (reflecting longer epidural exposure during labor) had a lower NACS at two hours.[103]

Another study assessed NACS among the newborns of mothers randomized into different epidural drug regimes. Researchers found that babies exposed to epidural fentanyl had the lowest NACS at twenty-four hours, suggesting that fentanyl, which crosses easily to the brain may have especially negative and persistent effects;[100] see the following discussion for more about fentanyl and breastfeeding.

Hormonal and Autonomic Effects

A recent study has suggested that exposure to epidurals in labor may effect newborn body processes (physiology). Jonas and colleagues measured the skin temperature of newborns during skin-to-skin breastfeeding two days after birth. Researchers found that epidural babies had elevated baseline temperatures that actually declined in response to breastfeeding, in contrast to unexposed babies whose temperatures rose and plateaued during this time.[104]

The authors speculate that epidural drugs may mis-set the temperature regulation system in the newborn, which can also occur for women laboring with an epidural, as above. The observed lack of temperature increase with breastfeeding may be due to a reduction in oxytocin levels in the baby's brain, which ordinarily will increase with skin-to-skin contact, reducing stress hormones and producing physical warmth along with a calm and connected feeling.[105] According to the authors, these physiological disturbances, occurring at a very critical period, may interfere with attunement of the baby's autonomic nervous system, perhaps even producing effects through to adulthood. Researchers conclude: "Given the large numbers of women receiving these treatments, even minor effects on newborns might have important future physiological and behavioural consequences for the human population."[106]

One small study has looked at epidural effects past six weeks in human babies. Brackbill assessed the orienting response—the initial response to novelty as measured by heart rate response—among eighteen exposed and unexposed babies at one, four, and eight months. Babies exposed to regional or general anesthesia at birth displayed an abnormal "defense" response at eight months, but not before this.[107]

Taken together, these two studies suggest that exposure to epidural drugs around the time of birth may produce short- and possibly longer-term shifts in the functioning of the autonomic nervous system, which regulates bodily functions in relation to internal and external changes. If the longer-term effects are valid, this suggests a developmental or imprinting effect that may have lifelong consequences (see chapter 6). More research into the long-term effects of epidural drugs on the infant's developing nervous system is critically needed.

Animal Studies

Animal studies suggest that these difficulties for epidural mothers and babies may be due to disruption of maternal hormones at birth and early postpartum. As described in chapter 6, maternal labor hormones peak around the time of birth and/or during the hour postpartum; this peak is designed to optimize maternal behavior and maternal-infant attachment, which is crucial for infant survival in all mammalian species.

As also described in chapter 6, French researchers administered epidurals to laboring sheep and found that the epidural ewes had difficulty bonding with their newborn lambs, especially those in first lambing, with an epidural administered early in labor.[108] Subsequent studies showed that this lack of maternal behavior and attachment was associated with lower brain levels of oxytocin.[10] This effect was substantially (but not totally) reversed when ewes had oxytocin administered directly into the brain.[10] Researchers conclude that disruption of the oxytocin system may contribute to these epidural maternal-infant effects. (Note that epidurals also reduce maternal levels of the other attachment hormones—beta-endorphin, norepinephrine, and prolactin—which would not be reversed with oxytocin administration.)

There are no substantial studies of the developmental effects of epidural analgesia on exposed human offspring. However, studies on some of our closest animal relatives give cause for concern. Golub administered epidural bupivacaine to pregnant rhesus monkeys at term, and followed the development of the exposed offspring to age twelve months (equivalent to four years in children). She found that milestone achievement was abnormal in these monkeys; at six to eight weeks they were slow in starting to manipulate, and at ten months the increase in "motor disturbance behaviors" that normally occurs was prolonged.[109]

Based on these animal findings, the same author concludes, "These effects could occur as a result of effects on vulnerable brain processes during a sensitive period, interference with programming of brain development by endogenous [internal] agents or alteration in early experiences."[46]

Breastfeeding

As with neurobehavior, effects on breastfeeding are poorly studied, and studies comparing exposure to epidurals and opiates are especially misleading because opiates have a well-recognized negative effect on early breastfeeding behavior and success.[110–114]

Epidurals may affect the experience and success of breastfeeding through several mechanisms. First, the epidural-exposed baby may have neurobehavioral deficits caused by drug exposure, as already described. These deficits are likely to be greatest in the hours following birth, when the newborn is normally alert and primed to initiate breastfeeding. The quoted studies suggest that epidural drugs can depress newborn neuro-behavior, which may impact breastfeeding.

One study measured the breastfeeding abilities of 129 babies, using the Infant Breastfeeding Assessment Tool (IBFAT) and found scores highest amongst unmedicated babies, lower for babies exposed to epidurals or IV opiates, and lowest for babies exposed to both. Infants with lower scores were weaned earlier, although overall similar numbers in all groups were breastfeeding at six weeks.[115]

In other research, babies exposed to epidurals and spinals were more likely to lose weight in the hospital, which may reflect poor feeding efficiency.[116] Other research has suggested that newborn breastfeeding behavior (assessed by the Preterm Infant Breastfeeding Behavior Scale, PIBBS) may be not be altered, on average, at two and twenty-four hours when ultra-low-dose epidural is used, although in this study, babies of unmedicated mothers tended to be held for longer, to latch on for longer, to suck more, and to swallow.[117] Note that all mothers and babies in this study were skin to skin for one hour following birth, which is likely to enhance newborn adaptation, suckling behavior, and breastfeeding success.[118]

A large prospective cohort study of infant feeding at six months postpartum found that women who had used epidurals (bupivacaine and low-dose fentanyl) were more than twice as likely to have stopped breastfeeding by twenty-four weeks compared with women who used nonpharmacological pain relief.[94]

Two recent studies have implicated epidural fentanyl as especially harmful to the initiation of breastfeeding. A group of UK researchers observed that newborns exposed to fentanyl in epidurals or spinals were the most likely to be formula fed at discharge: 54 percent compared with 52 percent with morphine epidural/spinal, 44 percent with local anesthetic epidural/spinal, 41 percent with intramuscular opioid, and 32 percent with nitrous oxide gas only.[119]

Perhaps the most compelling study is a randomized trial of different epidural fentanyl doses involving 177 experienced breastfeeding mothers who were intending to breastfeed again. Successful breastfeeding at six weeks was less likely among mothers randomized to high epidural doses of fentanyl. At six weeks, 19 percent of mothers assigned to high-dose fentanyl were not breastfeeding, compared with 6 percent exposed to low-dose fentanyl and 2 percent without fentanyl exposure. Babies with higher fentanyl exposure had lower neurobehavior scores (NACS) and at six weeks all mothers who had ceased breastfeeding reported that it was their babies, not themselves, who had difficulty.[120]

Epidurals may also affect the new mother, so that breastfeeding is more difficult. This is likely if she has experienced a long labor, an instrumental delivery or cesarean, or separation from her baby, all of which are more likely following an epidural. Hormonal disruptions may also contribute, as oxytocin is a major hormone of breastfeeding.

In an observational study of 131 vaginally birthing mother-baby pairs, Baumgarder found that babies born after epidurals were more than twice as likely to be receiving formula supplement on hospital discharge; this was a special risk for those epidural babies who did not feed in the first hour after birth.[121] A Finnish survey records that 67 percent of women who had labored with an epidural reported partial or full formula-feeding in the first twelve weeks compared with 29 percent of nonepidural mothers; epidural mothers were also more likely to report having "not enough milk."[122]

An Australian study of 992 first-time mothers randomized to epidural or continuous midwifery support found that epidural mothers weaned their babies earlier than mothers who had used alternative labor analgesia.[123] An observational U.S. study also found earlier weaning by epidural mothers.[124]

Two groups of Swedish researchers have looked at the subtle but complex breastfeeding and prebreastfeeding behavior of unmedicated newborns. Righard has documented that, when placed skin to skin on the mother's chest, a newborn can crawl up, find the nipple, and self-attach.[110] Newborns affected by opiate drugs in labor or separated from their mothers briefly after birth lose much of this ability. Ransjo-Arvidson found that newborns exposed to labor analgesia (mostly opiates, but including some epidural-affected newborns) were also disorganized in their prefeeding behavior—nipple massage and licking and hand sucking—compared with unmedicated newborns.[112]

Several other studies have not found overall detrimental effects of epidurals on breastfeeding.[103, 125, 126] In one of these studies babies were skin to skin with mothers for an hour after birth,[103] and in another, early skin-to-skin contact and suckling were regarded as institutionally normal.[125] However, even in these studies, babies with a lower NACS,[103, 126] associated in one study with higher drug levels,[103] were more likely to have difficulties with breastfeeding.

Note that, in one of these positive studies,[125] hospital policies were strongly supportive of breastfeeding—including not separating mothers and babies after birth—and this hospital boasted an exceptional rate of breastfeeding in all groups: over 70 percent at six weeks, which would make it more difficult to find statistical differences. It is also possible that early, uninterrupted skin-to-skin contact and institutional breastfeeding support (also components of the Baby-Friendly Hospital Initiative [BFHI][127]) may modify the impact of epidurals on breastfeeding. More research is obviously needed.

Women choosing epidurals may enhance their chance of successful breastfeeding by choosing an accredited BFH (baby-friendly hospital), or by negotiating for uninterrupted contact after birth, with breastfeeding support if necessary.

Satisfaction with Birth

Obstetric care providers have assumed that control of pain is the foremost concern of laboring women and that effective pain relief will ensure a positive birth experience. This belief has resulted in the development and promotion of obstetric techniques that very effectively relieve pain, but these developments have not necessarily led to improvements in women's overall satisfaction with the experience of birth.

In fact, there is evidence that the opposite may be true. Several studies have shown that women who use no labor medication are the most satisfied with their birth experience at the time,[128] at six weeks,[129] and one year after the birth.[130] In a large UK birth survey, the authors concluded that "epidural analgesia does not confer an improved maternal experience even when technically satisfactory and giving good analgesia."[131]

A recent review of satisfaction after childbirth found that personal expectations, support from caregivers, the caregiver-patient relationship, and involvement in decision-making are the most important factors in determining satisfaction with the experience of childbirth.[5] Note also that, contrary to medical belief, women with high expectations are more likely to be satisfied. The reviewer also notes that the highest rates of dissatisfaction are among women who had an emergency cesarean or an instrumental birth.

Finally, it is noteworthy that caregiver preferences may dictate, to a large extent, the use of epidurals and other medical procedures for laboring women. Klein found that women under the care of family physicians with a low mean use of epidurals were less likely to receive monitoring and Pitocin, to deliver by cesarean, and to have their baby admitted to newborn special care.[132]

Summary and Conclusions

Epidural analgesia offers the most effective form of pain relief, and its use is widespread. However, epidurals, spinals, and combined spinal-epidurals also cause major disruptions to the processes of birth, increasing the chances of slower labor, administration of Pitocin, instrumental birth, and possibly cesarean, and causing significant unwanted effects including dissatisfaction with the birth experience.

Other possible side effects for the mother include low blood pressure, itching, shivering, fever, sedation, need for urinary catheter, postpartum hemorrhage, and breathing difficulties. For the baby, risks include abnormal FHR reflecting lack of blood and oxygen, toxic effects from drugs, the need for early separation from the mother for a sepsis evaluation, and increased chances of jaundice, which may also involve separation and treatment.

There is evidence that epidurals can cause subtle neurobehavioral effects that may have ongoing negative effects for the newborn, for the infant-mother relationship, and for breastfeeding. These important areas urgently need more high-quality research.

In conclusion, epidurals have possible benefits, but also significant risks, for the laboring mother and her baby. Women who wish to avoid the use of epidurals are advised to choose caregivers and models of care that promote, support, and understand the principles and practice of natural and undisturbed birth.

chapter 8

LEAVING WELL ENOUGH ALONE
Natural Perspectives on the Third Stage of Labor

The third stage of labor—the time between birth of the baby and when the new mother births her baby's placenta—is an often overlooked but critical time for mother and baby. Both are making enormous transitions. For the baby, this involves major physiological changes to adapt to a radically new environment; for the mother, this shift transforms her from pregnant to nonpregnant within a few minutes. Fortunately these changes are usually smooth, being refined over millions of years for optimal maternal and infant well-being and survival.

These transitions and transformations can be enhanced by knowledge of the physiology of third stage for both mother and baby; by skilled care, predominantly "leaving well enough alone"; and by informed choice. This chapter provides information to help ensure an easy, safe, and pleasurable transition for mother and baby, as well as important information in regard to decisions such as cord blood banking.

The medicalization of pregnancy and birth has become deeply ingrained in our culture, making its influence difficult to unmask and culturally complex to challenge. Social and personal exposure to medicalized birth as "the norm" has left most of us ignorant and even mistrustful of the natural processes of labor and birth.

However, these processes remain encoded in every cell of our bodies, making modern women as superbly designed for giving birth as any of our ancestors. Our genetic code for birth is rich and accurate; it has evolved to reflect the most efficient and effective means of human reproduction, including optimal outcomes for mother and baby in the short, medium, and long term.

These ideal outcomes are mediated by the mother's hormones and instincts, which influence her emotions and behaviors, from preconception (with her choice of mate) through pregnancy, birth, and mothering. Above all, her genetic code, and the events that it triggers, are directed toward the formation of a secure bond between mother and offspring. A secure maternal-infant bond ensures optimal nourishment through breastfeeding, as well as optimal care, protection, and development for the growing baby, who is the most immature and incapable of any species. (See chapters 11 and 12 for more about the long-term benefits of attachment and breastfeeding).

Although well intentioned, modern obstetrics has not honored this genetic code. In the rush to protect mothers and babies from misfortune and death, obstetrics has ignored the powerful influences of the birthing mother's hormones, emotions, and instinctive behaviors, even as researchers struggle to understand their complexity.

Our culturally unprecedented neglect of the emotional and instinctive aspects of pregnancy and birth has major consequences for mothers and babies. During the third stage of labor, when mother and baby meet for the first time, the gap between our instincts and genetic code, and our culture's usual birthing practices, is especially wide.

At a time when Mother Nature prescribes awe and ecstasy, we have injections, examinations, and clamping and pulling on the cord. Instead of body heat, skin-to-skin contact, and the baby's innate instinct to find the breast, we offer separation, wrapping, and outside assistance to "attach" the baby. When time should stand still for those eternal moments of first contact, as mother and baby fall deeply in love, we have haste to deliver the placenta and clean up for the next case.

Medical management of the third stage has been taken even further in recent years, with the popularity of "active management of the third stage." Although much of the activity is designed to reduce the risk of maternal bleeding (postpartum hemorrhage, or PPH), which is certainly a serious event, it seems that, as with the active management of labor, the medical approach to labor and birth may actually lead to some of the problems that active management is designed to address.

Active management also creates specific difficulties for mother and baby. In particular, active management can lead to the deprivation of one-third, on average, of a newborn's expected blood volume. When active management is used, this extra blood, intended to perfuse the newly functioning lungs and other vital organs, is discarded along with the placenta. Possible consequences include breathing difficulties and anemia, especially in vulnerable babies; long-term effects on brain development are also very plausible.

The drugs and procedures used in active management may introduce extra risks for the mother, which are further explored here. Active management may pose other risks to the baby, as we will describe, and we do not know the long-term effects of the drugs used during the third stage, which may cross the placenta and reach the baby during an extremely sensitive stage of brain development.

Hormones in the Third Stage

As a mammalian species—defined by our mammary glands and the milk that they produce for our young—we share almost all features of labor and birth with our fellow mammals. We also have in common the complex orchestration of labor hormones, produced deep in our middle (mammalian) brain, which coordinates these processes and ultimately ensures the survival and well-being of mother and baby.

For example, the hormone oxytocin causes the uterine contractions that signal labor. After birth this hormone's effects within the limbic (emotional) brain help us to enact our instinctive mothering behaviors. Endorphins, the body's natural opiates, produce an altered state of consciousness and aid in transmuting pain, and the fight-or-flight hormones epinephrine and norepinephrine (adrenaline and noradrenaline, also known as catecholamines or CAs) give us the burst of energy that we need to push our babies out. Prolactin, the mothering hormone, is important in adapting our brain and bodies, including our breasts, to new maternity. These hormones continue to play crucial roles for mother and baby during the third stage.

At this time, the new mother's uterus continues to contract strongly and regularly under the continuing influence of oxytocin. Her uterine muscle fibers shorten (retract) with each contraction, leading to a gradual decrease in uterine size, which helps to shear the placenta away from its attachment site. Efficient uterine contractions are also necessary to slow bleeding from the placental site, which is initially a large and raw surface. These contractions cause a tightening of the interlacing muscle fibers (also called living ligatures) in the new mother's uterus, which seal off the maternal blood vessels and stop the bleeding. Third stage is complete when the birthing mother delivers her baby's placenta.

For the new mother, the third stage is a time of reaping the rewards of her labor. Mother Nature provides peak levels of oxytocin, the hormone of love, and endorphins, hormones of pleasure, for both mother and baby. Skin-to-skin contact and the baby's first attempts to breastfeed further increase maternal oxytocin levels,[1] strengthening the uterine contractions that help the baby's placenta to separate and the mother's uterus to contract down. In this way oxytocin (and the mother-newborn interactions that cause its release) act to prevent hemorrhage, as well as to establish, in concert with the other hormones, the positive first impressions that will help develop a secure bond between mother and baby.

The CAs are also important at this time. These hormones are normally produced under conditions of fear, stress, anxiety, hunger, and cold, when they divert blood to skeletal muscles, heart, and lungs to prepare the body for flight or fight. If the mother is fearful or anxious in labor, she will release these hormones, which will reduce the blood supply to her uterus and baby. Epinephrine and norepinephrine have also been shown to act directly on uterine muscle, slowing or even stopping contractions.[v]

During an undisturbed birth, however, the mother's CA levels will substantially increase with the transition from first to second (pushing) stage, giving her the extra strength that she needs to be upright and to push her baby out. Paradoxically, at high levels CA hormones have been found to cause an increase in the strength of uterine contractions,[2] which, along with a peak of oxytocin, will help the mother give birth quickly and easily. The effect of this hormonal outpouring has been called the fetus ejection reflex,[3] and it is thought to be the usual mechanism for birth in other species. High CA levels ensure that the new mother is wide-eyed and alert as she meets her baby for the first time.

Within minutes of birth, the new mother's CA levels start to decline[4] and, at these lower levels, revert to their original negative influence on her uterus.[2] A warm and calm atmosphere is needed to keep her CA levels on the decline and, therefore, her uterus well contracted.

If the new mother feels cold or fearful (perhaps due to separation from her baby), her CA levels may remain sufficiently elevated to reduce the ability of her uterus to contract and stop bleeding at this critical time. She may shiver, giving warning of this danger, and urgent action is required to warm her up. Elevated CA levels at this time have been linked with a higher risk of PPH[5, 6] and, in one small study, women with lower oxytocin levels were more likely to have third-stage problems.[7] In past decades, drugs that counteract the effects of epinephrine have been successfully used to prevent postpartum hemorrhage.[8]

The postpartum mother also enjoys an ongoing elevation in the hormone prolactin, the major hormone of breastmilk synthesis, which also adapts the mother's whole metabolic system for breastfeeding and her brain for new motherhood.[9] Maternal levels of this "hormone of tender mothering" remain high for up to six hours after birth, as measured in the blood,[10] and brain levels may be elevated for even longer.

In the minutes after birth the newborn also enjoys peak hormone levels, including elevations in oxytocin, beta-endorphin, and catecholamines. As with the mother, high levels of fight-or-flight hormones around the time of birth ensure that the baby is alert and wide-eyed at first contact with the mother, but levels of epinephrine decline in the following minutes. This parallels a reduction in newborn stress and an increase in stress-reducing hormones such as oxytocin and beta-endorphin, mediated through skin-to-skin mother-baby contact.

Studies of newborn babies who have enjoyed skin-to-skin contact after birth have found measurable signs of lower stress, including lower respiration rates, higher blood glucose, and lower base excess (reflecting reduced metabolic stress), compared with newborns separated and placed in cots or bassinets.[11] One study showed that this improvement in newborn physiology continues for many hours after birth, with higher foot temperatures (reflecting lower CA levels) at twenty-three hours among babies who had been skin to skin after birth compared with newborns who had been placed in a cot. Researchers suggest that skin-to-skin contact may reduce the negative consequences of the stress of being born.[12]

It is easy to forget that, during the third stage of labor, the new mother is still in labor and in fact, from a hormonal perspective, we could say that mother and baby are more "in labor" than ever at this time. The hormonal peaks enjoyed by mother and baby after birth reflect ongoing labor processes and adaptations that are crucial for the survival of both. Further, this hormonal situation is unique, and will never again occur for this mother and her baby, representing our best (and most evolved) opportunity to ensure successful attachment and breastfeeding and therefore species survival.

Maternal-Newborn Separation

There is a growing body of scientific evidence documenting the long-term harm that maternal-infant separation after birth can cause in all mammalian species, including humans.

Newborn separation from mother elicits an initial protest/hyper-arousal (fear-terror) response, involving the fight-or-flight hormones, with newborn activity (movement, noise) designed to attract the mother's attention. If reunion does not occur, fear-terror is followed by despair-dissociation, with metabolic and emotional shutdown and quieting, associated with high levels of numbing opiates, although the fight-or-flight system remains maximally activated.[13, 14] These powerful responses, designed to enhance survival for offspring lost in the wild, interfere with programmed brain development at this time. Despair-dissociation, in which fight-or-flight and metabolic shutdown overlap, may be especially toxic to the developing brain.[13, 14] (See also chapter 11.)

Documented long-term effects of newborn-maternal separation in animal studies include abnormalities in brain structure and function[15–17] and heightened responses to stress throughout life.[15] South African public health physician and skin-to-skin advocate Nils Bergman notes, from animal research, that the ability of newborns to tolerate separation from the mother is measured in minutes, and suggests that human babies may be even more sensitive to maternal deprivation.[18]

Although this vulnerability has not been formally tested in human studies, one might regard the routine separation of mother and newborn, which has become ingrained since the institutionalization of childbirth in the last century, as a large uncontrolled experiment with major psychological and perhaps physiological effects for most of our population. Bergman and other perinatal scientists equate this to the "violation of an innate agenda."[13]

One might also wonder whether the modern epidemic of stress (a term that was first applied to humans by researchers in the 1950s) and stress-related illness in our culture is a further outcome of maternal-infant separation after birth. There is increasing scientific evidence suggesting that our entire hypothalamic-pituitary-adrenal (HPA) axis, which mediates short-term fight-or-flight reaction as well as long-term stress responses and immune function, may be permanently misprogrammed by the continuing high stress-hormone levels that ensue when newborn babies are routinely separated from their mothers. Bergman believes that current epidemics of illness, including the ubiquitous metabolic syndrome, may be programmed by early separation.[18]

Carter comments, "There is increasing evidence for tuning or programming of neuronal [brain/nerve] systems by early experiences, in some cases by endogenous [internal] or exogenous [external] hormones."[19] This concept of vulnerability, in early life, to permanent misprogramming of central nervous system function because of experiences that are outside our genetic blueprint, is supported by Csaba's work on hormonal imprinting, described shortly. (See also chapter 6.)

Research by Jacobson and colleagues[20–22] and Raine and colleagues,[23] among others, suggests that contemporary tragedies such as suicide, drug addiction, and violent criminality may be linked to problems in the perinatal period such as exposure to drugs, birth complications, and separation from or rejection by the mother.

These findings lend support to experts such as Joseph Chilton Pearce, who believe that maternal-infant contact is crucial after birth and that separation of newborn from the mother prevents the activation of specific brain functions that are Mother Nature's blueprint for this time.[24] Michel Odent notes that almost every existing culture has rituals that disturb the early postnatal time—most often by separating mother and baby—and he believes that such rituals have predominated because they instill aggressive, and therefore more dominating and successful, traits in the offspring and culture. For example, Spartan warriors-to-be were apparently thrown on the floor after birth.[25] (See chapter 6 for more about maternal-infant separation after birth.)

One must also wonder about the effects on the newborn male, and on our society, of the postnatal ritual of circumcision, which involves extreme and measurable stress for the newborn, even when anesthetic techniques are used.[26–28]

With these understandings, the role of birth attendants in the hours following birth becomes clear. This role is to ensure unhurried and undisturbed contact between mother and baby; to adjust the temperature to ensure warmth for mother and baby; to facilitate skin-to-skin contact, mutual gaze, and prebreastfeeding and early breastfeeding behavior, with no other expectations for mother or baby; and to keep mother and baby together, except in extreme emergency. These measures can also include sensitively practiced observations, resuscitation (which can be done next to the mother or, for a baby with an intact cord, on the mother's thigh), and other safety measures.

Such priorities are sensible, intuitive, and safe, and help synchronize our hormonal systems with our genetic blueprint, giving maximum success and pleasure for both partners at this critical beginning of child rearing.

Placental Transfusion and the Baby

Adaptation to life outside the womb is the major physiological task for the baby in the third stage. In the mother's womb, the wondrous placenta fulfills the functions of lungs, kidney, gut, skin, and liver for the baby. Blood flow to these organs is minimal until immediately after birth, at which time huge changes begin in the organization of the newborn circulatory system. Within the baby's body, blood becomes diverted away from the umbilical cord and placenta over several minutes, and as the baby's lungs fill with air, blood is sucked into the pulmonary (lung) circulation.[29] Mother Nature ensures a reservoir of blood in the cord and placenta that provides the additional blood necessary for the perfusion of these pulmonary and organ systems; this is known as the placental transfusion or redistribution. The transfer of this reservoir (transfusion) of blood from the placenta to the baby happens in a stepwise progression.

According to research by Dunn,[30] during the second stage of labor, 66 milliliters (2.23 ounces) of blood is transferred from the baby and retained in the placenta, probably because the umbilical vein (which returns blood from placenta to baby) is compressed, and temporarily blocked, as the baby comes through the mother's vagina. This extra volume makes the placenta fuller and more rigid, which may help it remain attached to the mother's uterus in the minutes after birth, despite the sudden reduction in uterine size, and so continue to oxygenate the newborn until effective breathing is established. As the baby emerges, this pressure is released, allowing a bolus of warm, oxygenated, pH-balanced, placental blood to perfuse the newborn in the seconds after birth.

This transfusion is augmented during each of the mother's third-stage contractions, which are as powerful as those during labor. With each contraction, the in-utero placenta is compressed, squeezing blood into the newborn's body. Between contractions, the mother's uterus relaxes and some blood can return from baby to placenta through the low-pressure umbilical vein. Several studies have documented this process graphically by recording newborn weight gain in the minutes after birth.[31, 32] According to Gunther's observations, crying slows the baby's intake of blood,[32] which is also controlled by constriction of the vessels within the cord, both of which imply that the baby can regulate the transfusion according to individual need.

The majority of the placental transfusion is typically transferred to the newborn within three minutes, but it may take longer or, alternatively, it may be complete in only one minute,[33] with a quicker transfusion occurring when oxytocic drugs are administered to the mother to contract her uterus,[34] as will be discussed.

Gravity can also affect the transfer of blood, with transfer occurring most rapidly when the baby remains at, or slightly below, the level of the uterus.[35] However, the baby's position is likely to be important only if it is held very high above the uterus before clamping, or if the cord is clamped before pulsations cease: a skin-to-skin newborn with an unclamped cord can continue to redistribute blood volume, receiving or sending back blood to the placenta until an ideal blood volume is reached.

This elegant and time-tested system—which ensures that an optimum, but not a standard, amount of blood is transferred—is rendered inoperable by the current practice of early clamping of the cord, which usually occurs within thirty seconds of birth, and often within the first ten seconds.[36]

Early Clamping and the Baby

Early clamping has been widely adopted in western obstetrics as part of the package known as active management of the third stage, designed to reduce the risk of maternal hemorrhage after birth. Active management includes the use of an oxytocic agent—a drug that, like oxytocin, causes the uterus to contract strongly—usually given by injection into the mother's thigh as the baby is born; early cord clamping; and controlled cord traction, which involves pulling on the cord to deliver the placenta as quickly as possible.

Active management proponents have believed that immediate cord clamping is necessary because if the cord is not clamped before the oxytocic effect commences, the baby is at risk of having too much blood pumped from the placenta by the stronger uterine contractions. This area has been poorly studied. One early study using the ergot drug methylergometrine (methylergonovine) suggested that use of an oxytocic will hasten the baby's placental transfusion from three minutes to one minute; however, in this study, blood and red cell volumes were equivalent for babies with and without oxytocic exposure.[34] In contrast Dunn found that babies whose mothers received syntometrine (a combination of Pitocin and ergometrine/ergonovine) with cord clamping at three minutes, received an average of 40 milliliters (1.35 ounces) in excess of the normal placental transfusion.[37]

A recent review has analyzed maternal and infant outcomes according to the timing of cord clamping relative to oxytocic drug administration (cord clamping before and after oxytocic) and found no differences in any outcomes.[38] This may reflect the newborn's ability to avoid overperfusion by sending blood back to the placenta, as long as the cord remains unclamped. This is the blueprint among all other mammals, none of whom, obviously, clamp the cord before the placenta emerges. This finding is reassuring for recent policies that encourage the use of oxytocic drugs soon after birth along with delayed clamping.[39] However, there may be other negative effects for the newborn when an oxytocic drug is administered to the mother before the cord is clamped: see the following section on synthetic oxytocin and the baby.

And although the aim of active management is to reduce the risk of hemorrhage for the mother, "its widespread acceptance was not preceded by studies evaluating the effects of depriving neonates [newborns] of a significant volume of blood."[40]

Usher estimated that early clamping deprives the baby of 54 to 160 milliliters (1.8 to 5.1 ounces) of blood,[41] which, at the upper limits, is almost half of a baby's total blood volume at birth. The average placental transfusion is 100 milliliters (3.5 ounces, or almost half a cup), which is one-quarter to one-third of an average newborn's 350-milliliter total blood volume. Premature babies are likely to lose an even greater proportion of their blood through early clamping, because the placenta is relatively bigger in relation to the baby's body and contains more blood.

Morley comments,

> Clamping the cord before the infant's first breath results in blood being sacrificed from other organs to establish pulmonary perfusion [blood supply to the lungs]. Fatality may result if the child is already hypovolemic [low in blood volume].[42]

Peltonen recorded on film an early clamped newborn's heart function as the baby took a first breath.[43] This film showed that, for several cardiac cycles after the first breath, the baby's left heart had insufficient blood. Peltonen concludes,

> It would seem that the closing of the umbilical circulation [cord clamping] before the aeration of the lungs has taken place is a highly unphysiological measure and should be avoided.[44]

In recent decades, early clamping has been performed in order to obtain cord blood for analysis of blood gases and pH (acid-base) value. This is intended to provide evidence (or not) of lack of oxygen (hypoxia) during or before birth. This procedure has medicolegal implications, although, as one review concludes: "We found no evidence that this measurement is needed to conduct any treatment."[45]

According to Wiberg, blood samples for cord blood gases can be taken immediately after birth, followed by delayed cord clamping.[46] These researchers have also documented the changes in blood gas and pH values in later-clamped babies, which may help establish "normal values" when blood gas sampling is really necessary.[46]

Ironically, babies who are compromised in labor and/or birth are in most need of the extra blood and oxygen that delayed clamping will provide,[47] and are also the most likely to have a blood sample taken, making it important for caregivers to create policies and procedures that allow late clamping when cord blood gas sampling is performed.

Note also that a nuchal cord—the cord around the baby's neck—does not necessitate cord clamping, except in extreme situations. A nuchal cord occurs in 20 to 30 percent of births, and is usually easily loosened, or the baby can be "somersaulted" through, as described by Mercer.[48] Cutting a nuchal cord removes the baby's blood and oxygen supply, which can have devastating effects if the baby's first breath is delayed by shoulder dystocia or other birth difficulties.[49, 50]

Cesarean Babies

When the baby is lifted well above the uterus before clamping—for example, during cesarean surgery—the mother's uterus is unable to pump blood against the upward gradient, and the baby's blood may even flow back to the mother's uterus with gravity. Cesarean babies also miss the pressure-reperfusion effect, described earlier, which shunts an extra 66 milliliters of placental blood at birth, and they are also very likely to have their cords clamped and cut immediately, as a routine practice. All of these factors make cesarean newborns especially unlikely to receive their expected blood volume, or indeed any placental transfusion.[51] The consequence of this may be an increased risk of respiratory (breathing) distress. Several studies have shown that respiratory distress can be eliminated in cesarean-born babies when a full placental transfusion is allowed.[43, 52]

UK pediatrician Peter Dunn recommends that the cord of a cesarean baby remain unclamped, and that, after removal from the mother's uterus, the baby and conjoined placenta remain level until the cord stops pulsing in five to ten minutes, allowing the newborn to equilibrate its final blood volume.[53] The naked baby and (wrapped) placenta can also be placed on the mother's chest. Morley has similar recommendations for cesarean babies.[54] Another researcher found respiratory benefits by hanging the cesarean baby's placenta like a transfusion bag until the cord stopped pulsating.[52]

Gravity can also be used to assist a cesarean newborn's placental transfusion, with more blood transferred when the baby is held below the level of the placenta. Allowing the baby to breathe repeatedly before cord clamping may also promote placental transfusion for a cesarean baby.[55] Similarly, Weeks recommends that caregivers "wait a minute" before clamping the cesarean baby's cord, with the baby kept warm on the mother's legs.[47]

These techniques may be especially important for premature cesarean babies, whose survival may be greatly enhanced by allowing a full placental transfusion.[53]

Reduced Iron Stores and Other Early Clamping Consequences

The baby whose cord is clamped early also loses the iron contained within that blood. An average placental transfusion contains 30 to 35 milligrams of additional iron, which is equivalent to the iron contained in 100 liters (26 gallons) of breast milk.[56]

Not surprisingly early clamping has been linked with an increased risk of anemia in infancy. A recent meta-analysis suggests that early cord clamping increases the risk of anemia by five times at one to two days and doubles the risk at age two to three months, compared with clamping at two minutes or later. In this analysis early clamped infants also had lower iron stores at six months.[56] Other studies have suggested that the hazards of early cord clamping are even greater for babies of anemic mothers.[57] Early cord clamping has also been linked with elevated blood lead levels at six months, as a consequence of lower iron stores.[58]

Anemia in infancy has been associated with deficits in intellectual, visual, motor, and social-emotional development, even among otherwise seemingly healthy infants, with effects on the developing brain that may be permanent.[59]

The negative consequences of early clamping were recognized as far back as 1801, when Erasmus Darwin wrote:

> Another thing very injurious to the child is the tying and cutting of the navel string too soon; which should always be left till the child has not

only repeatedly breathed but till all pulsation in the cord ceases. As otherwise the child is much weaker than it ought to be, a part of the blood being left in the placenta which ought to have been in the child.[60]

In one randomized trial premature babies who experienced a delay in cord clamping of only thirty seconds showed a reduced need for transfusion, less severe breathing problems, better oxygen levels, and indications of improved long-term outcomes, compared with those whose cords were clamped immediately.[61]

Premature babies whose cord clamping is delayed also gain protection from intraventricular hemorrhage (IVH),[62] a form of bleeding in the brain that is not uncommon in this group. The increased risk with early clamping may reflect the fact that early cord clamping causes a sudden (but transient) increase in the baby's blood pressure,[63] which may particularly affect the premature baby's immature brain. As we will explore further, the early clamped baby may subsequently suffer from insufficient blood to supply the brain, a further risk factor for IVH.[64]

One must also wonder about the effects of the deprivation of a significant amount of blood on the full-term baby's brain. Some have suggested that some of our children's developmental problems, such as cerebral palsy,[65] autism,[66] and learning difficulties,[67] may be related to the practice of early cord clamping, which has become widespread in only the last fifty years or so.[68]

Early researchers Jaykka and colleagues,[69-72] and more recently, Mercer and Skovgaard,[73] have documented the elegant unfolding of the newborn lungs that occurs as the placental transfusion fills the small capillaries that support the alveoli (air sacs), reducing the pressure needed by the newborn to inflate their lungs and ensuring a safe transition to breathing. This paradigm also explains the wet lungs that are more likely when cesarean babies are deprived of their full placental transfusion; this is another powerful argument for leaving well enough alone in the third stage of labor.

Polycythemia and Jaundice

Some studies have shown an increased risk of polycythemia (an increase in the number of red blood cells in the blood) and jaundice when the cord is clamped later. Research shows that late clamped newborns may have up to a 60 percent increase in red cell volume (RCV) compared with early clamped babies.[74] Polycythemia may be beneficial because more red cells will be able to carry more oxygen to the newborn's organs and tissues. The higher level of protein contained in this extra blood is also advantageous in drawing fluid from the newborn lungs (by colloid osmotic pressure, or COP), and so preventing wet lungs and respiratory distress.[73]

The idea that polycythemia due to delayed clamping will cause the blood of otherwise-healthy newborns to become too thick (hyperviscosity syndrome), which is often used as an argument against delayed cord clamping, was suggested in an older trial that involved small numbers of babies, some of whom were premature. These authors described "symptomatic neonatal plethora," which was said to include cyanosis, breathing difficulties, low blood pressure, and low blood sugar.[75] This finding has not been substantiated in more recent high-quality research[76] and reviews.[36,77] It is also illogical, as a healthy newborn can easily compensate by dilating the blood vessels to accommodate higher-viscosity blood.[77,78] As with all mammalian species, our babies' circulatory systems are designed to balance this normal adjustment to life outside the womb.

Jaundice is caused by the breakdown of hemoglobin in excess red blood cells to produce bilirubin, the pigment that causes the yellow appearance of a jaundiced baby, and is highly likely when a baby gets the full quota of blood. Physiological jaundice—that is, jaundice due only to the normal breakdown of excess red blood cells—is present in almost all human newborns to some extent and may be prolonged by breastfeeding (hence the term breast milk jaundice).

Our understanding of jaundice has expanded recently, with bilirubin—which has been called a "born-again benignant pigment"[79]—now recognized as an important antioxidant, more powerful than vitamin E.[80] Bilirubin is produced in all mammals by a complex and seemingly deliberate pathway,[80] and it may have a critical role in protecting the newborn baby from oxidative stresses associated with adjustment to significantly higher oxygen levels outside the womb. Recent research confirms that mildly to moderately jaundiced newborns have better antioxidant status, which deteriorates when phototherapy is used to reduce bilirubin levels,[81] and an older study found that bilirubin has antibiotic properties sufficient to kill the pneumococcal bacteria.[82]

Studies do not show an excess of severe jaundice (such as would cause kernicterus, or brain damage) in babies who have had late clamping. Two recent reviews, including more than one thousand late clamped babies in total, both concluded that phototherapy or exchange transfusion for jaundice were no more common among late clamped compared with early clamped newborns.[36, 57] (See below for more about phototherapy and delayed clamping.)

The Compromised Newborn

Early cord clamping carries the further disadvantage of depriving the baby of the oxygen contained in the placental blood, intended to tide the baby over until breathing is well established. In situations of extreme distress—for example, if the baby takes several minutes to breathe—this reservoir of oxygenated blood can be lifesaving. Standard practice is to cut the cord immediately if resuscitation is needed, but resuscitation can be performed on the mother's thigh with the baby's placental circulation still intact.

UK obstetrician Andrew Weeks advocates allowing compromised newborns at least one minute for placental transfusion. He comments, "In these days of advanced technology, it is surely not beyond us to find a way of keeping the cord intact during the first minute of neonatal resuscitation."[83]

Garrison, a family physician from Canada, reports resuscitating a newborn who was unable to breathe for seven recorded minutes due to thick meconium and who survived without disability with an intact cord and placental circulation.[84] Other authors agree that clinically useful placental gas exchange continues for some minutes after birth, which is important because the newborn's early breaths are actually inefficient at gas exchange.[85]

When the cord is intact and the placenta still in the mother's womb, any drug given to the mother can pass to the baby, even during the third stage. Garrison reports a positive use for this conduit.[84] He notes that naloxone (Narcan)—which is sometimes administered to a newborn baby to counteract the sedating effects of opiate drugs such as pethidine (meperidine, Demerol) given to the mother in labor—can alternatively be administered effectively intravenously (IV) to the mother in the third stage, flowing to and waking up the baby in a matter of seconds. This provides further evidence of an ongoing metabolic pathway from mother to baby in the third stage.

Synthetic Oxytocin and the Baby

The baby exposed to active management may also be affected by maternal administration of synthetic oxytocin (Pitocin) during the third stage. This is most likely if new protocols advising early administration of an oxytocic drug with late clamping are followed.[39]

Carter and colleagues administered a single dose of synthetic oxytocin to prairie voles within twenty-four hours of birth and found disturbances in adult sexual and parental behavior. She suggests that small amounts may cross the human placenta, or alternatively there may be indirect effects;[86] she therefore cautions, "The assumption that perinatal oxytocin manipulations are without effect is largely untested, although the small but growing literature in animals suggests that this may be an invalid assumption."[87] (See chapter 6, Undisturbed Birth, for more on hormonal imprinting.)

A final consideration is the possibility that, as Edwards cautions, "though very rare, injections can be mixed up."[88] There are case reports of oxytocic drugs accidentally given to newborns instead of Vitamin K.[89, 90]

Cord Blood Banking

The recent discovery of the amazing properties of cord blood, and the hematopoietic (blood-making) stem cells contained within it, heightens the need to ensure that a newborn baby gets a full quota. Newborn hematopoietic stem cells are unique to this stage of development and will migrate to the baby's bone marrow soon after birth, transforming themselves into various types of blood cells.

Newborn cord blood—which is actually the placental trasfusion—was first collected and publicly banked in the United States in 1993,[91] with the aim of benefiting children with conditions such as leukemia, whose medical treatment (chemotherapy), aimed at destroying cancer cells, also destroys bone marrow. The marrow can be repopulated with the child's own blood cells, taken by bone marrow harvest before treatment (a surgical procedure) or bone marrow from a closely matched or related donor. When this is not possible, cord blood transfusion can provide a less-exact match. The availability of public banks, with a large number of donations, has increased the chances of a suitable allogenic transplant (from another individual) for many ill children.

There are now public non-profit cord blood banks in at least twenty-three countries around the world. In the United States, public cord blood banks sell cord blood for allogenic transplantation to matched recipients for US$15,000 to $20,000, which is usually covered by health insurance.[92]

Biological Insurance?

In many places private cord blood banks are persuading parents to pay large sums of money (US$1,000 to $2,000 initially plus an annual fee of $100 to $150, according to http://parentsguidecordblood.org) to store their baby's blood as "biological insurance," although the chance of actually using the blood is very remote.

For example, the likelihood of low-risk children needing their own stored cord blood (autologous transfusion) has been estimated at 1 in 15,000 to 20,000 at best,[91, 93] and a single cord blood donation is unlikely to be effective for treatment beyond childhood because the number of stem cells is too low.[94]

Autologous cord blood is unsuitable for children who develop leukemia because it may contain preleukemic changes and it doesn't produce the beneficial "graft versus leukemia" effect associated with allogenic stem cell transplants. For these reasons autologous cord blood transplant is associated with an overall increased risk of leukemia relapse.[91, 93] Autologous cord blood is also not clinically used for treatment of solid tumors (such as brain tumors) and cannot cure inherited conditions such as thalassemia and bone marrow failure.[91, 93]

According to a review by children's cancer researcher Michael Sullivan, "in most cases in which an autologous stem cell transplant is indicated for cancer, stem cells can be harvested from bone marrow or peripheral blood before transplant and in this case autologous umbilical cord blood has no known clinical advantage over standard bone marrow-harvested stem cells."[95]

Up to 2003, there have been only three published reports of treatment with autologous cord blood transplants from private banks, including one girl who recovered from leukemia in 2007 after a transfusion of her own cord blood and whose story is apparently widely used by private banks. However, according to experts, she would have done at least as well with conventional treatment involving bone marrow transplant.[95] Another case involved a child with acquired bone marrow failure, for which treatment with autologous cord blood is recognized as the only unequivocally beneficial use; however, the condition is very rare (around 1 in 200,000) and is curable with conventional therapy in over 70 percent of children, according to Sullivan.[91]

The European Group on Ethics in Science and New Technologies to the European Commission states, "indications to store cord blood at birth in view of a future autologous graft are for the present time almost nonexistent."[96]

Private cord blood banking is not recommended by the American Academy of Pediatrics, who advise members in their 2007 policy statement, "Cord blood donation should be discouraged when cord blood stored in a bank is to be directed for later personal or family use, because most conditions that might be helped by cord blood stem cells already exist in the infant's cord blood."[97, 98]

Note that many companies increase their business by offering a financial incentive to maternity care providers (around US$50) for each family who signs up with their blood bank. The American College of Obstetricians and Gynecologists (ACOG) notes: "Physicians or other professionals who recruit pregnant women and their families for for-profit umbilical cord blood banking should disclose any financial interests or other potential conflicts of interest."[99]

Cord blood banks use emotional advertising with highly improbable scenarios—for example, implying that banked cord blood may help to treat the child if they develop conditions such as stroke and Alzheimer's disease in old age. These hopeful scenarios are virtually impossible, given that the use of cord blood for such conditions is speculative according to current research; a single cord blood donation is currently inadequate for adult treatment; and cord blood has not been proven storable for decades, especially by private companies who are not regulated at present and who may not have the storage standards necessary to ensure prolonged viability of stem cells.[100] Public banks report that cord blood can be stored for fifteen to twenty years.[101]

It is also highly likely that other sources of stem cells, and other therapies, will be developed in the coming years: for example, recently stem cells have been discovered in breastmilk.[102]

Impact on the Baby

Although cord blood harvesting is promoted by both public and private institutions as harmless to the baby, it involves collecting the newborn's placental transfusion and requires early clamping—ideally within thirty seconds of birth—so that an adequate number of stem cells is obtained. Delayed cord clamping, which allows this blood to transfer to the baby, as discussed earlier, is likely to lead to an inadequate volume of blood harvested.

For example, in one study the volume of cord blood obtained was reduced from 75 milliliters, collected when the cord was clamped at 30 seconds after birth, to 39 milliliters collected when clamping occurred between 30 and 180 seconds. A low-volume collection indicates insufficient stem cells to be usable for transfusion.[103] Public cord blood banks generally discard collections below 40 milliliters,[104] with overall one-third to one-half of collections discarded, mostly because of low volume.[96, 105] Private banks, which are paid by parents to collect and store their baby's blood, do not generally discard the collections, and some may have a policy to accept lower volumes, although this may not guarantee usefulness.

Some centers collect residual blood from the placenta after it is delivered, although the amount is usually less than that obtained from the cord straight after birth, and still requires early cord clamping for an adequate collection.[103] Contamination is also more likely with a placental collection.

A cord blood collection of 100 milliliters from a full-term newborn (almost one-third of the 350-milliliter average newborn blood volume) is equivalent to the loss, in an adult, of 1.7 liters (3.5 pints) of blood, or three to four times the volume of a usual adult blood donation.

The American Academy of Pediatrics states,

> If cord clamping is done too soon after birth, the infant may be deprived of a placental blood transfusion, resulting in lower blood volume and increased risk of anemia in later life . . . There may be a temptation to practice immediate cord clamping aggressively to increase the

volume of cord blood that can be harvested for cord blood banking. This practice is unethical and should be discouraged.[97]

Experts have also expressed concern about the effects of the loss of hematopoietic stem cells,[106] and suggested that "Obtaining cord blood for future autologous transplantation of stem cells needs early clamping and seems to conflict with the infants best interests."[107]

Researchers have discovered other beneficial components and effects of cord blood, further emphasizing its importance for the newborn. These include neurotrophins that protect brain cells from death related to oxygen deprivation[108] and help to repair areas of brain cell damage;[109] epithelial progenitor cells that repair damaged tissue and produce new blood vessels;[110] stimulation of vascular endothelial growth factor (VEGF) by stem cells, which protects and repairs brain cells;[111] and the formation of glial cells and astrocytes from stem cells,[112] which repair damage to the white matter of the brain and may protect from cerebral palsy. Newborn stem cells may also have a general beneficial role in healing damaged tissues.[113]

It is ironic that cord blood has been recently suggested as a treatment for autism[113]—a condition that some experts believe may be due, at least in part, to the early cord clamping that would be necessary for collecting cord blood.[66]

International Perspectives on Cord Blood Banking

Private, for-profit cord blood banks exist in most European countries, with this "business based on hope"[114] spreading to developed and developing countries around the world.[92]

However, the European Group on Ethics in Science and New Technologies states, "The legitimacy of commercial cord blood banks for autologous use should be questioned as they sell a service, which has presently no real use regarding therapeutic options . . . The activities of such banks raise serious ethical criticisms."[115] The European Health Committee of the Council of Europe recommends that private cord blood banks should not be supported by member states or their health services.

Similarly, the UK Royal College of Obstetricians and Gynaecologists "remains unconvinced about the benefit of storing cord blood with a private bank for families who have no known medical reason to do so"[116] and notes, "Cord blood collection could jeopardise the mother's or the baby's health."[117]

The International Federation of Gynaecology and Obstetrics (FIGO) Committee for the Ethical Aspects of Human Reproduction and Women's Health concluded, in 1998:

> The information mothers currently receive at the time of requesting consent (for the collection of umbilical cord blood) is that blood in the placenta is no longer of use to the baby and this "waste blood" may help to save another person's life. This information is incomplete and does not permit informed consent. Early clamping of the umbilical cord following vaginal delivery is likely to deprive the newborn infant of at least a third of its normal circulating blood volume, and it will also cause a haemodynamic disturbance. These factors may result in serious morbidity [illness]. For consent to be informed, the harmful effects of early cord clamping should be disclosed and the mother assured that the collection of cord-blood will not involve early clamping. In summary, permission to collect blood from the cord for banking should not lead to clamping the cord earlier than 20–30 seconds after delivery of the baby.[118]

In summary, private cord blood banking involves taking a significant amount of blood at birth (blood the baby needs for optimal transition and iron stores), and paying thousands of dollars to store it away, with a very remote chance of later use by that child or the family. Public cord blood banking is perhaps more justifiable, but both involve the loss of around one third of the newborn's blood volume, with negative consequences, as described earlier, that may persist into infancy. As Diaz-Rossello concludes, "All the evidence shows that the best bank for that blood is the baby."[119]

Active Management and the Mother

Active management (oxytocic drug, early clamping, and controlled cord traction) represents a further development in third-stage interference, which began in the mid-seventeenth century when male birth attendants confined women to bed and cord clamping was introduced to spare the bed linen.[120]

Pulling on the cord was first recommended by the Frenchman Mauriceau in 1673, who feared that the uterus might close before the placenta was spontaneously delivered.[120] In fact, the bed-bound horizontal postures increasingly adopted under medical care meant that spontaneous delivery of the placenta was less likely: an upright posture, which women and midwives have traditionally used, encourages the placenta to fall out with the help of gravity.

The first oxytocic to be used medically was ergot, derived from a fungal infection of rye. Ergot was used by seventeenth and eighteenth century European midwives; its use was limited, however, by its toxicity. It was refined and revived as ergonovine (ergometrine) in the 1930s, and by the late 1940s some doctors were using it preventatively, as well as therapeutically, for postpartum hemorrhage.[120]

Potential side effects from ergot derivatives include a rise in blood pressure, nausea, vomiting, headache, palpitations, cerebral hemorrhage, cardiac arrest, convulsion, and even death. Ergot derivatives should not be administered to any woman who already has high blood pressure.

Ergot derivatives may have other unwanted effects, including suppression of prolactin, the hormone of breastmilk synthesis. According to Jordan, "Midwives need to consider that syntometrine [which combines ergonovine/ergometrine with Pitocin/Syntocinon] may adversely impact on breastfeeding."[121] Note that the lactation-suppressing drug bromocriptine is also an ergot derivative.[122]

This opinion is supported by the results of an Irish randomized controlled trial comparing active management using ergometrine/ergonovine with physiological management. Although prolactin levels on day two were similar between groups, significantly more women who had received ergonovine/ergometrine had stopped breastfeeding by one week; most women who gave up before six weeks cited "hungry baby/insufficient milk" as the reason.[123–125]

According to Hale, the ergot derivative methylergonovine (methylergometrine, methylergonovine maleate, MEM, Methergine) may not have this effect,[126] although one older study found lower prolactin levels soon after third-stage administration,[127] and another found that daily postnatal administration of this drug had negative effects on lactation and milk production.[128]

The paucity of research on the effects of third-stage drugs on lactation is troubling, given these concerns about ergot derivative and the fact that oxytocin is also a major breastfeeding hormone. Major reviews of drugs used in third stage management have also omitted this important outcome.[129–131]

Synthetic oxytocin, as used in the third stage, mimics the effects of natural oxytocin on the uterus; it was first marketed in the 1950s. Synthetic oxytocin has largely replaced ergometrine/ergonovine for use in the third stage, although the combination drug syntometrine is widely used in the UK. Syntocinon causes an increase in the strength of contractions, whereas ergonovine causes frequent high-pressure contractions, referred to by Dunn as "uterine fibrillations,"[30] which may increase the risk of trapping the placenta. Ergonovine/ergometrine may also interfere with the process of placental separation, increasing the chance of partial separation.[132]

In recent years misoprostol, a synthetic prostaglandin, has also been researched for use in the third stage. It is cheap and can be given orally, which makes it attractive for low-resource settings. Evidence suggests that it is less effective as a preventative, with more side effects such as nausea, vomiting, diarrhea, fever, and shivering.[133] However, it may be a useful drug for emergency treatment of PPH, and less misoprostol is transferred to breastmilk compared with ergot derivatives.[134] More research is needed before this drug is recommended for widespread use.

Active Management Trials

Active management has been declared "the routine management of choice for women expecting a single baby by vaginal delivery in a maternity hospital,"[135] by the influential UK Cochrane Collaboration, largely because of the results of the 1998 Hinchingbrooke trial[136] comparing active and expectant (nonactive, or physiological) management.

In this trial, which involved 1,500 women at low risk of bleeding, active management was associated with a rate of postpartum hemorrhage (blood loss greater than 500 milliliters, or around one pint) of 6.8 percent, compared with 16.5 percent for expectant management. Rates of severe PPH (blood loss greater than 1,000 milliliters) were low in both groups: 1.7 percent of active and 2.6 percent of expectant.

The authors note that, based on these figures, ten women would need to receive active management to prevent one PPH; they comment,

> Some women . . . may rate a small personal risk of PPH of little importance compared with intervention in an otherwise straightforward labor, whereas others may wish to take all measures to reduce the risk of PPH.[137]

Reading this paper, one must wonder how it is that almost one in six women bled after physiological management, and whether one or more components of Western obstetric practices might actually increase the rate of hemorrhage.

Botha, who attended more than twenty-six thousand Bantu women over the course of ten years, reports, "a retained placenta was seldom seen . . . Blood transfusion for postpartum hemorrhage was never necessary."[138] Bantu women deliver both baby and placenta while upright and squatting, and the cord is not attended to until the placenta is delivered by gravity.

PPH and the Mother

Some evidence suggests that clamping the cord, which is not practiced by indigenous cultures (nor by other mammals), contributes to both PPH and retained placenta by trapping extra blood within the placenta. This increases placental bulk, against which the mother's uterus cannot contract (and retract) efficiently, and which can lead to increased blood loss.[139]

A recent review by the Cochrane Collaboration has examined cord blood drainage (that is, clamping and cutting the cord, then letting the maternal side drain to reduce placental bulk); reviewers found that this reduced the length of third stage, and they recommended more research.[140]

Other Western practices that may contribute to PPH include the use of oxytocin for induction and augmentation of labor;[141–144] epidural pain relief;[145–148] episiotomy; perineal trauma; forceps delivery; and cesarean and previous cesarean, which increase the risks of placental problems such as placental abruption and placenta previa.[149–151]

Epidurals increase the chances of a long second stage and use of forceps, and they also reduce the oxytocin peak at birth,[152] all of which may increase PPH risk. The prolonged use of Pitocin during labor (for induction or augmentation) has been shown to desensitize the laboring mother's uterus to the effects of oxytocin by reducing her oxytocin receptor numbers.[153]

As noted, Western practices neither facilitate the production of a mother's own oxytocin nor direct attention to reducing catecholamine levels in the minutes after birth, both of which can be expected to physiologically improve the new mother's contractions and therefore reduce her blood loss. The routine practice of separating mother and baby deprives the mother of important opportunities to increase her natural oxytocin release.[1] Kennell and McGrath note, "Before the availability of medications such as Pitocin, the newborn's touches were probably crucial for the survival of mothers by raising oxytocin levels to cause strong, repeated uterine contractions, which prevented a fatal hemorrhage."[154]

The active management trials have not incorporated these important physiological factors. For example, in the Hinchingbrooke trial, only 8 and 1.7 percent of expectant and actively managed women, respectively, had their babies at the breast within ten minutes of birth, rising to 57 and 63 percent by two hours.[155]

It is also interesting to note Logue's finding of a significant difference in PPH rates according to the practitioner.[156] In the hospital that she surveyed, PPH rates ranged from 1 to 16 percent for midwives and 1 to 31 percent for registrars. She notes that doctors and midwives who were considered "heavy handed" had significantly higher rates.

Early Clamping and Feto-Maternal Hemorrhage

Clamping the cord can have other detrimental effects. Immediate clamping traps the placental transfusion—around a hundred milliliters of blood—in the placenta, which is then squeezed by the mother's uterus during third-stage contractions. With this extra volume, even the pressure of a normal contraction may force a significant amount of placental blood through the barrier that usually keeps mother's and baby's blood separate, and into the mother's bloodstream.[156, 157] This is called a feto-maternal hemorrhage (FMH).

An FMH therefore allows the baby's blood, which is immunologically different from the mother's, into her bloodstream, where her immune system can recognize it as foreign and form antibodies to destroy it. This occurs when an Rh-negative mother—a mother whose blood does not contain the Rhesus D (RhD) factor—is exposed to the blood of her Rh-positive baby (whose blood has the RhD factor) via FMH. This can cause the mother to make antibodies against the RhD factor (sensitization). There are many other less-common blood factors that can trigger sensitization following FMH.

If FMH occurs in third stage, this will not harm the newborn baby. However, these antibodies can be reactivated if the mother has a subsequent pregnancy with an Rh-positive baby and can pass through the placenta to her baby, destroying fetal blood cells (which are coated with the RhD factor) and causing anemia or even death.

Major blood group reactions between RhD-negative mothers and their RhD-positive babies can be very effectively prevented by the routine use of anti-D products such as Rhogam after birth, but because they are pooled blood products, these products carry the potential risk of transmitting unrecognized blood-borne infections.

All components of active management may increase FMH risk. The use of oxytocic drugs, either during labor or in third stage, has been linked to an increased risk of FMH and blood group incompatibility problems,[158, 159] because the stronger uterine contractions can cause microfractures in the placental barrier.[158] Recent case reports have also noted FMH with the use of oxytocin stress test during pregnancy[160] (which can cause significant harm to the baby) and with oxytocin induction.[161]

Early clamping, by increasing placental bulk, may also contribute to FMH. Early work by Dunn found an increased pressure in the placenta following early clamping, which was further increased when ergometrine (ergonovine) was administered, leading to rupture of visible placental blood vessels.[37] A recent randomized trial of "placental drainage" at cesarean found less FMH, as measured by fetal cells found in the maternal circulation, among mothers whose newborn's placenta had been drained,[162] an effect that would likely also apply when the placenta is allowed to "drain" into the baby.

Cord traction has been shown to damage the delicate placental vessels, producing an increased FMH risk.[163]

Avoiding active management is therefore likely to reduce the risk of FMH and sensitization to RhD and to other blood components. RhD sensitization is also less likely if mother and baby are incompatible in ABO blood groups[164] (for example, mother O, baby A, B, or AB; Mother A, baby B; mother B, baby A) because the mother has preformed antibodies and her immune system will destroy any of the baby's cells that enter her circulation. However, a moderate risk of significant FMH may exist (possibly around 10 percent[165]) even under ideal circumstances. For a more detailed discussion, see Sara Wickham's excellent book.[165, 166] Note that prevention of FMH at delivery has been poorly researched since the widespread use of anti-D after birth.

Cord traction carries other potential hazards. When the placenta is not yet separated, strong cord traction can actually pull the cord off, making placental delivery more difficult and surgery for removal more likely. Cord traction is also a painful procedure for the new mother. Strong cord traction can also rarely cause an inversion of the new mother's uterus, producing a state of profound maternal shock.

The World Health Organization (WHO), in its 1996 publication *Care in Normal Birth: A Practical Guide*, considers these risks and concludes,

> In a healthy population (as is the case in most developed countries), postpartum blood loss up to 1,000 mL may be considered as physiological and does not necessitate treatment other than oxytocics . . . [167]

In relation to routine oxytocics and controlled cord traction, WHO cautions,

> Recommendation of such a policy would imply that the benefits of such management would offset and even exceed the risks, including potentially rare but serious risks that might become manifest in the future.[168]

Recent Developments in Thinking about the Third Stage

In recent years there have been some welcome developments in the thinking and practice of third stage. U.S. authors Morley,[54] Mercer,[73, 77] and others have published papers that have deepened our understanding of neonatal physiology during third stage and of the risks of early clamping for the baby.

In the UK, the Cochrane Collaboration has reviewed the literature on maternal and neonatal outcomes in relation to the timing of umbilical cord clamping and has concluded that delayed cord clamping is advantageous for newborn iron stores, with, according to this review, no statistically significant difference in overall rates of jaundice but a small increased risk of jaundice requiring phototherapy for delayed-clamped babies (5 percent versus 3 percent early clamped).[38]

This finding is debatable, being substantially based on two studies, one of which had twice as many women using Pitocin in the delayed-clamping group, which likely accounts for the increased jaundice in their babies.[169] The second study is unpublished and therefore difficult to assess, but did not in itself find significantly more delayed-clamped babies requiring phototherapy for jaundice.

In relation to premature babies, the Cochrane reviewers unequivocally state, "Delaying cord clamping by 30 to 120 seconds, rather than early clamping, seems to be associated with less need for transfusion and less intraventricular hemorrhage."[62]

The Canadian Pediatric Society has also recommended delayed cord clamping in premature babies to reduce the need for blood transfusions.[170]

Opinion and research on early versus delayed cord clamping in full-term newborns, published recently in major journals, have also sided with delayed clamping. Hutton and Hassan's systematic review and meta-analysis in the Journal of the American Medical Association (JAMA) 2007, concluded that "Delayed cord clamping for a minimum of two minutes following birth is beneficial to the newborn, extending into infancy."[36] In the British Medical Journal (BMJ) in 2007, Weeks states, "There is now considerable evidence that early cord clamping does not benefit mothers or babies and may even be harmful" and recommends a delay of three minutes, with the baby on the mother's abdomen.[83]

In the influential U.S. *Journal of Perinatal Medicine*, Levy and Bliskstein comment, "the balance of available data suggests that delayed cord clamping should be the method of choice."[107]

It is also heartening to read the recent joint statement by the International Confederation of Midwives (ICM) and the International Federation of Gynaecologists and Obstetricians (IFGO), as part of the Safe Motherhood project.[39] This statement advocates routine active management, but, in a major shift for ICM/FIGO, now recommends that the baby's cord should not be cut until pulsation has ceased.

Choosing a Natural Third Stage

A woman's choice to forgo preventative oxytocics, to clamp late (if at all), and to deliver the placenta by her own effort, all require forethought, commitment, and the selection of birth attendants who are comfortable and experienced with these choices.

A natural third stage is more than this, however. We must ensure respect for the emotional and hormonal processes of both mother and baby, remembering how unique and critical this time is. Odent stresses the importance of not interrupting, even with words, and advises that the new mother should feel unobserved and uninhibited in the first encounter with her baby.[6]

This level of noninterference requires skill, experience, and confidence, as well as support from mentors and institutions. However, as I argue, attention to these nonmedical elements is essential for a safe natural third stage.

Lotus birth, in which the placenta remains attached to the baby until the cord separates naturally over several days, gives us another way to "slow the fire drill" after birth,[171] and allows our babies the full metaphysical, as well as physical, benefit of prolonged contact with the placenta. Like a good midwife, lotus birth secludes mother and baby in the early hours and days, ensuring rest and keeping visitors to a minimum.[172] (See the essay "Jacob's Placenta," page 185, for more about lotus birth.)

Third stage represents the first meeting between mother and baby, creating a powerful imprint on their relationship. When both are undrugged and quiet, fully present and alert, new potentials for love and trust are invoked for mother, baby, family, and the world we share.

Suggestions for a Natural Third Stage

For the mother:

- Choose caregivers who have skills, confidence, and trust in the natural processes of birth and third stage.
- Enjoy an undisturbed birth (see suggestions, page 127).
- Ensure a warm (even hot) room immediately after birth.
- Use the following suggestions for the caregiver.

For the caregiver

- Arrange resuscitation facilities that can be brought close to the mother after birth.
- Delay cord clamping ideally until after the mother has birthed her baby's placenta or even longer. If this is not possible, consider waiting for one of the following, in order of increasing benefit:
  - Until the baby takes a first breath
  - Until thirty seconds after birth
  - Until three minutes or so after birth
  - Until the cord stops pulsing
- If the baby does not breathe, or is "flat" at birth, do not clamp the cord. The baby needs the placental transfusion, which can supply essential oxygen for several minutes, protecting brain and organ systems. The baby can almost always be resuscitated on the mother's thigh with the cord intact.
- Facilitate uninterrupted skin-to-skin contact between mother and baby, ideally for the first hour after birth. An undrugged baby can find the mother's nipple and attach in this time.
- Allow at least one-half to one hour for the mother to deliver the placenta. A longer interval is safe, if there is no bleeding.
- Allow the mother to deliver the placenta by her own effort. The mother can squat, cough, and/or blow into the neck of a bottle, if necessary.
- If necessary, and a delay is safe, oxytocics are better given after delivery of the placenta.
- The cord can be cut after placental delivery, if desired. Clamping is likely unnecessary at this stage. In making this decision, parents may wish to observe their baby's reaction to handling the cord.

- If a cesarean is necessary, keep the baby's body close to, or slightly below, the level of the mother's uterus immediately after delivery. Keep the cord unclamped; baby and joined placenta can then be cared for on the same level (mother's chest, resuscitation trolley) until pulsation stops. Support skin-to-skin contact between mother and baby. (See chapter text for more information.)

Jacob's Placenta: A Love Story

In our culture, we call the baby's placenta the afterbirth and regard it as a waste product. However, the placenta performs a myriad of essential functions for the developing baby, and in many cultures it is respected—and even venerated. This essay explores the role and context of this amazing organ during pregnancy and birth, through the before-birth story of my third child, Jacob.

Jacob's conception was unexpected, and unknown to us for several weeks. We'd been on holiday in Tasmania, Australia's small southern island, and on the ferry trip home had carried not only Emma (four years) and Zoe (one year), but also their brother-to-be—a tiny mass of cells, barely a week past conception. As I slept fitfully on my bunk, Jacob's blastocyst, looking like a tiny blackberry just 1/12 inch (2 millimeters) in diameter, had already rolled down one of my fallopian tubes and was busy burrowing into the dark, thick lining of my womb.

For the next two weeks, Jacob-to-be obtained his nourishment directly from this rich lining, and I was oblivious to his presence. Quiet he may have been, but he was not quiescent; it was during this important time that Jacob's cells first became specialized, and he began to form his placenta. Deep inside this blackberry-shaped blastocyst, some of his cells clumped together to form an inner cell mass that would later become Jacob's body, umbilical cord, and amniotic sac. Other cells migrated outward to form the surrounding trophoblast that would become Jacob's placenta.

Once created, his trophoblast began infiltrating my womb more deeply, releasing enzymes to dissolve my uterine cells and blood vessels. In this way, Jacob created lakes of my blood—the placental lacunae—for his sustenance. Even as I attributed my overdue period to intensely breastfeeding Zoe while on holiday, Jacob's villi—finger-like projections from his developing placenta, each containing a newly formed blood vessel—were growing and dipping into my lacunae, our bloodstreams separated by the thinnest, most permeable of membranes.

Through this membrane I would, for the rest of the pregnancy, pass on all of the nutrients and growth factors that Jacob's body needed, and he would pass his wastes back to me. Furthermore, this membrane would prevent our blood cells from mixing, and my immune system from rejecting Jacob as a foreign invader.

As well as this, Jacob's villi were anchoring his developing placenta, acting as his roots in the firm soil of my womb-garden, and his body stalk—the tissue that would later become his umbilical cord—was keeping his embryonic body alive and attached to his placenta, like a floating astronaut's lifeline. At this time his body was smaller than a kidney bean, and just beginning to form limb buds—his future arms and legs.

Jacob's developing placenta had another important early task—the production of placental hormones—and it was this that revealed his presence. Under the influence of human chorionic gonadotropin (HCG), which his placenta had been producing in increasing amounts since a few days post-implantation, I was beginning to feel decidedly queasy. I finally realized that I was pregnant when this nausea visited me in the middle of the night. HCG was also the hormone that turned my pregnancy test predictably positive the next day.

Over the next few weeks I had intense, all-day morning sickness. It might have been more tolerable had I known at the time that this shift, which put me off spicy and bitter foods as well as tea and coffee, was actually caused by Jacob's placental hormones working to protect him from the high levels of natural toxins that such foods contain. Furthermore, my heightened sense of smell—another trigger for nausea—was ensuring that I ate only the freshest foods and avoided pungent aromas and cooking smells, which could also contain inhalable toxins. My nausea began to subside as Jacob grew beyond the embryonic stage (about eight weeks after conception), and was almost gone by the fourth month of pregnancy, when his organ systems were essentially fully formed and therefore less vulnerable to toxic damage.[1]

This two-month milestone (equivalent to ten weeks from the last menstruation) marked the beginning of Jacob's life as a fetus. By this time, his body had reached four to five centimeters in length and, thanks to the nourishment delivered by his placenta, his weight had increased to a creditable four grams, or one-seventh of an ounce—220,000 times greater than his weight at conception.[2] The trophoblast that had originally surrounded him had by now formed a near-mature placenta on one side and, on the other, a protective bubble—the chorion—that would eventually form part of Jacob's double-layered membranes.

Over the next two months, Jacob's placenta grew and spread. By the middle of my pregnancy, his placenta covered about half the wall of my uterus and was heavier than his body. Later in the pregnancy Jacob's body would grow much more, so that at birth his placenta would weigh about a sixth as much as his body. Jacob's versatile placenta was also able to migrate during pregnancy, moving slowly toward the best blood supply and away from areas of diminished supply. (This mechanism, known as *trophotropism,* is thought to explain many irregularities in placental shape and structure, as well as the healthy upward movement of most placentas that are low-lying (placenta previa) in early pregnancy.[3]) Although external to his body, Jacob's placenta was his most essential organ, performing all the functions that his immature gut, lungs, immune system, kidneys, liver, and skin were not capable of in my womb.

Working in place of his gut, Jacob's placenta enabled him to extract all the nourishment that he needed from my blood in exactly the right amounts—and his placental hormones could ensure that what he needed was available. For example, if there was an insufficient blood supply for his needs, he could, through producing the right hormones, order my body to increase my blood pressure and so increase the amount of my blood that was delivered to his placenta. Similarly, if he needed more glucose, he could ask for it—and, as a side effect of raising my blood glucose levels, I might end up with a diagnosis of gestational diabetes.[4] Jacob's placenta— like every baby's—was a tireless advocate for his own health and well-being.[5]

With his lungs full of amniotic fluid and with no access to air, Jacob obviously could not breathe in my womb, but he was able to obtain all the oxygen he needed from my oxygenated blood, delivered via his placenta. Along with my oxygen, Jacob also ingested any toxins that I inhaled into my bloodstream, most of which were transferred through his placenta as efficiently as the nutrients from my blood. My early nausea had again protected him by making me averse to polluted air and giving me a craving for cool, fresh air. Later in the pregnancy, when we decided to pull up the carpets in our bedroom—our version of preparing the nest—we kept Jacob's air fresh by choosing a floor varnish that would not emit toxic fumes.

Jacob's close attachment to me—the closest possible in human existence—presented some problems that his placenta could at least partly solve. If any bacteria had invaded my pregnant body and gained access to my bloodstream, his placenta could, to some extent, have filtered them out. Smaller particles, however—including toxoplasmosis and viruses such as rubella and herpes, all potentially harmful to Jacob because of his immature immune system—would be more likely to slip through his placental filter. Luckily, Jacob's placenta also allowed some of my antibodies to pass through, giving him ready-made immunity to almost all of the diseases I had encountered over my lifetime.

Jacob's placenta was also unable to filter out drugs or other chemicals, so that anything that was administered to me was also administered to him. Fortunately for both of us, neither my pregnancy nor my labor was complicated, and we avoided prescription drugs and painkillers of any kind. However, it is very likely that some of the chemicals in my diet—which was substantially but not entirely organic—would have found their way into Jacob's body, as well as other toxins, such as heavy metals (for example, lead and mercury) that I might have accumulated before my pregnancy. During his last few weeks in utero, his placenta transferred a rich and healthy store of iron—an essential metal—that would last him well into infancy.

Jacob's placenta was also an important site for detoxifying and expelling his bodily wastes, which could flow easily back into my bloodstream and be excreted through my body. This kept a light load on his kidneys and liver—both immature organs in utero—while keeping mine busy. Not only was I eating and breathing for him—I was peeing for him as well.

Like all unborn babies, Jacob had practical difficulties with cooling off, enveloped as he was in my warm body. His placenta was therefore doing what his skin could not: offloading his excess heat into my cooler circulation. Luckily, Jacob's was a winter pregnancy and this extra heat, which I positively radiated, kept me warm at night.

But, of course, neither Jacob nor I needed to spare a thought for these feats, performed continuously by his wondrous placenta as naturally and as necessarily as the beating of his heart. Jacob's placenta was his constant companion, a warm pillow humming gently with the flow of blood.[6] For me, his placenta was an idea rather than a tangible reality, but it was an integral part of how I imagined him in my belly and of the pictures I drew during my pregnancy.

As Jacob's due date approached, we made some special preparations for his placenta. We planned a lotus birth[7] for Jacob, as we had for his sister Zoe, which involved not cutting the cord at all: Zoe's placenta had remained attached until her cord came away from her navel on the sixth day. This had been a beautiful ritual, allowing Zoe a gentle transition between womb and world, and keeping us also in a serene, timeless space. Lotus birth had been fairly simple for us—I had sewn a red velvet bag to envelop her cord and placenta, which we bundled up with her for those few days.

Jacob's due date came and went, with several revisions and a lot of waiting. I enjoyed my three supposedly overdue weeks, and my instinct was always that my baby was thriving. My doctor offered me tests of placental function—essentially checks of the levels of hormones such as human placental lactogen (HPL) and estriol, which are produced or processed by the placenta—and we discussed scans and heart monitoring to check my baby more directly.

The conventional thinking has been that the placenta "ages" past term, potentially compromising the baby's growth, well-being, and ability to cope with labor. However, placental anatomists have shown that the placenta continues to expand and increase in surface area beyond forty weeks, and that a healthy, well-embedded placenta has a large "functional reserve."[8]

So Jacob's stalwart placenta was still growing and supporting him. Although the way that Jacob signaled his readiness for birth is still not known for certain, that message was no doubt relayed through his placenta. One likely messenger is corticotropin-releasing hormone (CRH), ordinarily a stress hormone secreted by the brain but produced in pregnancy by the baby's placenta. Placental CRH production rises steeply in late pregnancy, when it acts to prepare the baby's lungs for breathing and the mother's womb for labor.[9]

I was expecting a nighttime labor—I'd had a few "false starts" during the previous nights—and sure enough, labor began around 1 A.M. It proceeded slowly and gently, giving Jacob ample recovery time between my contractions, each of which squeezed his placenta and so temporarily cut off his blood supply. Fortunately, Jacob, like all mammalian young, was superbly adapted to these periods of low oxygen supply (hypoxia) in labor and birth, as evidenced by the quick recovery of his heart rate after each contraction.

After eleven hours or so, Jacob was born into the water in a tub in our back room, witnessed by his amazed sisters. Around thirty minutes later I stood up to deliver his placenta into a plastic bowl. Jacob's unclamped cord and attached placenta created a few minor difficulties—my doctor had a rather difficult time collecting a sample of the cord blood (to check Jacob's blood group), and we had the challenge of keeping his placenta bowl afloat when Emma and Zoe climbed into the tub.

Because we didn't clamp or cut his cord, Jacob received his placenta's final gift to him-a transfusion of an extra 3.5 ounces (100 ml) or so of his own blood. This blood had been stored in his placenta and was designed to assist him at birth by filling the blood vessels in his lungs, kidneys, liver, gut, and skin—all the organs he hadn't used in the womb—with oxygen-rich blood. Jacob's placental transfusion was also a safety net, able to tide him over if his breathing was not established right away.

If we had clamped Jacob's cord immediately after birth, he would also have missed out on the extra iron—about a month's supply—contained in his placental transfusion, as well as his own rich store of stem cells, which would later develop into new blood and immune cells. Some experts in this area would add that we may have given Jacob protection from cerebral palsy, attention deficits, and perhaps even autism, because we allowed his brain to receive the full blood supply intended for him by Mother Nature.[10]

All other mammals, and attendants in most traditional cultures, wait to cut (or bite) through the baby's cord until after the placenta has been delivered—and with good reason. Jacob's placental transfusion reduced the size of his placenta by 100 milliliters, and my uterus was able to contract more efficiently around it, thus decreasing my chances of hemorrhaging. Jacob's less bulky placenta was also easy—and pleasurable—to birth. (See chapter 6 for more about delayed cord clamping and the placental transfusion.)

After we left the water, we took a closer look at Jacob's placenta, still attached to him. It was a beautiful, round, full placenta: dark red on one side—the villus side, which had been attached to the wall of my womb—and glistening silver on Jacob's side, due to the covering of his membranes. Stretching out these membranes, we could almost reform the watertight sac that had enveloped and protected Jacob for nine months; it might even have been possible to guess from its shape where his placenta had been attached to my womb. We marveled at Jacob's triple-vesseled cord, twenty-four inches (60 cm) or so from his belly to his placenta, and branching out under the placental membranes like the trunk of his "tree of life," as the placenta has been called.

Had we measured Jacob's placenta, it would have been eight to ten inches (20 to 25 cm) in diameter (a little smaller than a dinner plate), around one inch (2.5 cm) thick, and about one pound (500 g) in mass. We did check it to ensure that it was complete before we patted it dry and placed it gently in a sieve to drain for a few hours. If placental fragments had remained in my womb, I could have risked hemorrhage or infection in the hours or days following birth.

For the next three days we dried and salted Jacob's placenta every twelve hours or so, then wrapped it carefully in a cloth diaper, and then in the red velvet bag I had sewn. Jacob's "breaking forth" time—the time between his birth and the separation of his cord—was quiet and still as we honored his original wholeness, and we respected his integrity by not choosing circumcision. We watched as his cord dried out and hardened from his umbilical end; it separated without any fuss on the fourth morning. We kept Jacob's placenta in our freezer, even through a move between states. When Jacob was four, he chose a jacaranda tree to plant over it.

Lotus birth is a new ritual, having only been described in chimpanzees before 1974, when clairvoyant Clair Lotus Day began to question the routine cutting of the cord. Pregnant with her third child and living in San Francisco, she found an obstetrician who was sympathetic to her wishes and her son Trimurti was born in hospital and taken home with his cord uncut. According to Day, there are many references to this practice in holy texts including, in the Bible, Ezekiel 0.10: "In the beginning, thy navel was not cut."[11]

Almost all traditional cultures have beliefs and rituals that highlight our relationship to this extraordinary organ. In Bali, for example, the placenta, or *ari-ari*, is said to live on in spirit as one of the child's four siblings or guardian angels, which can be called on in times of need. A Balinese child greets his or her placenta on rising in the morning and prays to it for protection at night. Every new moon and full moon, and on each holy day, offerings are placed at the burial site of the placenta. After death, the placenta is believed to accompany the soul of the deceased to heaven to testify as to whether the person fulfilled his or her duty in this lifetime.[11,12]

The place of placental burial is important in many cultures. Among some peoples, the placenta must remain hidden from evil spirits to safeguard the newborn baby; other burial practices emphasize the lifelong connection between placenta and child. For example, villagers in Zimbabwe believe that burying the placenta in the family home will ensure that their offspring will always return home.[13] Sir James Frazer, writing in the early twentieth century, noted that "Even in Europe many people still believe that a person's destiny is more or less bound up with that of his navel-string or afterbirth." Frazer reports that German midwives would give the dried navel-string to the father, telling him to preserve it carefully in order to keep the child healthy and free from illness.[13] One modern-day lotus birth advocate, the late Jeannine Parvati Baker, believed that we all have a strong connection to the place where our navel-string and placenta are buried.[14, 15]

The relationship with our placenta does not end with its disposal, whether by ritual burial or by hospital incineration. Placental symbolism is everywhere in our culture, from the handbags that we carry—holding our money, diary, and other items of survival—to the soft toys that we cram into our babies' cribs. Some believe that much of our culture's discontent, and our urge to accumulate possessions—including all of the aforementioned—come from the traumatic loss of our first possession: our placenta.[16] And each year we honor our placenta by lighting candles on our birthday cake—in Latin, the word *placenta* means "flat cake."[17]

Jacob's placenta has been his conduit, passing life from my body to his. Now this placenta—his womb-twin, his primal anchor—has gone back to the earth. Seven years after his birth, Jacob told me "your placenta is like your heart," and I realized that he received more than physical nourishment through his placenta. Along with the oxygen, nutrients, hormones, and all the other placental gifts, Jacob also received my love, which was equally his sustenance in my womb, transmitted subtly but vitally by this amazing organ—the placenta.

chapter 9

CESAREAN SURGERY
The Whole Story

Giving birth via cesarean surgery is very new in human history. This operation can be a necessary and lifesaving intervention for mother and baby
in some situations, but current cesarean rates are extreme, and far higher
than the number of mothers and babies who are truly at risk. For healthy
mothers and babies, cesareans introduce the potential problems of major
abdominal surgery as well as extra risks because the normal processes
of birth are bypassed.

Women are often unaware of the potential problems, and may even
believe that cesareans are safer than normal birth. This chapter gives
medical evidence around cesarean safety to help women considering this
option—including those who have had a previous cesarean—to make an
informed choice. Suggestions are also given for when a cesarean is truly
necessary.

The first documented cesarean occurred in 1581, when Swiss swine-
herd Jacob Nufer used his own instruments on his wife, who had
been in labor for many days. Not only was the operation successful, but
Madame Nufer subsequently gave birth to four other children, including
twins. Other isolated cases occurred through to the nineteenth century,
although mortality was as high as 75 percent at this time due to lack
of anesthesia, ignorance of hygiene, and the unavailability of effective
treatment for postoperative infection.[1, 2]

Cesareans were usually performed for obstructed labor: this was common in women up until the 1950s because of poor nutrition in childhood
causing rickets and pelvic deformities. Although most cesareans took
place in a hospital, textbooks from the 1930s give advice for performing
cesareans at home, including a recommendation to use electric lighting

rather than candles, which could be ignited by the volatile ether anesthetics that were used.[2, 3]

Advances in anesthesia and antiseptic techniques, the use of blood transfusions, and, particularly, the discovery of antibiotic drugs in the 1940s have all contributed to increased cesarean safety, which has expanded the "indications": conditions for which a cesarean is held to be medically appropriate. Lower segment ("bikini scar") cesareans were first described by John Munro Kerr in 1926, making cesareans safer for subsequent births.[4]

In the United States, cesarean rates have increased dramatically over recent decades, from 5.5 percent in 1970[5] to around 22.8 percent in 1993[5] and 31.1 percent in 2006.[6] The Canadian national cesarean rate was 26.5 percent,[7] and the English rate was 23.5 percent,[8] in 2005–2006.

High cesarean rates add substantial burdens to the health care system: initial cesarean costs are around US$4,372 per planned primary cesarean, compared with $2,487 for planned vaginal birth[9] (2003 figures), which does not take into account increased costs due to higher likelihood of special care for the baby and rehospitalization for the mother. Equivalent UK estimations are £3,200 for a cesarean and £1,698 for a vaginal birth, which incorporates some of the costs of care for two postnatal months.[10, 11]

Cesarean rates have increased significantly in many other developed and developing countries. Those with extreme national rates include: China (40.5 percent in 2000); Mexico (39.1 percent in 2002); Brazil (36.7 percent in 1996); Italy (36 percent in 2002); and Portugal (30.2 percent in 2002).[12] Higher rates have been recorded in the private, compared to public, medical systems in Madras (Chennai) India (47 percent private versus 20 percent public in 1997–1999),[3] Australia (40.3 percent private versus 27.1 percent public in 2005),[14] and Brazil, where the rate in private hospitals was over 80 percent in 2004.[15]

The World Health Organization (WHO) states, "There is no justification for any region to have a higher rate [of cesareans] than ten to fifteen percent"[16] This figure is supported by a recent analysis of international cesarean rates against maternal and perinatal mortality, which also suggests that, at rates above 15 percent, the risks to mother and baby begin to outweigh the benefits.[12]

Risks to the Mother

A cesarean involves major abdominal surgery, which carries unavoidable risks. Studies show that the risk of the mother dying after cesarean surgery, although low overall, is around four times higher than after vaginal birth, even considering maternal health conditions.[17-19] For example, the risk of the mother dying after elective (nonemergency) cesarean is estimated at two in ten thousand—four times higher than normal vaginal birth.[18] Major causes of death are infection, blood clots, and anesthetic accidents.[19]

In addition, 20 to 40 percent of women have post-cesarean complications—infections of the uterus, wound, or urinary tract are most common.[20-23] Cesarean mothers are twice as likely to have severe complications and five times more likely to require antibiotics after birth compared with women giving birth vaginally.[24] Up to one in ten women may experience an accidental laceration (cut) elsewhere in their uterus[23] or other pelvic structure. A recent Canadian review found that serious complications such as major infection, hysterotomy, or cardiac arrest were overall three times more likely among low-risk cesarean mothers than for women giving birth vaginally: 27 per 1,000 versus 9 per 1,000, respectively.[25] Another recent study found a more than 50 percent increased risk of stroke in the year following cesarean.[26]

Studies of psychosocial outcomes show that, after a cesarean, women are less satisfied with their birth experience,[27] more likely to be rehospitalized,[9] less confident with their babies,[27] less likely to breastfeed,[27] and more fatigued[28] even up to four years later.[29] Research into the impact of cesarean on postnatal depression (PND) is not consistent, with some studies showing increased PND rates following an emergency cesarean[30] and others no effect.[31, 32] Lobel and DeLuca analyze the literature and conclude that cesarean mothers more often have depressed mood, but may not fulfill the full criteria for actual PND.[27] A depressed maternal mood after cesarean delivery may relate to delayed contact with their babies: in one detailed study, cesarean mothers were more likely to experience a delay in first contact and to have a lower mood in hospital and also eight months later, compared with vaginally birthing mothers.[33] In other research, over half of mothers who experienced an unplanned cesarean had some symptoms of post-traumatic stress.[34]

Cesarean delivery has been portrayed as advantageous to women's pelvic floor function, especially in terms of avoiding urinary incontinence. However, recent reviews have concluded that the protective effects of cesareans in this regard are small and short-lived,[27, 35] and statistically nonsignificant for anal incontinence.[36] Large population studies have also shown that cesareans do not significantly protect the mother's pelvic floor in the long term.[37]

Risks for Future Pregnancies

A woman will continue to experience the effects from a cesarean through all of her reproductive life. Many studies show reduced fertility,[38] both voluntary[39] and involuntary,[40] following a cesarean, with one in four cesarean mothers still fearful about giving birth five years later.[40]

Ectopic pregnancy, a life-threatening condition of early pregnancy, is more likely among women with a previous cesarean,[41] and several large, comprehensive studies have found an approximately doubled risk of unexplained stillbirth following a cesarean first birth.[42 43, 44] A previous cesarean may also double a woman's chances of a breech baby in subsequent pregnancies[45] and increase the risk of uterine rupture, as will be discussed.

The risk of placental problems (placenta previa or low-lying placenta; placental abruption, in which the placenta separates early; and placenta accreta, in which the placenta won't separate after birth) are all increased by two to four times in mothers with a previous cesarean.[46, 47] All are potentially life-threatening and increase the risk of death for both mother and baby. Placental complications after the birth are the major reason for the seven to fifteen times increased risk of emergency hysterectomy after a cesarean[48, 49] and a previous cesarean.[50] Note that the risks of many or most of these complications increase with the number of previous cesareans.[51]

Cesarean Risks to Healthy Babies

Large population surveys have found cesarean newborns to be two to five times more likely to need intensive care treatment compared with low-risk vaginally born babies.[24, 52] This may partly relate to an increased risk of iatrogenic (medically caused) prematurity; even when a supposedly accurate due date has been estimated by ultrasound scan, around 10 percent of cesarean babies are born more than two weeks early.[53]

Studies have found that cesarean babies have an increased risk of breathing difficulties after birth: one survey found minor problems for around 6 percent of cesarean babies compared with 3 percent after vaginal delivery.[52] In other studies, serious breathing problems were double (for example, from 0.8 percent following vaginal birth to 1.6 percent for cesarean babies, in one study[54]) even for those born at term.[53, 55] Persistent pulmonary hypertension, a potentially fatal condition, is more common in cesarean babies[56] and may affect up to 3 to 4 per 1,000 elective cesarean babies compared with 0.8 per 1,000 vaginal births.[57] Breathing problems may reflect lack of hormonal stimulation, especially the catecholamine surge (see chapter 6) and loss of the placental transfusion (see chapter 8).

Overall, it has been estimated that a low-risk cesarean newborn may be 70 to 90 percent more likely to die before hospital discharge[24] and two to three times more likely to die in the first year, compared with vaginally born babies,[58] for all of the reasons just given. There is also a 1 to 2 percent risk that the baby may suffer laceration by a surgical knife during the operation.[59, 60]

Some of these findings may be due to cesarean babies missing the labor-induced activation of organ and hormone systems (including the catecholamine surge just mentioned), which prepare the newborn for life outside the womb. Body systems that have been found to differ between cesarean and vaginally born babies include thyroid,[61, 62] adrenal,[63] kidney,[64] lung,[52] gut,[65] blood,[66] and immune system.[67, 68] Changes in the immune system have been shown to last at least six months[69] and may be explained by lack of normal exposure to the mother's healthy gut flora during the birth process, producing long-lasting and perhaps permanent abnormalities in the baby's own gut flora.[70] These shifts in gut flora, which prime the immune system, can lead to allergies and asthma, and have also been linked with later health problems such as diabetes (which is more common among cesarean-born children[71–73]) and obesity.[74] (See chapter 4 for more about the importance of gut flora.)

Other aspects of cesarean delivery may also compromise newborn gut flora, including: the high likelihood of preoperative antibiotics (which can change maternal gut flora[75]); exposure to detrimental bacteria present in a large hospital, including those carried by staff;[70, 76] lack of early skin-to-skin contact right after birth; higher chance of separation and of a longer stay due to illness; higher likelihood of receiving antibiotics;[76] and reduced chance of successful breastfeeding,[29] which is important for optimal gut flora.[76]

Successful breastfeeding is less common following cesarean birth,[29] likely due to factors including delayed contact between mother and baby; loss of the ecstatic hormones, which are also important for breastfeeding for both; less newborn alertness; and ongoing sedating drug effects for mother and baby. Studies have shown abnormalities in the hormone prolactin, the major hormone of breast milk synthesis, in the hours following cesarean;[77] and in the patterns of release of prolactin and oxytocin, the letdown hormone, for cesarean mothers breastfeeding on day three.[78] (See chapter 6 for more about hormones following cesarean.) When breastfeeding is not successful, there are significant and lifelong disadvantages for the health and well-being of offspring and possible detrimental effects to the mother's health. (See chapter 12.)

In all pregnancies following a cesarean, the baby is at increased risk of prematurity, low birth weight, stillbirth, poor condition at birth, and death, for the reasons just stated.

Several studies have linked cesarean birth with longer-term problems. Researchers have found increased risks of type 1 diabetes,[79] asthma[80, 81] through age thirty,[82] allergies,[83] and food allergies[84, 85] for cesarean offspring, as well as abnormal oral bacteria associated with dental cavities.[86] Abnormalities in gut flora may contribute to these effects.

Vaginal Birth after Cesarean

Women who are pregnant after a previous cesarean need good-quality information in order to decide whether they would prefer to undergo an elective repeat cesarean section (ERCS) or to attempt a vaginal birth after cesarean (VBAC). In most studies, around three-quarters of women attempting a VBAC are successful, with excellent outcomes for mother and baby.[51, 55, 87, 88]

Both choices involve some additional risks. For a VBAC mother, the most serious is rupture of her uterus, with estimated risk around 1 in 200 with attempted VBAC[88, 89] and 1 in with 600 with ERCS.[89] Uterine rupture may manifest as a mild wound dehiscence, in which the scar begins to separate, or less commonly it may have life-threatening effects for mother and baby. The UK Royal College of Obstetricians and Gynecologists summarizes, "Women considering planned VBAC should be informed that this decision carries a 2 to 3/10,000 additional risk of birth-related perinatal death when compared with ERCS. The absolute risk of such birth-related perinatal loss is comparable to the risk for women having their first birth."[90]

The risk of serious illness in a VBAC baby is also increased by around eight to ten per thousand overall compared with a baby born by ERCS, mainly due to problems for babies whose mothers have an emergency cesarean.

Administering Pitocin for induction or to speed a VBAC labor increases rupture risk by three to four times,[88] with the risk as high as one in fifty for women given the highest doses of Pitocin, according to one study.[91] Induction with misoprostol (Cytotec) is even riskier and is not recommended for women with a previous cesarean.[92] For the mother planning a VBAC, there is an added 1 percent risk of endometritis (uterine infection) and blood transfusion.[51]

Balanced against this are increasing risks of maternal complications with every additional cesarean. These include placenta accreta; injury to bladder, bowel, or ureter; intensive care unit admission; hysterectomy; blood transfusion requiring four or more units; and a longer duration of operative time and hospital stay.[90]

Most institutions recommend continuous fetal heart rate (FHR) monitoring in a VBAC labor in order to detect signs of rupture as early as possible; they may also recommend delivery in a center equipped to perform immediate cesareans. An ACOG recommendation for the latter has severely restricted VBAC options in the United States,[93] even though the risk of the baby dying has been estimated, as already mentioned, to be no higher than for a woman having her first baby.

Some women have found that alternative birth environments such as homebirth and birth centers, are the most amenable to VBAC, with benefits that include a higher chance of normal birth.[94] This must be weighed against the small (but significant) additional risks associated with VBAC in an out-of-hospital setting, (especially, according to one study, for women past forty-two weeks or with more than one previous cesarean),[95] but the final decision must always rest with the woman herself.

Reasons for Unnecessary Cesareans

Many commentators have recognized a link between high cesarean rates and routine use of obstetricians as primary birth attendant: Wagner notes that countries with high numbers of obstetricians caring for healthy women (Australia, Canada, United States, Greece) have high cesarean rates, but no better outcomes.[96]

Higher cesarean rates for women under an obstetrician's care may reflect "The higher level of comfort that obstetricians feel with the risks associated with cesarean deliveries compared with those associated with vaginal deliveries . . ."[97]

In contrast, low-technology models of care (midwifery, birth center, homebirth) are at least as safe, involve fewer interventions, and have lower cesarean rates—typically below 10 percent,[98–100] with a recent large, prospective homebirth study showing a 3.7 percent cesarean rate.[100] In the UK, national guidelines recommend increased access to homebirth as a means of reducing the cesarean rate.[101]

Although there is much discussion of cesarean for primary maternal request,[97] this is a very uncommon reason for cesarean. The U.S. Listening to Mothers II survey found that only one mother out of 252 reported requesting a cesarean with no medical reason, whereas two women reported that their practitioner decided they should undergo a cesarean without a medical indication.[102]

Other studies have found similarly that only 1 to 2 percent of pregnant women request a cesarean without medical reason.[103] Women preferring cesarean were more likely to have had a cesarean or an "awful" or "unpleasant" prior birth, and nominated "safety for the baby" as a major reason.[104] There is a lack of good quality research in this area.[105]

Further Cesarean Consequences

Normal, undisturbed birth is associated with peak levels of at least four feel-good hormones that contribute to mother-infant bonding as well as safety for mother and baby. In animal studies these hormones are important for instinctive mothering behaviors, and in humans these hormones also enhance ease, safety, and reward in birth. (See chapter 6 for more details.)

Studies show that cesarean mothers have a different hormonal pattern during breastfeeding three days after birth, which implies that there may be longer-term effects on this delicate system.[78] An Australian study found that after having a cesarean, women were more likely to have a loss of self-esteem, whereas after a vaginal birth, women generally experienced an elevation in self-esteem.[106]

And for the baby, "We do not yet know the subtle but long-term effects of depriving the baby of the full processes of labor."[107]

Good Reasons for a Cesarean

Cesareans have, as described, significant risks, but sometimes these risks are outweighed by the risks of vaginal birth or by the need for immediate delivery of an at-risk baby. Circumstances in which a cesarean is likely to benefit mother and/or baby include placenta problems, including severe placenta previa and placental abruption; HIV infection; a first episode of herpes virus at the end of pregnancy; and severe fetal distress or other significant complications in labor.

The comprehensive and evidence-based UK National Institute for Clinical Excellence (NICE) guidelines recommend against a scheduled cesarean for estimated large baby and/or small pelvis (cephalopelvic disproportion or CPD), women who are more than one week overdue (post dates) without other complications, hepatitis B for which the baby can be treated after birth to reduce transmission, and uncomplicated infection with hepatitis C.[10]

NICE guidelines recognize that there is insufficient evidence, and do not recommend a routine cesarean except as part of research, for multiple births, small-for-date babies, premature babies, and mothers with a recurrence of herpes virus.[10]

Cesarean surgery for breech birth is controversial, and currently medical opinion is swinging back toward the option of vaginal birth in certain circumstances.[108–111] Many experts, NICE included, suggest an attempt at external cephalic version (ECV) to turn a breech baby to head-down.[10]

Having a Good Cesarean

Sometimes a cesarean is truly necessary, and we can be grateful that this lifesaving technology has become so much safer and more accessible for many women around the world. Usually a necessary cesarean will be scheduled as an elective procedure, although some obstetricians are recognizing the benefits, for the baby, of an in-labor nonemergency cesarean.

Having a good cesarean requires forethought and planning, and usually a good relationship with caregivers who are open to discussion and negotiation. Issues that may need to be considered include waiting for labor to begin to ensure the baby's readiness for birth; epidural or spinal anesthetic rather than general anesthetic (usually standard and preferable except in emergencies); asking if the drapes can be lowered so you can see your baby's birth; requesting that the baby's cord be clamped late or not at all (see chapter 8); asking to see, or even take home, your baby's placenta; and allowing immediate skin-to-skin contact between mother and newborn. In some places women have had the pleasure of receiving their baby from the hands of the surgeon immediately after delivery, with ongoing skin-to-skin contact as a priority. These changes in cesarean routines (e.g., providing a dedicated nurse or midwife to support the mother and ensuring uninterrupted mother-baby contact) can be applied in most situations, as described in a recent publication.[108]

Requests concerning the environment at the time of birth, which are usually reasonably easy to negotiate, might include bringing your own music, asking for a verbal description of the operation as it proceeds so you are fully involved, requesting silence at the time of birth, and allowing the mother's voice to be the first heard by her baby.

Another important request is to keep your baby close and ideally skin to skin in the hours following birth. This will require assistance and supervision, as you may be affected by anesthetics and post-operative painkillers, but it will keep your baby warm, help to activate newborn abilities including breastfeeding, optimize the release of "ecstatic" hormones for you and your baby, transfer beneficial bacteria, and reduce stress and trauma for both of you. Breastfeeding and mood may also improve with immediate and ongoing mother-baby contact, a fact recognized by the World Health Organization (WHO) and their Baby-Friendly Hospital Initiative (BFHI).

Under the BFHI, cesarean mothers and babies generally are reunited skin to skin within ten minutes of arrival in the recovery room, and skin-to-skin contact is continued for at least an hour, unless there are complications for mother or baby. If you have the option, consider choosing a BFHI-accredited hospital for your cesarean.

If you are unable to hold your baby, your partner or support person could have skin-to-skin contact until you are able to. This is a task that most new fathers will relish, and it may begin an enduring bond between father and child. In the days after birth you could also request to have the lowest dose possible of painkillers to reduce effects on yourself and your baby (via breast milk) and to participate as much as possible in the care of your baby. You may also need some extra help with breastfeeding in the early days due to cesarean effects, and you may also appreciate the near-constant emotional support of your partner, friends, or relatives, especially if you have had an emergency cesarean.

Summary

We are fortunate to live in times when a cesarean is available for those few mothers and babies who truly need it. However, a cesarean represents major abdominal surgery for the mother and is also a major deviation from normal for the baby. Risks and benefits must always be discussed by all involved. The ultimate decision, in almost every circumstance, belongs to the mother. When a cesarean is truly necessary, both mother and baby require special care, with personal and institutional support for early and ongoing skin-to-skin contact and breastfeeding.

chapter 10

CHOOSING HOMEBIRTH

Homebirth has been portrayed as a radical and perhaps even unsafe choice in modern times. However, many studies conducted over many years in many different countries confirm that homebirth is a safe option for modern families. Women choosing homebirth have the lowest chance of needing drugs and intervention and the highest chance of a normal birth. of any modern birthing option. This chapter provides medical information and support for those who choose to maximize their chance of a gentle birth by having their baby at home.

Throughout human history, women have always given birth in a familiar place, with familiar and trusted companions. Globally most babies are still born at home, and even in westernized countries, homebirth was the norm until the last fifty years or so. Many of our grandparents were born at home, and even some of our parents—including my own mother and father.

A Brief History of Hospital Birth

The move from home to hospital began in the eighteenth century, when male midwives—the equivalent of today's obstetricians—needed a captive population to practice their skills in childbirth and began offering free hospital care for poor (and sometimes homeless) women. The first lying-in hospital was established in Dublin in 1745, and lying-in hospitals were subsequently established in other parts of Europe and the United States.

Hospital birth under the care of the male midwives was initially exceedingly dangerous. As de Costa records,

> . . . the crowding of patients, frequent vaginal examinations and the use of contaminated instruments, dressings and bed linen spread infection in an era when there was no knowledge of antisepsis.[1]

This new disease—"childbed fever"—killed, for example, 13 percent of women under the care of doctors in the Vienna Lying-In Hospital in 1846, compared with 2 percent of women under the care of midwives.[2] Its contagious nature was identified by Ignaz Semmelweis in Vienna, Thomas Watson in London, and Oliver Wendell Holmes in Boston, but there was strong resistance to the idea that childbed fever could be due to doctors' negligence of hygiene. It was not until the end of the nineteenth century that the need for attention to basic antisepsis was appreciated and became part of routine care.[1]

Although the mortality for women giving birth in hospital is now equivalent to that of homebirth, there remain increased risks of infection—especially antibiotic-resistant infection—for mothers and babies in the hospital. In addition, there are other major iatrogenic (medically caused) risks in the hospital that can make homebirth a good choice.

Birth Interventions and Homebirth Safety

Perhaps the major risk of hospital birth is the risk of unnecessary intervention. As described in chapter 6, Undisturbed Birth, medical interventions have been shown to interfere with the delicate hormonal orchestration of birth for mother and baby, with unknown long-term effects. Cesarean surgery, which is much more likely for women who choose a hospital birth, increases the risk of maternal death, even among healthy mothers (see chapter 9), and a traumatic birth can make the transition to motherhood more difficult and painful for mother and baby, with major impact also possible for the partner, family, and friends.

In the United States, Childbirth Connection's (formerly the Maternity Center Association) 2002 and 2006 Listening to Mothers surveys found "virtually no natural childbirth" in either survey, which included over three thousand women in total.[3, 4] In the 2006 survey, around one-half of women were induced; almost three-quarters had an epidural administered; and one-third gave birth by cesarean.

In comparison, women who plan homebirth have, in most reported studies, around a 70 to 80 percent chance of giving birth without intervention. Cesarean rates for women who plan to give birth at home are generally 5 to 10 percent.[5-8] Because of the low use of drugs (most homebirth practitioners do not carry pain-relieving drugs), home-born babies are more alert and in better condition than those born in the hospital. Official U.S. figures give the out-of-hospital birthrate (including birth at home and in freestanding birth centers) as 1 percent.[9]

In terms of outcomes for mothers and babies, most studies of planned homebirth show perinatal mortality figures (the numbers of babies dying around the time of birth) that are at least as good as the hospital figures, with lower rates of complications and interventions. For example, Johnson and Daviss's landmark 2005 study of over five thousand U.S. and Canadian women intending to deliver at home under the care of certified professional midwives (CPMs) showed equivalent perinatal mortality, with rates of intervention that were up to ten times lower, compared with low-risk women birthing in the hospital. Rates of induction, intravenous drip (IV), rupture of membranes, fetal monitoring, epidural, augmentation, episiotomy, and forceps were each less than 10 percent, and 3.7 percent of women required a cesarean.[8]

In a review of the safety of homebirth for the authoritative Cochrane Collaboration, Olsen states:

> There is no strong evidence to favour either home or hospital birth for selected low-risk pregnant women. In countries where it is possible to establish a home birth service backed up by a modern hospital system, all low-risk women should be offered the possibility of considering a planned home birth . . . [10]

In the Netherlands, where around one-third of babies are born at home under the care of a midwife, outcomes for first babies have been shown to be equivalent to those of babies born to low-risk women in the hospital, and outcomes for second or subsequent babies have been shown to be better.[11]

UK statistician Marjory Tew has analyzed some of the largest data sets of home and hospital birth in the Netherlands[12] and the UK (before the advent of hospitalization).[13] Her conclusion, accepted by UK Government policy makers, is that birth at home or in small GP (family physician) units is safer than birth in obstetric hospital for mothers and babies in all categories of risk.[14] She also concludes that modern obstetric interventions, applied to the whole birthing population, have made birth more dangerous, not safer.[15] Her book, *Safer Childbirth? A Critical History of Maternity*

Care documents the false information that was used to promote a shift from home to hospital birth in the UK in the 1950s to 1980s.[14]

Why Homebirth?

Homebirth is often an instinctive choice for expectant couples , although this instinct can also be backed up by good-quality information and research. Some prefer homebirth because of a previous negative experience in the hospital or because they have witnessed (or heard stories of) bad experiences.

Others come to homebirth because they have heard positive homebirth stories or even, like my partner and me, have had the privilege of supporting friends birthing at home. Others may want to make choices that are very difficult in the hospital—such as vaginal birth after cesarean—and some families want their children, or other family members, to be more involved than is possible in a hospital birth room. Some homebirthers have been born at home themselves.

Women who choose homebirth tend to be older and better educated than the general population and include many health professionals—including midwives and a few doctors, such as my partner and myself.

Homebirthers are generally more trusting of their bodies and of the natural processes of birth, and they tend to be more self reliant and self-responsible in other aspects of their lives. The experience of giving birth in one's own time, in one's own space, also reinforces these attitudes, giving the new mother a solid confidence in her abilities and those of her baby, and laying a firm foundation for pleasurable mothering.

For the homebirth father, being fully present and involved at the birth of his child can be a life-changing event. The father's experience is usually very different at a hospital birth, where hospital staff may treat him as peripheral or may conscript him to recommend interventions to his wife.

Making an Uncommon Choice

Homebirth is still a minority choice in western countries. Couples who choose homebirth may encounter negative attitudes from friends, family, doctors, and media, many of whom are unaware of the good outcomes associated with homebirth. It may also be difficult to find a caregiver, especially outside metropolitan areas, and in some places—including where I live, in Australia—homebirth may be an expensive choice, with all costs borne by the family.

However, the one-on-one midwifery care that most women will receive through homebirth is, as the chief medical officer of health in Brisbane puts it, the "Rolls Royce" of maternity care, shown to give equally good or better outcomes compared with care from a doctor or obstetrician, and higher rates of satisfaction.[16] One study has also shown better outcomes; in particular, 33 percent lower newborn mortality and 31 percent less risk of low birth weight, among babies born under midwifery care.[17]

The midwife who provides this type of care becomes intimate and knowledgeable about the woman, her partner, and family, building a trusting relationship that will provide real support through labor, birth, and early parenting. This level of support may help reduce stress, and stress hormones, for the pregnant woman, contributing to the better outcomes just mentioned. Many midwives create a birthing community, formally or informally, in which expectant and new mothers and families can meet and socialize.

Outside such supportive circles, however, homebirthers may find a lack of support for their informed choice. It may be useful to remember that these anxieties are often expressed by people who have a genuine and appropriate concern for the family's welfare, such as prospective grandparents. Sometimes we may choose to engage in dialogue and education to counter others' worries, and at other times we may save our energy and remain confident internally. Sometimes keeping our plans to ourselves may be the best option, especially around people who are likely to share their horror stories of birth.

Homebirth in Other Countries

The Netherlands has the highest rate of homebirth in the Western world, which is consistent with its philosophy of protecting low-risk women from unnecessary interventions.[18] In the Netherlands, specialist obstetric care is provided by the state only to women who need it, whereas midwifery care (for home or hospital birth) is free to every pregnant woman. The Netherlands has some of the lowest rates of intervention (including low rates of cesareans and epidurals) in the Western world, with good outcomes for mothers and babies.

Midwifery care for homebirth is also provided free in the UK, although in the public system women are not able to choose their own midwife and may not have the same caregiver through pregnancy and birth. Some mothers report that there are biases against homebirth within the system, although homebirth has been recognized at a governmental level (by the Changing Childbirth Report), and UK policy makers have been working toward offering homebirth as a choice for all women. The UK National Institute for Clinical Excellence (NICE) cesarean guidelines recommend encouraging homebirth to help reduce cesarean rates,[19] and one UK survey found that, given a free choice, 22 percent of women would opt for homebirth.[20]

In New Zealand there has been a renaissance of midwifery care in the last twenty years, which has increased the homebirth rate to an estimated 7 percent[21]—although rates vary widely among regions. Women can choose their own midwife, who will care for them at home or in the hospital and is paid by the government. Nationwide, outcomes for mothers and babies have continued to improve with this choice of care.

There has also been a resurgence of midwifery care and homebirth in Canada, with the first training and recognition of midwives in 1999 in some provinces where practice was previously illegal. Midwifery care is also increasing in the United States, with the number of births attended by midwives (mostly in the hospital) increasing from 1 percent in 1975 to 7.9 percent in 2005.[22]

Setting up a Homebirth

How do you go about organizing a homebirth? This varies from country to country, but generally your first task will be to find a midwife.

In the United States, certified nurse-midwives (CNMs), who have trained as a nurse as well as a midwife, may work with obstetricians or family physicians and may also offer care for hospital births. "Direct entry" midwives have trained through an apprentice or educational system and may be accredited as a certified practicing midwife (CPM). Availability of homebirth services and accreditation (and legality) of midwives varies between states.

In Canada, some provinces have government-regulated midwifery, including Alberta, British Columbia, Manitoba, Ontario, and Quebec, with free midwifery in most of these places. Midwives attend births in the hospital, home, and/or birth centers, depending on the province.

In the UK, almost all homebirth midwives are employed by the National Health Service; women wanting this option will need to access a midwife through her local general practitioner or supervisor of midwives. Access should improve following the UK government's recent commitment to offer every woman the option of homebirth. The availability of independent midwives who work outside the NHS in the UK is limited and this option is generally expensive.

To find a homebirth midwife, you can look in the phone book under medical, birth, or childbirth services. Also search online for "midwife" and your local area. See also the links and resources section at www.sarahjbuckley .com. Even better, ask around for personal recommendations or look for a local homebirth group who can give you more advice and a list of names.

Even in areas where homebirth and/or midwifery is either illegal or not legislated, there may be midwives (although they may not be able to use this title) who can care for you at home. Ask among natural birth or parenting groups, or use chat lists such as www.mothering.com to post your question.

When you find a prospective midwife—or even better, a list of prospective midwives—consider asking the following questions by phone or, ideally, in person. Your gut feeling about the midwives you interview may be as important as the information they give you.

Questions to Ask Your Midwife

- What training and experience do you have?
- What is your basic philosophy of birth care?
- What prenatal care do you provide?
- Do you work with other midwives? Am I likely to meet them or to have them care for me during labor?
- What backup arrangements do you have?
- What care and observations will you do during labor?
- Are there laws or regulations that may influence the care that you can offer?
- What equipment do you carry?
- What assistance can you give if labor is difficult or prolonged?

- Are you experienced and trained in resuscitation of mother and baby?
- Can you suture (stitch) tears at home?
- What happens if I need to transfer to the hospital?
- What postnatal care do you provide?
- What are your rates of transfer to the hospital, of interventions, and of complications such as perineal tears and postpartum hemorrhage?
- Do you have children yourself and, if so, what was your experience of birth?
- Do you offer any alternative skills such as herbs, homeopathy, or acupuncture?

Consider, too, how flexible and accommodating your interviewees seem: your situation may change or you may change your mind about various aspects of your care later in pregnancy, and it is good, in any planning for birth, to keep your options as open as possible.

You can get a sense of how calm, confident, and nonjudgmental the midwife is, and how much she allows the interview to center around you and your needs. This tells you that she will stand back during labor, allowing you and your labor to take center stage, although she will be observing you and attending to your care. Some of the best midwives may seem quiet and unassuming at first meeting.

A Homebirth Support Group

Attending a homebirth support group, or just getting together with a few experienced homebirth mothers, is one of the best ways to prepare for homebirth. You can share stories of birth, ask questions, and most important, have the experience of being with mothers and babies, which sadly has become uncommon in our culture.

If there is no local group, you could consider starting a homebirth support group yourself. Choose one day per month that suits you, and ask local midwives to get the word out for you. My local (Brisbane, Australia) homebirth support group always begins with a short introduction around the circle, then we ask one mother to share her birth story. After this, we have a general discussion, particularly inviting questions from new members, and we finish with a short evaluation from everyone. After the meeting we enjoy a shared lunch, with plenty of time to chat and pass the babies around!

Homebirth and the Sacred Cycle

Birth is not an isolated event in our lives, but rather a part of our feminine sexual cycle. As mothers we move from menstruation to conception, pregnancy, birth, postnatal, and breastfeeding, and then back to menstruation. When this cycle is honored as a life-giving continuum, each of these experiences can be deep and satisfying.[23]

Homebirth ensures that these sacred events stay within our own space, keeping the circle whole and inviolate. Homebirth can bless our homes and our families many times over, creating a luminous atmosphere in the early weeks and months, and giving us memories and experiences that can sustain us—mothers, babies, fathers, and children—for a lifetime.

Jacob's Waterbirth: Perfect Timing

My third pregnancy was unexpected, teaching me about trust and timing and increasing my capacity for surrender. Jacob's home waterbirth was an exquisite experience, although not without challenge, and gave our family a blissful start to life as a family of five.

I remember it as though it were yesterday. We were driving down Hoddle Street in Melbourne, heading for the ferry that would take us south to the island of Tasmania for a family Christmas. Buckled up in the back seat were Emma, just four, and Zoe, fourteen months.

I turned to Nicholas and said, "You know, I have definitely not wanted another baby until now, but now I'm feeling it would be okay if it happened."

"Yes," he concurred, and with his medical mind added, "I'd really like you to have another baby before you get past thirty-five."

Thinking back, I can almost feel a shimmer in the air; some solidification of the spirit that would become our third child Jacob, who had now found the smallest crack in a previously closed door and was heading toward earth—toward us, his new family—at the speed of light.

I was truly surprised, and actually rather fearful, when I did conceive. It took me several weeks to realize that I was pregnant, and several months to trust Jacob's timing. I was especially afraid of the two-year gap there would be with Zoe, which was exactly the gap between me and my younger sister.

My body was in good shape, though, and I was active and healthy through the pregnancy. We chose again to have a homebirth with the midwife-family physician team that had supported us so beautifully with Emma and Zoe's homebirths.

I had a strong urge for water in this pregnancy and spent a lot of time swimming. As a family, we relished our weekly family swim sessions with Cookie Harkin, Zoe's "Baby Swim" teacher. I also attended Cookie's prenatal sessions, in which we floated face down in her pool using snorkels and buoyancy rings, with dim lights and relaxing music. It was blissful to share my baby's experience, being softly suspended in warm water with soothing noises.

Later in the pregnancy, I began to use a monofin, a large flipper that holds both feet and enables a dolphin-like swimming movement under the surface. While monofinning, I could feel my baby's exhilaration as well as my own, and I wondered, in retrospect, if my baby chose to stay extra weeks in my womb to get his fill of this pleasure.

I decided to use a birthing tub during this labor, with the possibility of giving birth in the water. I figured that water would give me privacy and space in what could be a full house: Emma and Zoe, a good friend to care for them, my doctor, my midwife, and Nicholas. I was also curious to experience waterbirth, which some of my friends described enthusiastically.

The tub I hired from my midwife had been custom-made from hollow metal pipes (actually, car exhaust pipes) that fitted together, with a liner that was laced over the frame. It was quick to set up and not too high, so I could step into the pool relatively easily. We had a practice run to see how many tanks of hot water we would need to fill it and how long it would take, allowing for time for the hot water tank to reheat (three tanks, and about four hours). During the practice run I managed to cook the waterbed heater that kept the tub warm onto a piece of foam, and I had to buy a new heater!

The tub, set up and ready to be filled, kept vigil in our back room as I went one, then two, then three weeks past my original expected date. I was blessed to have caregivers who were happy to revise these (rather uncertain) dates, so that I was able to enjoy this waiting without undue pressure. My only concern was to fit in with my parents' timetable; they were coming to help after the birth and had to reschedule their flight from New Zealand several times.

Labor started for me at one in the morning, and I woke Nicholas to fill the tub around two-thirty. This labor was very slow and gentle from the start, and I spent time both in and out of the water. I found that I couldn't sway my hips as well in the tub—at least not without causing a tidal wave—but I certainly relished the water as I rested between contractions. Zoe, who had woken before dawn and was naked from early on, spent much of early labor trying to get in with me and then contented herself with floating her dollies in the water.

We had the tub in our family room, and Nicholas had thoughtfully grown some beautiful cinerarias in the adjoining garden, which I could see through the window. My task in this labor was to slow down and go with the gentle pace. Getting out and walking around didn't speed up labor for me, as it does for some women after a few hours in the tub.

When the contractions became challenging later in the morning, I found the water soothing and supporting. I had a feeling that this baby would be born in the water, but it was important to me that I was not fixed on this idea. I remembered how important it had been to me to have my feet on the earth and allow gravity to help me give birth to my second baby Zoe, who was born posterior (face up).

At transition, before the urge to push was strong, I felt the reality of this baby, who I would soon be holding in my arms. I felt a wave of fear followed by a strong connection and commitment. As my baby's head came lower, we saw a mass of white in the water; the soft creamy vernix that covered his skin was floating out as I pushed.

I was kneeling, supported by the side of the tub, as he was born. At 8 pounds 4 ounces (3.75 kg), Jacob was my biggest baby, and I could feel my pelvic bones open as he emerged. Chris, my midwife, caught him in the water and passed him to me. Unlike some waterborn babies, he cried quickly and vigorously. In the exhilaration of the moment we didn't think to check his sex, and we had another wave of joy when we discovered, some minutes later, that we had a son.

I stood up out of the water to deliver Jacob's placenta, and we chose not to cut the cord. (See the essay "Jacob's Placenta," page 185, for more about this practice, called lotus birth). My doctor took a small sample of Jacob's cord blood (to test his Rh blood group) and then we floated his placenta in an ice-cream carton until I was ready to get out, about an hour after the birth. Before this, Emma and Zoe climbed in and said hello to their new brother. After the birth, we siphoned the water onto the garden, which made cleaning up very easy.

Jacob's cord separated the day before my parents arrived: perfect timing! My mother and father gave us wonderful household support, allowing me to rest and settle into new motherhood, and providing superb grandparenting to my older children. Our house radiated calm and completion, blessed by another beautiful Birth, with a white camellia tree blooming outside our window.

Jacob's pregnancy and birth taught me to trust my children's timing, to trust life to support us, and to surrender and accept love and outside assistance. Jacob's birth inspired me to write and speak publicly about birth, sharing my stories and knowledge to support others, so that mothers, babies, fathers, and families can create their own exquisite start.

Part 2

gentle mothering

chapter 11

LOVE, ATTACHMENT, AND YOUR BABY'S BRAIN
How Gentle Early Parenting Promotes Lifelong Well-Being

Our ideas about infant development have radically changed in recent decades. Previously, babies were considered blank slates; now we know that human infants have their own inbuilt programs, even from birth, and require specific care for optimal development, especially brain development. This chapter blends the neuroscience of infant development with practical information for new parents, providing support and suggestions for the instinctive and attachment-style parenting that will benefit our babies and children all their lives.

Human babies, like the babies of all our mammalian cousins, are born in a very incomplete state. In fact, human babies are even more immature at birth than other mammals, because several million years ago our female ancestors began to walk upright (bipedally). The changes in pelvic shape necessary for bipedalism created less space for our baby's heads to come through the mother's birth canal, requiring our offspring to emerge with smaller heads, and therefore less mature brains, at birth.[1]

However, this does not mean that our babies are incapable or stupid, as many have believed until recently. The capacities of our newborns are perfect for the environment that they will inhabit—the mother's body—and for the learning and growing that will eventually make them perfectly adapted for their adult environment.[2, 3]

For example, your newborn baby has a focusing distance of around ten to twelve inches: perfect for looking at your face, when held in your arms or at your breast. The first time your newborn looks at your face, brain cells (neurons) will be activated and will electrically fire in the brain areas concerned with vision and with facial recognition. As your baby gazes at you again and again, repeated firing will lead to the formation of wiring—connections that link the vision and the facial recognition areas of the brain—and your baby will gradually begin to recognize your face.

This firing and wiring in response to experience, and especially experiences during social interactions, is very important for early brain development. Our babies are born with a huge number of neurons—around two hundred million—but with very few connections (synapses) between these neurons. These synapses will form according to the baby's experiences, because, according to neuroscientific principles, "cells that fire together, wire together." This makes our babies' immature brains very pliable, designed to be sculpted by early experiences;[4] as neuropsychologist Allan Schore comments, ". . . early experiences with the social environment are critical to the maturation of brain tissue."[5]

The experiences that will begin to fire and wire your baby's brain start in your womb, with the physical sensations that provide the earliest learning. These include being physically supported by the womb and amniotic fluid, being kept warm by your body warmth, being gently rocked as you walk, being exposed to different tastes from your diet via the amniotic fluid,[6] hearing your voice and the voices of other family members, and feeling calm and settled when you are calm and settled. Conversely, high levels of stress during pregnancy can fire and wire your baby's brain for dysfunctions in learning and overreactivity to stress. These robust human findings emphasize the need for rest and nurture during pregnancy.[7]

After birth, different experiences will fire and wire other areas of your baby's brain. These experiences, which still primarily concern your physical interactions with your baby, include warmth and the tactile and olfactory stimulation from touching your body, especially your skin; bodily support and movement from being held; the sensations and tastes that your breast milk provides, including tastes from your diet; listening to your voice; and, as you hold your baby close, hearing your heartbeat, which will be already connected to (fired and wired with) pleasurable and soothing feelings from the womb.

Mutual Regulation

These physical inputs from your body will provide optimal experiences for your baby's brain development in other ways. The physical interactions between you and your baby will contribute to the physiological stability—also known as *homeostasis*—for both of you by a process called *mutual regulation.* Mutual regulation involves you and your baby exchanging information and influencing each other's body processes for ongoing well-being and optimal development.

Mutual regulation is crucial for our young babies, who are less able to control their own body processes. For example, newborn babies have difficulty keeping themselves warm, but will be perfectly heated when skin to skin on the mother's chest. In fact, as mentioned in chapter 13, when your newborn is placed on your naked chest, your skin temperature will immediately increase to warm your baby,[8] making your skin-to-skin newborn warmer than a newborn who is dressed and placed in a crib (cot).[9]

Skin-to-skin contact with your body also regulates your newborn baby by reducing stress hormones. Lower levels of stress and stress hormones will reduce your baby's energy requirements, improve blood sugar levels, and stabilize temperature, among other beneficial effects.[10]

Your body's ability to regulate your baby's temperature, and the lowering of your baby's stress hormones while in physical contact with you, continue to benefit your baby throughout infancy. Contact with you, especially skin-to-skin contact, activates your baby's parasympathetic nervous system (PNS)—the "rest and digest" body program that switches off stress; enhances digestion, healing, and growth; and imprints calm and connection through the hormone oxytocin, discussed extensively in the first part of this book.

On the mother's side, contact with her baby enhances her mothering hormones, including oxytocin and prolactin, helping to regulate her maternal instincts and behaviors. In the same way, the baby's breastfeeding, especially when frequent both day and night, enhances the mother's health (and the health of her baby and any future babies) by regulating her fertility and increasing child spacing.

Our growing understanding of mutual regulation demonstrates that, in many important ways, mother and baby are one physiologic organism—

motherbaby—and underscores the importance of your ongoing presence to optimize your baby's body functioning and development.

Mutual regulation continues to benefit parents and growing offspring in many areas. For example, bed sharing mothers and babies experience mutually regulated sleep cycles, wherein both are in light sleep at the same time, which makes night feeding easier and more pleasurable. (See chapter 14 for more on the science of sleep.)

As our children grow, our input and regulation continue to benefit their emotional—and emotional brain—development. Through consistently providing our loving presence and support, especially in times of upset and anger, we help our children regulate their own emotional states, a skill related to neuronal wiring in parts of the limbic (emotional) brain.[11, 12]

An Ideal Environment

One of our most important roles as parents is to provide an ideal environment for our babies and children. In this consumer-driven culture, it is easy to assume that we will create this environment from things that we buy.

Perhaps we can remember that, for more than a hundred thousand human generations, our foremothers cared for their babies in the wild with no crib, carriage or stroller, diapers, or other accessories, and probably little clothing. Yet our minimalist forebears thrived because the mother's body was able to provide all that her baby needed, and her presence was obviously irreplaceable for infant survival.

In modern times our babies continue to be hardwired with an expectation that their needs will be met through constant maternal care and mutual regulation. And as modern mothers we continue to be hardwired to give this irreplaceable and life-sustaining care, which is reinforced by our maternal and breastfeeding hormones and also by our babies' behavior.

These factors—our hormones and our babies' behaviors—both activate the *maternal circuit* in our limbic system, the brain areas that stimulate maternal behavior in all mammals. The maternal circuit includes a powerful reward system: the mesocortico-limbic dopamine system, which motivates all mammalian mothers to give this necessary care to their offspring and rewards them for doing so.

For example, during breastfeeding the mother's pituitary releases pulses of oxytocin, which stimulates mothering behavior and reduces stress and stress hormones.[13] The calm and connected feelings stimulated by oxytocin[14] support nursing mothers in soothing and nurturing their offspring.

The nursing-related release of oxytocin also activates the mesocortico-limbic dopamine reward system,[15] as does the hormone beta-endorphin, also released by all mammalian mothers and babies with breastfeeding and intimate body contact.

As breastfeeding mothers we also release the hormone prolactin with each nursing episode. Mothers (and others, including fathers[16]) also release prolactin through infant care and especially infant carrying.[17, 18] High levels of prolactin from breastfeeding and infant carrying can help us to mother (and father) well by making us more "tolerant of monotony,"[19] reducing our need for external stimulation and supporting the "ordinary maternal preoccupation"[20] that our babies require. Although prolactin reduces our stress levels, it also increases "social desirability," making us more likely to submit our own needs to the needs of our vulnerable offspring.[21]

These benefits were demonstrated in a human study in which new mothers were randomized (or not) to receive soft baby-carrying slings. Researchers found that the babies who were carried in these slings in infancy were more secure at age thirteen months, which may at least partly reflect the beneficial effects of prolactin on maternal behavior.[22]

When we carry our babies we provide an ideal environment in other ways. In monkeys and other primates (of which we are a subset), movement in infancy is crucial for brain development.[23] Movement stimulates the vestibular (balance) center and the cerebellum, at the base of the brain, helping to establish brain-wiring connections that have major consequences for later brain development. For example, an area called the cerebellar vermis, which is stimulated by movement, is now thought to be a crucial region for mental health in adulthood. Some of the negative consequences of early stress or neglect are thought to be mediated by malfunctions of the cerebellar vermis.[24]

Developmental psychologist James Prescott found that, in the same way, mother-infant carrying (or not) in different human cultures can predict with 80 percent accuracy whether that culture is peaceful or aggressive.[25]

Prescott concluded that lack of carrying can cause somatosensory affectional deprivation (S-SAD) in mammalian babies, associated with hyperexcitability and aggression in adulthood. His cross-cultural research also links high rates of carrying, of physical affection toward infants, and of weaning at older than two and a half years with low rates of suicide and violence in adulthood. As he poignantly argues, "Only more mother-infant bonding can prevent cycles of violence."[26]

The importance of the "in arms" phase is also emphasized by anthropologist Jean Leidloff in her book *The Continuum Concept.*[27] Leidloff, who visited the Venezuelan Yequana tribe many times and observed their parenting practices, notes the infant's "soft muscle tone of ancestral well-being," which she relates to being constantly held or carried.

Note also that for most of human prehistory constant carrying was essential to protect our babies from predators. It is therefore logical that the urge to be carried would be hardwired into our infants' brains as a safety measure (explaining why babies will cry to be carried) and that infant carrying would be reinforced and rewarded as an integral component of maternal behavior.

An ideal environment for infancy also includes access to the mother's breast during the day and at night (see chapter 12); security at night through cosleeping (see chapter 13); protection from painful and traumatic events, including circumcision; and liberal touch, social interactions, and body contact (ideally skin to skin) with loving adults.

Building an Attached Brain

Our babies' brains, like those of all mammals, develop in a specific sequence that exactly matches the experiences that they expect to have at different stages.

In the first year, our babies expect to be physically close to the mother as primary attachment figure and, with time, to participate in an increasingly complex social environment that grows to include father, siblings, extended family, and friends.

Positive early social experiences trigger emotional and social learning, but more importantly, they create pathways by firing and wiring the affiliative parts of the brain—those areas concerned with relationships. Appropriate social and interactive experiences in infancy will wire our children's brains for ease and pleasure with future social interactions.

This gives our offspring more than good social engagement; ease in relationships brings with it major and long-term advantages. Studies with adults are showing lifelong health benefits to individuals who have good ongoing social connections, and conversely more illness and shorter lives among those who report less "social capital."[28]

For the first three years, the right side of a child's brain is dominant over the left side, with rapid right-brain growth from the last months of pregnancy through the end of the second year.[29] The right brain is involved with bonding and attachment[30] and is closely connected with the limbic system—the emotional brain— which also undergoes a growth spurt during the first two years.[31]

The creation of "an attachment bond of emotional communication" between mother and baby will build a healthy right brain and limbic system and is a major developmental task for the first two to three years.[32] This secure bond is built through the baby's repeated positive and attuned interactions with the mother (and later with others), including episodes of mutual gaze and smiles, experiences of heightened emotions such as laughter and joy, and temporary disengagements (pulling away) when the input is too intense for the baby.

These mother-baby interactions, which have previously been regarded as indulgent play, have been found to involve complex and highly syn-chronized behaviors, including synchronizing of facial expressions, body movements, and brain activity. From the perspective of brain activity, this could be seen as the baby mirroring, and actually downloading, the mother's brain patterns and behaviors, and incorporating them into their own brain structures and future behaviors.[33]

Emotionally smooth interactions or "affect synchrony" between mother and baby will build brain pathways that optimally wire the baby's brain. Conversely, when the mother is consistently emotionally unavailable to her baby, or when her reactions are most often unex-pected or out of synchrony, firing and wiring will be less than optimal, potentially leading to attachment problems that can affect the indi-vidual for a lifetime.[33]

According to Schore, "During the last 10 years, many studies have documented the enduring impact of the maternal visual, vocal, and tactile [touch] emotional stimuli on the infant's brain development and on the resulting emotional, social, cognitive, [thinking] and regulatory capacities in later life."[32]

Early interactions with our babies therefore not only sculpt their growing brains, but also act as a template for their future relationships. For our children the brain programs that are downloaded at this time will be available and likely imprinted during interactions with their own offspring—our grandchildren. This is one way in which parenting, experiences, and behaviors are transmitted across generations. (This phenomenon also explains the uncanny experience of repeating the exact words to our children that were said to us in childhood.)

Attunement also encompasses our role in regulating our baby's experiences and reactions. As with regulation of physical processes, our babies need help with adjusting their emotions and emotional reactions, especially when experiences are new or stressful. When we respond calmly, we are modeling with our brains and producing a brain program that the baby will download and integrate as a template for future stressful situations.

The emotional regulation that attuned caregivers provide is critical because young babies have no ability to self-regulate their emotions and so are easily overwhelmed by feelings such as sadness, fear, and even excitement. Our ongoing presence and availability will meet their need to learn emotional self-regulation. Conversely, when caregivers are consistently absent, or emotionally unavailable to help with regulation, babies can become overwhelmed and severely stressed, leading to the toxic brain chemistry described later, with possible long-term consequences.

The enduring impact of our early experiences is also imprinted through changes in brain hormone systems, which again center around the limbic system. For example, female rats who receive high-quality maternal care in infancy will give their babies the same high-quality care, even if they are genetically bred to give low levels of maternal care.[34] These well-mothered mothers have an increased sensitivity to oxytocin in their limbic systems,[35] making them more calm, connected, and rewarded in relation to infant care.

Similarly, human studies are increasingly linking secure attachment and good parental care in childhood with robust oxytocin function, giving individuals an effective "calm and connection"[13] response mediated by oxytocin when under stress.[36, 37]

Secure attachment, based on optimal maternal care, may be even more important for genetically vulnerable offspring. Primate researchers studied "high-reactive" rhesus monkeys: those individuals who were timid and overreactive to stress as juveniles and, in adulthood, were usually confined to low status within the troop. However, when these offspring were cross-fostered by experienced and exceptionally nurturing mothers, they became precociously confident, often rising to high-status positions in the troop, with high-reactive cross-fostered females becoming exceptionally nurturing mothers themselves.[38]

The right brain and limbic system pathways are also connected to the autonomic nervous system (ANS)—the system that keeps the body in balance (homeostasis) by adjusting our inner state in response to external changes. Positive experiences of bonding and attachment will fire and wire these systems optimally, giving our children the ability to adapt physically and psychologically to stress and change, and therefore building resilience in adulthood.[4, 33, 39]

Control, Compassion, and Touch

From ten months to two years, our children undergo a major growth spurt in another important brain structure. The orbitofrontal cortex (OFC), situated behind the forehead close to the eye sockets, acts as an executive controller of brain and body on many levels. For example, the OFC links to the amygdala—the fear center—and can modify our instinctive fear reactions, allowing us to be less fearful, more sociable, and more curious when we judge that our environment is safe.[29]

The OFC is also involved with emotional self-regulation, giving us the ability to maximize our pleasant emotions and minimize unpleasant feelings. In adults a healthy OFC can help reduce fear and anxiety, whereas malfunctions in the OFC have been found in adult anxiety and obsessive disorders[40] and major depression.[41] The right OFC is closely wired with the right brain and limbic system, and it also requires attuned early interactions for optimal development.

The right brain and OFC also give us the ability to interpret facial expressions, creating awareness of—and the possibility of empathy for—another's emotional state. Secure early attachment with a sensitive caregiver who has helped with emotional regulation will build the optimal brain wiring that provides this important human capacity.[42] These scientific understandings confirm the Dalai Lama's teaching: "We learn compassion mainly from our mothers."[43]

Recent attachment research has focused on analyzing face-to-face interactions between an attuned mother and her baby, as described in the previous section, perhaps because these episodes are easy to study in the laboratory. However, many other early experiences will fire and wire the baby's brain, thereby sculpting brain development.

For example, in the early weeks, before responsive smiling and other social interactions, the pathways that are developmentally ready for firing and wiring are those from the amygdala to the hypothalamus, which controls the autonomic nervous system and also produces many important hormones. The amygdala also processes olfactory information, so that olfactory stimulation, through close contact with the mother, may also be important for early brain development.[44]

Firing and wiring at this time occurs in response to touch and smell, which will help to regulate the oxytocin and arginine vasopressin (AVP) hormonal systems.[44] Liberal maternal-infant body contact will therefore imprint calm and connection (oxytocin) and minimize stress (AVP) during interactions, giving a good start to the pre-attachment phase.[33]

Touch is also important at this time because it regulates the future functioning of the stress system via the hormone CRH.[33] In rats, optimal levels of tactile stimulation provided by the mother in infancy enhance adult learning and social behavior and give resistance to stress in adulthood.[45] This is likely to be true for humans, as suggested by improvements in premature babies' growth, alertness,[46] and subsequent development[47] after receiving increased skin-to-skin contact in the hospital.

There are many other aspects of attuned early parenting that, although not yet studied, are likely to contribute to brain development. These may include episodes in which the baby is carried passively, observing other activities, as well as interactions and activities that stimulate multiple senses and bodily systems, such as breastfeeding and bed sharing.

Experts note that in humans, as in animals, high levels of parental care are required to optimally sculpt the offspring's growing brain and to confer resiliency to stress.[45] However, the rewards are commensurately large: as Teicher and colleagues comment, "adequate nurturing and absence of intense stress permit the mammalian brain to develop in a manner that is less aggressive and more emotionally stable, social, empathic, monogamous and hemispherically integrated [between left and right brain]. We believe that this enhances the ability of social animals to build more elaborate social structures and enables humans to better realize their creative potentials."[48]

Unloved, Unregulated, and Unwired

When we understand the necessity of attachment and social experiences for optimal brain development, we can also understand that neglect can be at least as harmful as abuse or trauma. If our children do not receive the appropriate stimulation during specific periods of brain growth, firing and wiring—and therefore their brain function—will be deficient in that particular area.

Young children who are not given the appropriate parental care and stimulation in the early years may have less than optimal functioning on the right brain, limbic system, orbitofrontal cortex, and other related areas. This may predispose them, as adults, to a host of problems, including: deficiencies in attachment that impact adult relationships; difficulties in emotional self-regulation that increase the chances of depression and anxiety disorders; lack of empathy for others; lower levels of happiness because of inability to maximize pleasant emotions and minimize negative emotions; and limitations in their ability to give their own children optimal care for brain and emotional development.[39, 48]

We can also consider that brain development follows a sequence, with new developments built on previous foundations. In this way, lack of wiring in critical, early-developing right-brain areas may also impact subsequent development, including cognitive development. This suggests that "early loving," which optimizes right brain and limbic development, is likely to be much more important than "early learning" in building a healthy, well-functioning brain.

While neglect can cause underwiring in crucial brain areas; abuse and trauma in the early years can have other long-lasting effects on our children's brain structure and function. Note also that lack of regulation is stressful to babies and young children, so that neglectful parenting is likely to be experienced as traumatic.

For babies (as for adults), traumatic events cause emotional distress. Emotionally distressed babies will cry, and our crying babies expect that we, as caregivers, will help them repair these dysregulated experiences. If we are not available, physically or emotionally, not only will the creation of regulating brain pathways be missed, but our babies' ongoing emotional distress can cause a cascade of stress hormones that is toxic to the brain and nervous system.

Initial distress activates the fight-or-flight sympathetic nervous system (SNS), releasing high levels of epinephrine (adrenaline) and norepinephrine (noradrenaline) into the brain and body. Within the brain, high levels of epinephrine and norepinephrine, along with the stress hormones CRH and cortisol and other activating (excitatory) brain chemicals, cause hyperarousal along with a hypermetabolic state, in which brain cells consume excess fuels, leading to metabolic stress and, if prolonged, brain cell death. A hyperaroused baby is physically active, moving and crying as a means of attracting caregiver attention.

As this state of hyperarousal escalates, our babies are not just stressed, but frantically distressed: researcher Bruce Perry calls this state "fear-terror."[49]

When hyperarousal is long-lasting, with no response from caregivers, distress gives way to a dissociative state, in which crying ceases and the baby shuts down, both emotionally and physiologically. The parasympathetic nervous system (PNS) is activated, slowing heart rate and decreasing blood pressure, which helps to conserve energy and body heat. However, the SNS remains activated, with ongoing elevations of epinephrine and norepinephrine. Within the brain, high levels of opiate chemicals lead to numbing of pain and emotion and inhibit crying.

This "despair-dissociation" state is an extreme but adaptive response that is hardwired into all mammalian babies as a safety mechanism in case of abandonment by the mother in the wild, where ongoing crying would increase risk from predators and also waste energy. In this state, the baby quiets down and conserves energy, and may even be able to feign death to escape predators, although the stress system is still maximally activated.

When babies are in this dissociated state, a toxic chemistry, involving high levels of cortisol in combination with the other brain-activating chemicals, can cause brain cell death, particularly in the limbic system. This can lead to abnormal functioning in this "emotional brain" and, according to some experts, may increase lifelong mental health vulnerability.[39, 48]

This sequence—from fear-terror to despair-dissociation—occurs with prolonged separation or ongoing unresponsiveness from caregivers, which is also experienced by the baby as a life-threatening separation. This reaction is also likely in situations such as sleep training, in which babies are left to "cry it out" with minimal or no comforting until they "fall asleep," which is more likely a dissociative state, with ongoing toxicity to the brain. (See chapter 13 for more about "crying it out.")

Studies have found many brain abnormalities in animals and humans who have experienced repeated or ongoing early stress and trauma, which likely reflects damage from prolonged and repeated toxic brain states.

In animals, researchers have used early maternal separation as a model of stress. In rodents, this leads to increased stress responsiveness in adulthood. In studies of nonhuman primates, early separation leads to higher resting levels of CRH, the executive stress hormone; lower resting levels of cortisol; abnormalities of brain chemicals such as dopamine, serotonin, and norepinephrine; and increased fearfulness in adulthood.[50]

Similarly, studies of severely neglected children have shown lower levels of cortisol, with an abnormal "flat" diurnal (daily) pattern of release, which may signal future vulnerability to post-traumatic stress disorder (PTSD).[50] One study of children adopted from Romanian orphanages, where early care was extremely inadequate, found exceptionally high cortisol levels over daytime hours six years after adoption.[51] However, researchers are not yet certain whether these abnormalities are permanent, and it is also unclear whether short-term changes in cortisol and the hypothalamic-pituitary-adrenal (HPA) stress system in response to stress and trauma will inevitably produce permanent brain changes[50] such as those described in the following section.

Teicher and colleagues have compiled a list of documented brain effects of early abuse, including early maternal-infant separation, in animals and humans and correlated these with possible effects on adult health. These authors note that exposure to early stress changes the molecular structure of the stress-response system, which "programs and primes the mammalian brain to be more fearful and to have an enhanced noradrenergic [involving norepinephrine], corticosterioid [cortisol], and vasopressin [AVP, another brain stress hormone] response to stress."[52]

These authors also suggest that increased cell death and reduced size in the hippocampus (the short-term memory center), as found in stressed or separated animals and maltreated children, predisposes to anxiety and dissociative states and increases vulnerability to PTSD in adulthood.[4]

Other mechanisms by which early trauma may damage the brain and predispose to adult psychiatric problems include:

- Increased and irritable brain activity in the amygdala due to prolonged or repeated episodes of fear-terror, which may lead to impulsive violence in adulthood
- Decreased wiring in the corpus callosum (which joins left and right brain), as found in women who had been sexually abused, which may cause anxiety
- Abnormal activity in the cerebellar vermis, as found in young adults who had been sexually abused in childhood, which has been associated with schizophrenia, autism, depression, and ADHD
- An overactive right brain and underactive left brain (found in abused children under psychiatric treatment), which has been linked with depression in adulthood[4]

Other researchers have shown that securely attached children have lower cortisol release in stressful situations, and that "subtle infant maltreatment"—spanking or use of maternal withdrawal as a control tactic—is associated with higher cortisol release under stress and higher resting cortisol levels, respectively.[53]

Attachment researcher and professor of child development Megan Gunnar summarizes: "Studies of variations in parental care within the normal range in humans strongly indicate that less sensitive and responsive caregiving is associated with poorer concurrent regulation of the HPA axis in childhood. Sensitive and responsive care and associated secure attachment relationships appear to provide a powerful buffer for the HPA axis during early development."[54]

This research does not imply that infrequent, short episodes of maternal absence or other mild stresses that are promptly repaired are harmful to babies and young children. In fact, brief episodes of dysregulation and repair teach our offspring that "negativity can be endured and conquered" and may confer resilience.[44] Note also that in nonhuman primates, caregivers apart from the mother (*alloparents*) can buffer the effects of maternal separation.[50]

It is also likely that even moderate traumas can be healed through prompt (and, if necessary, ongoing) regulation and repair. Our natural tendency to cry, babies and adults alike, when we recall traumatic events may represent an important mechanism to self-repair past traumas. Although not researched neuroscientifically, supporting our babies and children to express their emotions around past, present, or ongoing trauma, as advocated by experts such as psychologist Aletha Solter,[55] may provide important opportunities for emotional repair.

It is obviously impossible to fulfill all needs and avoid all stresses for our babies (who can even be upset by the texture of clothing!), but it is important to be available and to offer our sensitivity and presence most of the time. D. W. Winnicott, a UK child psychiatrist and pioneer in attachment research, reassures as that we only need to be "good enough mothers" to fulfill our babies' needs for secure attachment.[20]

Building Attachment:
Summary and Recommendations

This growing body of scientific and neuroscientific research, which validates the lifelong importance of attachment for our offspring, contrasts starkly with current parenting literature and advice, which includes encouragement to avoid holding our babies and to leave distressed babies alone to "cry it out."

The following recommendations are consistent with our understandings of infant brain development and are likely to enhance mothering ease and pleasure, and to optimize emotional and relational well-being for our offspring for a lifetime:

- Reduce stress in pregnancy. This will limit the negative effects of maternal stress hormones on fetal brain development. Consider regular gentle exercise, a wholesome diet, adequate sleep (including daytime naps if needed), yoga or other meditative activities, regular massage, liberal maternity leave, and building of support circles for early parenting. (See also chapter 6 for more suggestions during pregnancy and birth.)

- Plan a restful postnatal "babymoon." Prioritizing rest and recovery will give a relaxed (perhaps even transcendent) start to family life. Ideally allow six weeks of attentive support, without other obligations, for the new mother. Regular massage during this time, as practiced in some cultures is especially beneficial.

- Ensure uninterrupted mother-baby contact, preferably skin to skin, in the early hours and days after birth. This will reduce newborn stress, optimize temperature regulation, enhance early breastfeeding, and positively regulate infant stress systems.

- Promote continuous or near-continuous mother-baby body contact, including holding and carrying, in the days and weeks after birth. This will optimally wire amygdala-hypothalamic, vestibular, and cerebellar pathways, with possible long-term psychological benefits.

- Enjoy liberal body contact and breastfeeding in both daytime and nighttime. This will mutually regulate mother and baby; optimize hormonal systems for ongoing ease, pleasure, and well-being; and reduce separation-induced stress for the baby.

- Practice ongoing infant carrying and/or physical contact through the early years. This will soothe and regulate babies and young children, especially in times of stress and distress.

- Create ample opportunities for positive social interactions with attuned, attentive, and available caregivers. This will begin to optimally wire the right-brain and OFC, building emotional self-regulation, with possible long-term protection from anxiety and depression.

- Prioritize the ongoing and ready availability of a primary caregiver—ideally, the mother—through the first one to three years.

This will optimize attachment and ensure the smooth development of emotional and physical self-regulating capacities.

- Relish ongoing and liberal breastfeeding and cosleeping through the first year and beyond. This will optimize hormonal caretaking and reward systems (oxytocin, prolactin, beta-endorphin), enhance mutual regulation for mother and baby, and optimize breast milk supply and nutrition, with long-term health benefits for mother and baby.

- Avoid severe stress (including circumcision), as far as possible, especially in the first one to two years. This will reduce exposure to toxic hyperarousal/dissociation brain chemistry, which can lead to cell death in the limbic brain and possibly to lifelong mental health vulnerability.

- Commit to remaining calm and physically close to your child during episodes of unavoidable stress, distress, and anger (theirs or others') to help ensure rapid regulation (soothing).

- Offer repeated assistance during emotionally difficult times, which will help to fire and wire self-soothing brain pathways, leading eventually to self-regulation in these areas.

- Prioritize secure attachment in the early months and years, by attending to all the preceding items on this list. This will optimize development in the right brain, limbic system, and autonomic nervous system, which may increase lifelong resilience to stress.

- Build family, social, and community support for these choices, as much as possible. This will reduce parental stress and enhance the sustainability of all of these important parenting practices.

chapter 12

BREASTFEEDING
The Gift of a Lifetime

Breastfeeding is now recognized as giving optimal infant nutrition and nurture. Breastfed babies have major health benefits in the short, medium, and long terms. Conversely, nonbreastfed babies can experience many disadvantages to current and long-term health and well-being. This chapter provides information to support mothers in making this important choice, and includes specific medical evidence to support women who would like to nurse for more than one to two years.

Breastfeeding is one of the most valuable gifts you can give your baby. Breastfeeding will enhance health and development through the important first year and, if you choose, for the years beyond. Breastfeeding is also a wonderful asset for mothering, keeping nursing mothers connected and in love with their babies. Breastfeeding's substantial benefits apply to both short- and longer-term nursing, and some of the benefits will last for your child's entire life.

Breastfeeding involves more than the transfer of breast milk from mother to baby. Breastfeeding is an act of total nurture, involving holding, gaze, and bodily contact. Breastfeeding stimulates the release of loving and pleasurable hormones, which induce loving and pleasurable feelings for both partners; these hormones also reward and reinforce breastfeeding and at the same time enhance both infant brain development and maternal instincts and behaviors.

Breastfeeding past one year is increasingly accepted in our culture, and it has additional benefits for mother and baby.

Breast Milk: Perfect for the Whole Baby

Through millions of years of evolution, our female bodies have become perfectly adapted to feed our babies. The act of lactation is common to all mammals—those animals with the ability to nurture their young with breast milk produced from their mammary glands. Each species' milk is different, but is specifically constituted for its young and for the particular stage of development. For example, if birth is premature, the milk will be adapted for the premature baby, and the composition of milk changes as the offspring grows.

For most of human history, breastfeeding has been crucial for infant survival. Even in times and places where babies have been fed other first foods, breastfed babies were recognized as healthier and more likely to survive. This benefit persists today, and includes babies born in countries with relatively low infant mortality like the United States, where, according to one study, formula-fed babies are 25 percent more likely than breastfed babies to die in the first year of life.[1]

Breastfeeding is part of a complex immunological system that protects the growing baby from diseases to which mother or baby are exposed. When a nursing mother encounters infectious agents in her gut and lung—the main routes of human infection—the antibodies that she forms will travel to her breasts and will be transferred to the baby via breast milk, giving specific protection against infections that the baby is, or will soon be, exposed to. A breastfed infant receives a relatively high dose of maternal antibodies. up to 1 gram per day via breast milk, compared to a total of 2.5 grams produced daily in the body of an average adult.[2]

Other components of breast milk that enhance the functioning of the baby's immune system include lactoferrin, which has antibiotic, immunostimulatory, and anti-inflammatory properties; oligosaccharides (long-chain sugars) that block the mucosal attachment of bacteria such as Hemophilus influenza and pneumococci; and immune cells such as lymphocytes, which may even be taken into the baby's body.[2] Breastfeeding also stimulates the development of the thymus, an important component of the immune system in childhood. A nonbreastfed baby has a thymus that is only half the size of that of a breastfed baby.[2]

These factors are especially important for newborn babies, whose immature immune systems make them very vulnerable to infection. Early breast milk, also known as colostrum, is rich in antibodies and also includes protection via "memory lymphocytes" against illnesses that the mother has encountered over her lifetime.[3]

The newborn baby's immune system matures as the gut becomes colonized with healthy maternal bacteria (bowel flora). These bacteria are transferred during the process of birth and will influence the baby's gut and immune health throughout life. There are also factors in breast milk that enhance the establishment and growth of healthy gut flora, and "The effects on the intestinal microflora may be the most important protective capacity of breastfeeding against neonatal infections."[4] (See chapters 4 and 9 for more about the importance of gut flora.)

The act of breastfeeding causes secretion of important gut hormones for mother and baby. These hormones, which include cholecystokinin and gastrin, stimulate growth in the intestine, making digestion more efficient for both over the long term.[5]

All of these factors help explain the reduced risks of infection among breastfed babies, including decreased risks of septicemia, serious gut infections including necrotizing enterocolitis, diarrhea, and vomiting in the first year of life, respiratory illnesses including ear infections, urinary infections, bacterial meningitis, and, according to some studies, sudden infant death (SIDS).[6, 7]

A mature immune system not only is important for fighting infection, but also will help the individual to discriminate between self and not-self. This is an important part of immune competence and a protective factor against autoimmune diseases, in which the body makes antibodies against itself. Consequently, children who were breastfed in infancy are less likely in later life to have autoimmune diseases including allergies, asthma, celiac disease, insulin-dependent (type 1) diabetes, and juvenile rheumatoid arthritis.[6, 7]

Breastfed children are also less susceptible to inguinal hernias, childhood lymphomas (cancers), dental cavities and malocclusion; and have better speech, advanced social and motor development, higher IQ, and better school grades than their nonbreastfed peers. As they grow into adulthood, breastfed individuals are also at decreased risk of inflammatory bowel disease (Crohn's disease and ulcerative colitis), multiple sclerosis, obesity, and cardiovascular disease. Breastfed females are less likely to develop cancers of the breast, ovary, and endometrium (lining of the uterus) in adulthood.[6, 7]

In one large cohort study, adolescents who had been breastfed for at least seven months were 20 percent less likely to be obese than their nonbreastfed peers; this difference increased by 8 percent for every extra three months of breastfeeding.[8] This finding may relate to the more optimal bowel flora among children who have been breastfed.[9] Other studies have also shown better cholesterol and blood pressure profiles in offspring who had ever been breastfed.[6, 7]

A large prospective population study found that breastfed children had better psychosocial resilience at age ten, in relation to parental separation or divorce, than nonbreastfed children.[10] A recent study has confirmed previous findings of enhanced IQ among breastfed children, with an increase of 5.9 points overall and higher teacher's academic ratings at 6.5 years compared with their nonbreastfed peers. (This is the first randomized study of IQ and breastfeeding, and involved more than thirteen thousand children born to mothers randomized to give birth in baby-friendly or non-baby-friendly hospitals.[11])

Breastfeeding is now recognized as the perfect and complete food for babies up to six months of age, and exclusive nursing is recommended for this duration.[7, 12, 13] It has been estimated that exclusive breastfeeding to six months, and continued breastfeeding to at least one year, would prevent 13 percent of deaths of children under five worldwide, saving the lives of 1.3 million children every year.[14]

Benefits to Breastfeeding Mothers

Breastfeeding also offers major health benefits to nursing mothers. For example, the risk of breast cancer is reduced by 8 percent for every twelve months of breastfeeding over a lifetime.[15] Cancers of the uterus and ovary are also less common, possibly because of breastfeeding's suppressing effects on the nursing mother's menstrual cycle.[16] A Chinese study found that the risk of hip fractures in later life was reduced among those who had given birth by 13 percent for every six months of breastfeeding. According to this research, women who had breastfed for more than two years had a 70 percent reduced risk of hip fracture after menopause, compared to those who had breastfed for six months or less.[17]

Studies have shown other benefits to maternal health. These include, among women who lactated for more than three months, more rapid weight loss after birth along with favorable changes in HDL cholesterol that persisted after weaning, suggesting lower risk of heart attacks and stroke in later life.[18] Other researchers have found improved immune function, possibly dues to lower stress, among breastfeeding mothers compared with formula-feeding mothers.[19] Still other studies have followed breastfeeding women in later life and found reduced risks of type 2 diabetes[20] and of the "metabolic syndrome," which includes vulnerability to diabetes, obesity, high blood pressure, and detrimental blood lipids including cholesterol,[21] with more benefits associated with longer duration of nursing in both studies.

Breastfeeding also gives benefits by delaying the return of fertility. These include better iron levels because of delayed menstruation, and a lower chance of conception. For example, a breastfeeding woman who has not menstruated, and whose baby is younger than six months and is receiving only breast milk, has a very low chance of conception (1 to 2 percent per year), equivalent to the efficacy of the contraceptive pill. This contraceptive effect is known as the lactational amenorrhea method (LAM) and is the most common and effective method of child spacing in the world.[22] Ecological breastfeeding uses stricter criteria and reports an even better contraceptive effect.[23, 24] Breastfeeding therefore leads to wider child spacing, which enhances the survival and well-being of the mother and her subsequent babies.

Hormonal Highs for Mother and Baby

As well as all of the health benefits just described, breastfeeding offers other intrinsic rewards to mothers and babies. For all mammals, these include the effects of the breastfeeding hormones: oxytocin, the hormone of love; endorphins, hormones of pleasure; and prolactin, the mothering hormone. These hormones, which are released from deep within the brain with every breastfeeding episode, keep the nursing mother calm, relaxed, and lovingly focused on her baby. Babies also receive oxytocin and endorphins in breast milk, which explains the relaxation and pleasure that babies and children derive from breastfeeding.

Increased levels of beta-endorphin, which is present in breast milk and also released in the nursing baby's brain, may contribute to optimal brain development through enhancing the growth of brain cells in the orbitofrontal cortex.[25] (See chapter 11 for more.)

Both oxytocin and endorphins also activate the mesocorticolimbic dopamine pathways in the brain of mother and baby. The involvement of this powerful reward system, which is also associated with addictive and dependent behaviors, reflects the evolutionary importance of ongoing breastfeeding for the well-being of mother and baby. It also suggests that breastfeeding is designed to create a mutual dependency—what we might call a positive addiction—between mother and baby, which will optimize long-term well-being and survival for both partners.

Breastfeeding Beyond the Early Months

Although breastfeeding beyond the early months is still uncommon in most Western societies, it has been increasing in popularity in recent years. Sometimes called "extended," "long-term," or "full term" breastfeeding, nursing past one, and even two, years has endorsement from major organizations.

For example, the American Academy of Pediatrics now recommends breastfeeding for at least twelve months,[7] and the World Health Organization recommends that, for optimal growth, development, and health, breastfeeding should continue for up to two years or beyond.[26] The American Academy of Family Physicians (AAFP) states, "Breastfeeding beyond the first year offers considerable benefits to both mother and child, and should continue as long as mutually desired."[27]

Full-term breastfeeding also has strong historical and cross-cultural support. Mothers in most traditional cultures breastfeed into at least the second year, as did most mothers in western Europe until this century.[28] Even in medieval times, the dangers of early weaning were understood, and sickly infants, twins, and males were breastfed longer than the usual one to two years.[29]

Full-term breastfeeding continues to offer significant benefits for modern mothers and babies. Babies who are breastfed through the first year of life have fewer illnesses, both minor and major, [30, 31] and a lower chance of death[1] and serious illness—a protective benefit that extends to at least three years of age.[32] AAFP states, "If the child is younger than two years of age, the child is at increased risk of illness if weaned."[27]

Breastfeeding into the second year also gives a strong benefit in terms of nutrition. Research from Kenya, where the nursing mother's nutrition was judged to be marginal, has estimated that breast milk can supply up to one-third of a toddler's daily energy needs, as well as two-thirds of fat requirements, 58 percent of vitamin A requirements, and almost a third of calcium needs.[33] A U.S. study shows that breastfeeding through the first year has an ongoing dietary benefit, achieving a better food intake and less need for maternal persuasion to eat well in the second year.[34]

Breast milk also has continuing nutritional benefits for older children. After one year or so, the composition of breast milk changes, with increased amounts of the important long-chain fatty acids (LCFA) such as DHA that are critical in the formation and function of the brain and nervous system. Research shows that, although breastfeeding toddlers may receive a lower volume of milk, the increased concentration of LCFA makes their total intake, via breast milk, of brain-nourishing fats the same. The ongoing supply of LCFAs is optimal because, in humans, brain development continues through early childhood.

This rich fat content, along with the presence of the milk sugar lactose, also explains why older nursing children have described the taste of breast milk as "as good as chocolate" and "better than ice-cream."[35]

Newer studies that have looked at breastfeeding benefits in relation to duration of nursing have found that other protective effects, such as prevention of obesity and other illnesses, also increase with breastfeeding duration.[1] Researchers have also found that the immune benefits of breastfeeding actually increase as weaning approaches. Some have called this increase in antibodies, as breastfeeding declines, the "parting gift" to the baby, ensuring ongoing good health and strong immunity.[36, 37]

Full-term breastfeeding continues to give physical benefits to nursing mothers through the release of calming and rewarding hormones in her body as she nurses, as described earlier. As well as these immediate benefits, the nursing mother also receives longer-term protection against premenopausal breast cancer (more so with prolonged nursing),[15] ovarian cancer, and osteoporosis.[16] One study estimated that our current high rates of breast cancer in western countries would be reduced by almost half if we increased our lifetime duration of breastfeeding.[15]

Breastfeeding and Love

As a family physician, all of these benefits impress me, but as a nursing mother, the best aspects of breastfeeding have been the relationships with my nurslings. Breastfeeding has helped me to stay connected and in love, relaxed and open, and has reminded me that, as big as my nurslings may sometimes seem, they are in reality still young, with strong needs for nurture.

Through breastfeeding, we can promote heath and happiness in our families, and give our children the gift of a lifetime.

Bees, Baboo, and Boobies: My Breastfeeding Career

Bees, baboo, boobie. These are the words that my four children have used for my breasts and for their experiences of breastfeeding. Blissful, breast-full, intense, addictive. These are some of my experiences during my sixteen years of breastfeeding. Healthy, holistic, healing. These are just some properties of the liquid love that my breasts have generously produced, day in, day out, for my nurslings, and that every breastfeeding mother and baby enjoy.

My first child, Emma, was born in 1990, and as of this writing my youngest child, Maia, is recently weaned. Over this time—my "breastfeeding career"—I have discovered more about breastfeeding, and learned that it is actually designed to be blissful and addictive, and to reward both partners at each nursing episode through the flow of the hormones of love, pleasure, and tender mothering.

First Nursling

My story of breastfeeding begins with my birth in New Zealand in 1960. This era was a very low point for breastfeeding, and neither my three siblings nor I were breastfed. My mother was told that her ample breasts couldn't make enough milk, although I am sure that, given the right support, she could have breastfed as easily as her own mother, my grandmother, who nursed each of her three children for nine months.

When I became pregnant for the first time (then living in Melbourne, Australia), I had few concerns about breastfeeding; I simply presumed that it would be smooth and easy for me. Later in my pregnancy, I had a vivid dream that my baby was skinny in my womb but fattened up quickly on my breast. This was an accurate premonition; Emma was born at home after a short and sweet labor, one month early and weighing only 5 pounds 1 ounce (see the essay, "Emma's Birth—Sweet and Oceanic" on page 20). Her prematurity and low birth weight gave me and my partner Nicholas a beautiful opportunity to devote ourselves to her well-being, and she filled out within a few weeks, just as I had dreamt.

Breastfeeding Emma was an unexpected pleasure for me: holding her close by day and snuggling up with her for those long, milky nights. I returned to work part-time when she was four months old, leaving her in Nicholas's care. I learned the art of expressing, and of building up my milk to make it easy. For example, I would feed from one breast all night and express the other side in the morning. After a few months, Emma decided that she preferred to wait for my return, which I appreciated, being heavy with milk after a five-hour separation. I found expressing my milk to be rather a chore: luckily I was able to avoid it with my subsequent babies, who came to work with me.

Emma's first year came and went, and my contemporaries were weaning their babies. I enrolled in a women's health course and felt my focus begin to shift, all the while slowly cutting down Emma's breastfeedings. At this time, the idea of nursing a two-year-old was strange to me, and Nicholas thought it was positively warped (although his mother had breastfed him until he was eighteen months, in 1958!).

However, my revelation was soon to come. When Emma was fourteen months old, I came across a book called *Mothering Your Nursing Toddler*[1] at our local breastfeeding group. Here was one of the clearest expressions of what I wanted for my child—an inner sense of security, loving relationships, and good health—and it was as simple as continuing to breastfeed. Enthusiastically, I opened myself back up to Emma, and breastfed her right through my next pregnancy. When Zoe was born I tandem fed, and I finally weaned Emma when she was just over four—around the same time that I conceived my third child.

Second and Third Nurslings

Breastfeeding Emma through my second pregnancy wasn't always easy. My nipples were very sensitive, although this eased around twenty weeks. It was difficult, but necessary, to cut down on Emma's breastfeeding, and I noticed how much more solid food she ate; obviously she had still been substantially nourished through her five or six daily breastfeedings.

Zoe's birth was my most difficult. Like Emma, she was born posterior (facing up) and I had several challenging hours at the end of my labor (see page 33 for Zoe's story). Zoe was a very easy and content baby who lived in my front carrier—her outside womb—for quite a few months. Breastfeeding was again easy; Emma, at two years and ten months, was old enough to wait her turn, and I appreciated her help with my overabundant supply in the early days. I noticed with surprise that my toddler was gentler in her feeding than my chomping newborn.

When Zoe was just fourteen months old, I unexpectedly conceived again, while on a family holiday in Tasmania. It took me a while to realize that I was pregnant—I was sure that my delayed period was due to intensively breastfeeding Zoe, who had been sick with ear infections, fevers, and vomiting for the whole holiday.

I continued to nurse Zoe throughout this third pregnancy, supporting my body with traditional Chinese medicine and good nutrition. Toward the end of my pregnancy, when I really needed some space, I stopped nursing Zoe at night, and she moved to sleeping in another bed with Nicholas and Emma. Zoe had just celebrated her second birthday, and Emma was not yet five, when they saw their brother born—a beautiful waterbirth in the sunshine of our back room, overlooking the garden (see page 212 for Jacob's story).

Having three babies close together, and breastfeeding so intensely, was a big challenge for my body, and I learned a lot about looking after myself through this experience. One of the most nourishing rituals that I began was taking an afternoon rest. This hour or two in bed (or at least with my feet up) gave me a physical rest, and sometimes sleep too, and also quieted the house down. My children, if too old to sleep, could play with special toys, listen to tapes, or read books in bed with me. My afternoon rest kept my life simple by ensuring that major outings were confined to mornings, and also gave me the energy that I needed to get through the evening shift.

Having a regular massage also became a habit, and a wonderful way of thanking my body for the intense hands-on mothering that I have given to my children.

Jacob was another easygoing and delightful baby, adored by his big sisters. Feeding him was pleasurable, but I was stretched by feeding Zoe as well, and I often had to refuse her requests for "bees." When Jacob was around five months, Zoe stopped asking for regular breastfeeding, although I still nursed her occasionally until she was four or so. This was sad for me, but I really needed to look after myself at this time.

I had a great job to go back to, working with a homebirth family physician and his wife: I was able to choose my own hours, I could bring Jacob to work with me, and I was blessed with a wonderful caregiver for Zoe. However, work became less and less attractive, because of the organization and the shift in consciousness that I needed to make to be a good medical practitioner. I eventually went back to one half-day every two weeks when Jacob was nine months old, taking him with me, and I was relieved when our plan to move interstate allowed me to stop work altogether when he was around twenty months.

In Transit

We moved from Melbourne to Brisbane just before Jacob turned two, taking a month's camping vacation in the process. I spent most of the transition time feeding and carrying him, and it wasn't until we settled into our new home that I could pry him off my breast. After this I also stopped feeding him overnight (when he understood "no baboo until morning"), and later he moved in to sleep in a double bed with his sisters.

The next year was one of the most difficult times for me as a mother. We settled on the outskirts of Brisbane, where I had no friends or acquaintances, and I was at a low ebb physically, after eight years of continual breastfeeding (plus three pregnancies). I was lucky to find some wonderful natural health practitioners, who helped me rebuild my body with good nutrition and well-chosen remedies. (I took a lot of homeopathic sepia—the remedy for worn-out bodies!) Slowly I found my community of like-minded mothers and families, and I regained my vitality.

Jacob's late toddler age was replete with negotiation around "baboo," and my rule was "Baboo in the morning, baboo at rest time, baboo at sleep time"—a theme that I later repeated with Maia. Breastfeeding has, for me, naturally subsided as my nurslings have grown, due partly to their increasing interest in the outside world and partly to my own need to reclaim my space (and my breasts).

I was committed to breastfeeding Jacob until he was four and continued to nurse him happily twice a day or so. Going away for a day or two wasn't difficult, as we were both easy and flexible about it.

A few months before his fourth birthday, Jacob announced, "You can stop giving me baboo now, Mummy."

"Okay," I said, "but what if you change your mind?"

"Just say no," he advised me.

So the next time he asked, I did this, to which he replied, "I didn't mean it, Mummy!"

His fourth birthday was my limit, although there were maybe one or two breast-feedings afterward. I was also turning my attention to having another baby. One month after Jacob's weaning, I conceived Maia Rose; this delighted the children, especially Jacob, who told me, "Good Mummy for having another baby."

Fourth Nursling

Maia's was a very enjoyable pregnancy. We were all in a blissful state; the only tensions arose from negotiations between Nicholas and me about my desire for an unassisted birth. (See "Maia's Birth—A Family Celebration," page 128.) I enjoyed having a break from breastfeeding and began to wonder if I really wanted to go back to it. But after an ecstatic birth and beautiful baby, of course I loved every minute.

The early weeks with Maia were also blissful. I rested a lot—in fact, I stayed in pajamas for two weeks to mark this important respite, and Nicholas brought me lunch in bed every day. I knew, from experience, that this nourishment and rest would keep me centered for the whole of the following year. Our first outing was to take Maia to school as Jacob's "show and tell."

I did have some challenges at this time with baby Maia, who was unsettled at irregular times. With the help of a friend—a breastfeeding counselor and mother of five—I finally figured out that I had an oversupply problem; that is, my milk was let-ting down too quickly and in volumes too big for Maia's newborn digestive system. Once I adjusted my nursing techniques—feeding her in an upright position was especially effective—things settled down.

After this, breastfeeding was easy and enjoyable. I began practicing elimination communication (not using diapers) with Maia, which added another dimension to our relationship and increased my intuitive connection with her. (See my article at www.sarahjbuckley.com for more about this beautiful mothering practice.) She was very much an "in-arms" baby, and I barely put her down for the first six months. I carried her in my traditional Asian front pack during the day and nestled up with her for daytime and nighttime sleeps.

I stopped feeding Maia overnight at around two years of age, as I had with Jacob, and began to limit her daytime feedings to three or four. Our afternoon rests were simple, as she was usually eager to "have boobies, go sleep" after lunch. Her nighttimes have also been easy because our family members all go to bed together at around 8:30 P.M.

At age four—the time when my others had weaned—Maia continued to nurse occasionally, usually at sleep times. We continued to bed-share, and Maia had an acute awareness of my presence (or absence) at night, as she had as a baby. With time, her need for nursing decreased, and by five she was having only an occasional suckle. Her last breastfeed was a few weeks past her seventh birthday.

For me, breastfeeding has been meditative as well as pleasurable, and has contributed immensely to the mindfulness of my mothering. Breastfeeding has kept me soft, present, and surrendered, and with each episode I have consciously experienced the dissolution of my self, as "my heart melts, and flows into my baby as breastmilk" as Jeannine Parvati Baker so eloquently says.

My breasts have been all kinds of shapes and sizes over the years, and now, toward the end of my breastfeeding career, they are different again. They are softer and stretchier—more relaxed, as Emma kindly observed, especially my well-loved nipples. My breasts have been a source of pleasure and nourishment for my children, and through them I have also been pleasured and nourished.

Breastfeeding reminds us of the universal truth of abundance; the more we give out, the more we are filled up, and that divine nourishment—the source from which we all draw—is, like a mother's breast, ever full and ever flowing.

chapter 13

BABIES, MOTHERS, AND THE SCIENCE OF SHARING SLEEP

Sleep is a major issue for new parents in our culture: how can we get more sleep, how can our babies get more sleep, and how can we ensure their safety during sleep? There are a variety of answers to these questions, most of which are based on cultural assumptions rather than science—or even common sense. This chapter introduces both science and common sense into this vexed and emotive issue, and provides information to help parents decide what sleep arrangements will work best in their own families.

Babies and sleep. Sometimes it can seem that the two are mutually exclusive, and sleep issues can be worsened by those pervasive questions asked of all new mothers: "Is he a good baby?" and "Is she sleeping through the night?"

Although well-meaning, such questions can leave us wondering whether we, or our babies, are displaying early signs of misbehavior, even social deviance, by refusing to sleep through the night. We might worry that we are allowing long-term and perhaps permanent "bad habits" to develop from frequent waking that will perpetuate the bone-aching tiredness that we feel every morning. We worry that we ourselves might never again sleep through the night.

In the face of these worries, and the widespread pressure to conform to social norms of infant sleep, we are unlikely to confess our true nocturnal habits: that we sometimes bring our babies into bed with us because it's the only way we can begin to feel rested. Again we might worry that we are risking our baby's well-being—or even her or his life. We wonder if babies have changed in a generation, or if our foremothers, and mothers in other cultures, might have faced the same dilemmas.

And sometimes, when it's very dark and quiet, we may be comforted by the image of mothers and babies all around the world, sleeping and waking through the night: a vast blanket of nocturnal mothering spreading as the world turns to darkness, and folding away with sunrise.

Perhaps the nights aren't so bad after all.

Babies and Sleep

One of the problems that our culture creates for new mothers is the belief that infant sleep is, or should quickly become, the same as adult sleep. This makes "sleeping through the night" an important goal. However, this idea is based on a misunderstanding of normal infant sleep and is the source of much misinformation and even suffering for mothers, babies, and families.

Mothers will recognize that their babies do not follow adult patterns of behavior in other areas such as feeding, motor abilities, and daytime sleep, so it is logical that baby's nighttime sleep patterns will also be unique and evolving. All this is due to the extreme immaturity of our human baby's brain and nervous system: a baby's brain is only one-quarter of adult size at birth, compared with at least one-half adult size in other animals. This makes human babies the least capable and most dependent on parental care of any species.

Furthermore, as scientists have discovered, our babies' dramatic brain development does not automatically unfold with time, as was previously thought, but is crucially dependent on the context and care that surrounds them. As Rima Shore comments in the Families and Work Institute report, *Rethinking the Brain*,[1] "Early interactions don't just create a context; they directly affect the way the brain is wired."

This combination of nature and nurture will be enhanced when we follow our babies' cues, which tell us their developmental needs at every stage of parenting. It can be reassuring to know that we don't need a degree in child development to mother well, only the willingness to respond to our instincts and our babies in a way that brings peace, joy, and ease at each age and stage.

Evolutionary Perspectives
and Mutual Regulation

If we understand that our baby's sleep patterns have evolved over millions of years, and that, for the vast majority of this time, mothers and babies have lived in the wild, we can understand the logic of infant sleep.

In this context, sharing sleep has been a necessity for infant survival, giving babies not only safety from predators, but also warmth, easy access to mother's breast, and assistance with the function and maturation of developing bodily processes through mutual regulation.

Mutual regulation refers to the influence that mother and baby have on each other's physiology and behavior, helping to bring them into optimal function. One example is regulation of temperature. When a newborn is placed skin to skin with the mother, maternal body heat will increase, without her awareness, and her baby will be warmer than a newborn who is wrapped and placed in a crib.[2] Skin-to-skin contact between mother and baby, sometimes called "kangaroo care," also helps stabilize the baby's heart rate and breathing.[3]

Sleep laboratory studies of mothers and baby show similar effects, with babies that share the same sleeping surface (bed sharing) having warmer temperatures[4] and faster heart rates[5] compared with solitary sleeping babies. Bed sharing babies also move more, which may contribute to temperature and heart rate effects and which also reflects the richer sensory environment and extra stimulation of smell, touch, taste, and hearing that they gain through close proximity to the mother.

Babies who sleep in the same room as the parents (one form of co-sleeping) have been shown to have up to five times less risk of sudden infant death syndrome (SIDS) compared with babies sleeping in a separate room.[6] It is likely that this also reflects mutual regulation, with the parent's presence and regular breathing helping to regulate the baby's breathing. (See chapter 11 for more about mutual regulation.)

Separation and Stress

In psychological terms, physical closeness with the mother, by day as well as at night, also represents security and safety and is what all mammalian babies expect. A mammalian baby who is separated from the mother will utter a separation distress call that alerts the mother and motivates her to retrieve her young. This has also been observed in newborn human babies.[7]

The significant stress that occurs when mammalian babies are physically disconnected from their mothers, even for short periods of time, has been shown in animal research to have detrimental effects into adulthood and to increase susceptibility to stress for the rest of their lives.[8]

Similarly, when a human baby is left isolated (that is, with no sensory contact with the mother or other caregiver) the baby's nervous system will signal life-threatening danger, and the infant is programmed, through millions of years of evolution, to protest through crying. Crying is usually a very effective signal to elicit care and reconnection. This explains why babies will cry when we try to "put them down" in the day or night, and also explains their built-in, ongoing need for reassurance and security through physical contact.

It is possible that significant adverse effects may occur for human babies, as for other species, following separation from the mother, especially in the early weeks; if separation is prolonged and/or if the baby exhibits signs of severe stress. Severe stress is evident when a long bout of solitary distress and crying is followed by quieting, with emotional and physical withdrawal. This mammalian "despair-dissociation" response is designed for extreme circumstances in which crying fails to reestablish contact with the mother, and it becomes safer to shut down and feign death. The protest-despair response is associated with particularly high brain levels of the stress hormone cortisol. High cortisol levels can lead to permanent changes in important brain structures, including the amygdala and the hippocampus, which is involved with the formation of memory and is especially vulnerable to stress.[9] (See chapter 11 for more about the despair-dissociation response.)

These findings should make us very cautious about subjecting babies and young children to methods such as "controlled crying" and "crying it out," designed to make our babies to sleep for longer periods. These methods will almost certainly provoke the protest-despair response and high cortisol levels in our babies—and likely in ourselves, if we are listening to our babies crying for many minutes.

Controlled crying and crying it out are usually a last resort for parents who are desperate for sleep, as we all are at times. However, these methods not only are likely to be harmful, but also do not generally produce long-lasting results and must be repeated at regular intervals. This is not surprising when we consider that we are trying to shift hard-wired brain patterns that have ensured optimal infant care and survival for millennia.

The alternative to these methods is to work with our biology and instincts and consider giving our babies the security and happiness that they need, day and night. Our babies' nocturnal needs can be most easily met, as they have been for millennia, by some form of cosleeping.[10]

The Variety of Cosleeping

As implied, cosleeping is not one single arrangement for mother-baby sleep, but reflects a variety of possibilities used with different children, families, and cultures.

Technically, the term *cosleeping* refers to any arrangement in which mother (or caregiver) and baby are sleeping close to each other, but not necessarily on the same sleeping surface. Cosleeping practices can include baby sleeping in a basket, crib, or "side car" on or next to the bed; baby in a basket suspended from the ceiling over the bed; baby in a crib or cot in the same room as the parents (and possibly other children); baby in bed with mother and/or father; baby in bed with grandparents.

The term *bed sharing* is confined to practices whereby the mother (or other responsive adult) and baby are sleeping on the same surface, although this also can vary. In some cultures, the baby may have separate bedding or be placed on a specialized pillow, as in China.

McKenna and McDade suggest that we define safe mother-infant cosleeping as "a class of sleeping arrangements in which at least one responsible, safety-educated, adult co-sleeper (whether mother or not) sleeps close enough to actively monitor (and/or breastfeed) the infant using at least two sensory modalities simultaneously, i.e. tactile and visual, or auditory and visual, or auditory and tactile etc etc."[11]

Modern Sleep Arrangements

Although solitary infant sleep has become normal, even required, in many Western cultures, it is actually a very recent and culturally unique phenomenon. In Western cultures, bed sharing between mother and nursing baby (usually up to two years old) was standard practice until around

150 years ago. Older children would cosleep with siblings, with a member of the extended family, or, among the upper classes, with a servant or nursemaid.[12]

The 1800s saw the rise of the child-rearing expert, usually male, who emphasized self-reliance from an early age, with strict guidelines for breastfeeding, toilet training, and sleep. Newborns were expected to sleep with the mother, but they were to be removed to an unshared room before the age of one.[12]

With the Industrial Revolution in the late 1800s and the decline of the extended family, most mothers outside of the wealthy upper class became solely responsible for the house and children, and this was easier if each child required less of the mother's one-on-one time. Solitary sleeping was further encouraged by the discovery that diseases such as tuberculosis could spread via inhalation, and people were warned not to breathe the air of another.[12]

As the twentieth century advanced, smaller and increasingly affluent families began to build houses with separate sleeping quarters, so that each child could sleep alone. The myth arose that "crib (cot) death" was caused by mothers overlaying and smothering their babies; this misinformation further frightened mothers away from sleeping with their babies.[12] Recent recommendations in relation to Sudden Infant Death Syndrome (SIDS) and cosleeping[13] have maintained the cultural bias toward solitary infant sleep.

However, this shift to solitary sleep has not been a global phenomenon: worldwide, mother-infant cosleeping is still widespread.[14, 15] A 1971 anthropological survey of 186 cultures found that, in every culture, the baby slept in sensory proximity to a person, and that, in two-thirds of cultures, mother and baby shared a bed.[16] More recent studies show that cosleeping is still widely practiced; for example, around three-quarters of mothers in Singapore bed-share with their babies,[17] and bed sharing up to school age is considered a "normal family activity" in Sweden.[18]

An international survey from 2001 reports the highest rates of bed sharing in China, Sweden, Chile, and Denmark (88, 65, 64, and 39 percent respectively) and the lowest rates in Turkey, Ukraine, Argentina, and Hungary (2, 9, 15, and 16 respectively). In this survey, the cosleeping rate in Manitoba, Canada, was 23 percent, and 21 and 25 percent in Scotland and Ireland, respectively.[15]

A U.S. survey found that, in 2000, 47.3 percent of parents reported sleeping with their babies at some time, with around 13 percent of babies usually sharing an adult bed at night.[19]

Note that cosleeping, and especially bed sharing, is likely to be significantly underreported, as many parents who bring the baby into their bed at some time may not categorize themselves as bed sharing.[19] A UK study that asked more detailed questions found that 70 percent of parents had bed-shared with their baby at some time in the first three months.[20]

The Science of Bed Sharing

Early researchers in infant sleep research used solitary-sleeping babies as the norm. Little was known about the biological processes involved with cosleeping or bed sharing before professor of anthology James McKenna and his colleagues invited mothers and babies into their sleep laboratory to monitor their physiology (body processes) during sleep.

These researchers have subsequently conducted many studies, monitoring overnight sleep patterns as mothers and babies slept together or in separate rooms. They found that not only do bed sharing pairs get into the same sleep cycles, but babies who bed-share experience more frequent arousals, triggered by the mother's movements, and spend less time in deep sleep.[21]

As a researcher in SIDS, Professor McKenna believes that these low-level arousals, which do not actually awaken either partner, give the baby practice in arousing and may lessen a baby's susceptibility to some forms of SIDS, which are thought to be caused when a baby fails to arouse from deep sleep to reestablish breathing patterns. Professor McKenna speculates that our young babies are not developmentally prepared to sleep through the night in a solitary bed, which involves long periods of deep sleep, which is not a normal pattern for young babies.

Videos taken during these studies show that bed sharing mothers, even in deep sleep, are obviously aware of their baby's position, and move when necessary to avoid overlaying. At no time in the studies did bed sharing mothers impede the breathing of their babies, who had higher average oxygen levels than solitary sleepers.[21]

McKenna's conclusions—that bed sharing and other forms of co-sleeping may actually protect against SIDS—are supported by population studies in places where cosleeping is prevalent. Places such as Hong Kong[22] and China[15] have some of the lowest rates of SIDS in the world, along with high rates of cosleeping.

Bed sharing and other forms of cosleeping, especially when associated with breastfeeding, are also likely to enhance infant brain levels of beta-endorphin, a hormone of pleasure that is released during breastfeeding and other pleasurable social and physical infant-parent interactions. Beta-endorphin is thought to enhance growth in parts of the brain that regulate emotional states,[23] a finding that emphasizes the importance of pleasure and pleasurable interactions for young babies.

The Safety of Bed Sharing

In the developed world, SIDS is the most common cause of death for infants between one month and one year old, and peaks between the ages of two and four months. In the last few decades researchers have investigated many factors that may increase or reduce SIDS risk, including infant sleeping practices. One breakthrough has been the identification of prone (face down) sleeping as a major risk factor, and global "back to sleep" awareness campaigns have drastically reduced SIDS incidence, especially in those westernized countries where SIDS incidence has been high. More recent studies, discussed in detail shortly, have investigated the interactions between SIDS and bed sharing, and, although conclusions remain controversial, some light has been shed in this area.

Most SIDS researchers use a *case-control* technique, whereby factors possibly associated with SIDS are compared between SIDS babies (cases) and larger numbers of healthy babies (controls). For example, if 90 percent of SIDS cases were found in the prone position, but only 10 percent of controls, we would guess that the prone position could be a risk factor for SIDS. More sophisticated (multivariate) analysis is then used to tease out different influences and estimate the numerical risks of individual factors.

Research that describes only the number of cases and does not include a control group is not useful or accurate in assessing risks. This includes high-profile studies that have used the U.S. Consumer Product Safety

Commission and similar data (which lists the number of babies dying in adult beds, but with no comparison figures) to recommend against bed sharing.[24, 25]

Other studies have used inaccurately low bed sharing figures in comparison groups, leading to significant overestimation of risks. For example, one U.S. study based its extreme conclusions about the risks of infant suffocation in adult beds on a bed sharing rate of 9 percent,[6] whereas surveys mentioned previously found that almost half of U.S. babies bed-share at some time.[20] (This figure has increased from around 40 percent in the early 1990s[20] and may be underreported, as previously mentioned.)[20]

Several excellent large case-control studies have looked at the relationship between bed sharing and SIDS, controlling for many other factors known to influence SIDS risks. In a large and extremely detailed UK study, Blair and colleagues found that bed sharing was not a risk factor for SIDS once statistical consideration was made for maternal alcohol use, maternal smoking, use of duvets (comforters, continental quilts), extreme parental tiredness, and household overcrowding. These factors were especially important for infants under fourteen weeks of age.[27] Similarly, a large New Zealand study found that bed sharing was a risk factor for SIDS only if the mother smoked or had smoked during pregnancy.[28] A study from urban Chicago found no increased risks when a baby shared the bed with only the (nonsmoking) parents.[29]

Several studies have suggested that bed sharing may be unsafe for younger, but not older, babies. Two studies showed a small additional SIDS risk for bed sharing babies aged less than eight weeks[30] and fourteen weeks,[27] although in the latter study this risk was not significant when maternal smoking was taken into account.[27] A recent Scottish study is the only research to find a sizeable increase in SIDS risk for babies of any age (in this case, only babies less than eleven weeks) who were bed sharing with nonsmoking mothers.[1]

Other limitations of SIDS and bed sharing studies include a lack of differentiation between habitual and reactive bed sharing.[32] For example, a baby who is brought into the parent's bed because of illness or unsettled behavior may already be at increased risk of SIDS, because even mild illness is a risk factor for SIDS. In this way, bed sharing may be falsely associated with higher SIDS risk. The only study that has controlled for habitual/reactive bed sharing found no link between bed sharing and SIDS.[27]

Other researchers have also noted that bed sharing in SIDS cases seems to cluster with other risk factors such as adolescent mothers; poverty; black race; sleeping baby in prone position; presence of bedding hazards, including pillows that can overlay the baby and other children sharing the bed; and sleeping on a sofa or other unsafe surface.[33] Case-control studies that have found increased SIDS risks for bed sharing babies have generally not accounted for all of these factors, especially bedding hazards.

One small but detailed study from Alaska, where SIDS incidence has decreased and bed sharing increased in recent years,[34] found that only one out of forty bed sharing SIDS babies died without the presence of risk factors such as sleeping prone, parental intoxication, and/or sleeping on a waterbed or sofa.[35]

It is also likely, as will be discussed, that bed sharing practices associated with breastfeeding are different from, and probably safer than, those associated with formula feeding. This has been poorly studied, and feeding status has not been recorded in many of the large studies.

In spite of these controversies and a serious lack of high-quality data, in 2005 the American Academy of Pediatrics (AAP) issued a policy statement recommending against bed sharing.[13] This policy is likely to do more harm than good, given the strong links between bed sharing and breastfeeding, and the well-recognized benefits of breastfeeding. Bed sharing and other forms of cosleeping are also increasing in popularity, making it even more important to inform parents how to bed-share safely. This approach has been endorsed by organizations such as UNICEF,[36] the Academy of Breastfeeding Medicine,[37] and the Royal Australasian College of Physician and Surgeons, Pediatrics and Child Health Division.[38]

Safety in Perspective

To summarize the studies, "bed sharing may not be a risk factor per se but an environment in which specific risk factors may be present."[39] This statement highlights the importance of reducing known risks and hazards in the bed sharing environment (see "Ten Tips for Safe Sleeping" at the end of this chapter). Breastfeeding is likely to be an important and perhaps protective factor against SIDS, especially in bed sharing situations. McKenna comments, "No epidemiological study to date has included a sufficient number of exclusively breast feeding, nonsmoking, safe bed sharing mother-infant pairs to know if this arrangement can be, as has been hypothesized, protective . . ."[40]

It is also important to be aware of the actual magnitude of the issue. Although SIDS remains the leading cause of infant mortality beyond the newborn period, the overall incidence is low. Around 1 baby per 2,000 dies of SIDS in the United States and the UK, with the highest rate in any developed country (New Zealand) still fewer than 1 baby per 1,000.[41]

Bed Sharing and Breastfeeding

The combination of breastfeeding and bed sharing (or other forms of cosleeping) is ideal for both mother and baby. Studies show that bed sharing mothers breastfeed more often overnight, and bed sharing babies nurse for two to three times longer, than during solitary sleep.[10, 42] This ensures optimal infant nutrition and also optimizes the mother's milk supply.

Bed sharing reinforces breastfeeding because it is easier for a bed sharing (or cosleeping) mother to accomplish the more frequent feeding that a breastfed baby requires, because of the high digestibility of breast milk and the human baby's small stomach.[42]

As McKenna and McDade comment, "mother-infant cosleeping represents the most biologically appropriate sleeping arrangement for humans and is both ancient and ubiquitous simply because breast feeding is not possible, nor as easily managed, without it."[43]

UK researchers have built on McKenna's sleep-lab data by recording bed sharing mothers and babies in their own homes, finding some important differences between the bed sharing practices associated with breastfeeding and formula feeding.

Overnight filming has shown that breastfed babies almost always sleep facing the mother's body, with the baby's head at breast level. Breastfeeding mothers usually cradle their babies, with an over-arching arm preventing the baby from moving up and a curled-up leg preventing the baby from moving down. In these studies, nursing mothers and their babies spent three-quarters of the time actually touching each other.[44]

Bed sharing, breastfeeding mothers also frequently checked their babies during the night, visually and by touch, and acted to uncover their heads, if necessary, during the night.[44] Researchers speculate that maternal impairment by alcohol or extreme fatigue may increase SIDS risk by impairing this (or another) aspect of maternal responsiveness.[45]

In contrast, bed sharing, formula-fed babies tended to be placed higher in the bed, at eye level with the mother and sometimes on top of pillows, which is hazardous because the baby can move down and become overlaid by the pillow. Formula-feeding mothers and babies spent less time facing each other, and mothers also had fewer arousals and so spent less time available to monitor infant safety.

Formula-fed babies were more often on their backs, whereas breastfeeding babies spent more than half the time on their sides.[44] Although this is not the ideal position according to our current knowledge, and it has been found to increase SIDS risk generally, side-sleeping in the context of breastfeeding and bed sharing may give less, or no, added risk. Researchers observed that very few breastfeeding babies rolled forward into the unsafe prone position because this was prevented by the mother's proximity.[44]

In another study by the same group, 253 mothers and babies were followed over time with interviews and sleep logs. Researchers found that more of the non-bed sharing mothers abandoned breastfeeding in the early weeks. Lead investigator Helen Ball comments: "When mothers are not prepared to get up periodically in the night and breastfeed, they generally pursue one of three options: (1) feed the baby formula . . . (2) undertake a 'sleep training' program . . . or (3) sleep next to the baby . . ." [46]

These studies highlight the complex interrelationships between bed sharing and infant feeding as well as our need for more sophisticated research to increase our understanding. However, the information that we do have supports the belief that mother-baby breastfeeding and bed sharing are part of a mutually beneficial evolutionary system with significant benefits (especially the lifelong benefits associated with successful and long-term breastfeeding) that will balance any possible risks, which are not as yet clear from the research.[10]

This research also tells us that bed sharing formula-feeding mothers may need to take extra precautions, especially with regard to safe placement of the baby.

Simple Sleep with Tired Children

Bed sharing is widely practiced because parents are largely practical people. Bed sharing helps with nighttime parenting because it gives us more time horizontal in bed, helping us to feel rested even when nights are busy. Bed sharing also gives us less time vertical, feeding and settling our babies, which is how we might otherwise spend much of our nights. Mothers who breastfeed and bed-share also can, and usually do, fall asleep while nursing, helped by the calming effect of the breastfeeding hormones.

Bed sharing is not a holy grail of parenting, however safe and evolutionary it may be, and may not suit every mother and her baby. Many families (including those from other cultures) have adapted other forms of cosleeping to suit themselves.

For example, if parents need more space in the night than bed sharing allows, they can consider having a cot, crib, cradle, or "side car" next to the bed or in the same room. (Given the data presented, I would always encourage parents to at least bring their young baby into their bedroom.) McKenna and McDade suggest that safe cosleeping allows for supervision of the baby with at least two senses, and babies can be both heard and seen with these arrangements. Parents should always ensure that their cosleeping arrangement does not allow any gaps greater than one inch (2.5 centimeters, approximately two finger-widths) as recommended in "Ten Tips for Safe Sleeping" on page 263.

Babies and young children will usually fall asleep more readily when they have company and feel secure. Breastfed babies, like their mothers, also benefit from the release of relaxing hormones, including beta-endorphin and oxytocin, which together make breastfeeding Mother Nature's best sleeping potion. Many mothers, myself included, also find it easy and enjoyable to breastfeed older babies and even toddlers to sleep, especially for daytime naps.

In my own experience, the supposedly dire consequences of nursing my young children to sleep have not materialized, and all my children have developed healthy sleep habits. Our family likes easy evenings, so we have committed to provide adult company (and perhaps a lullaby) to help our older, weaned children fall asleep. We have also encouraged older siblings to share sleep, which seems to help their daytime relationships. And even though my children are used to company at night, this has not prevented them from enjoying "sleeping over" with friends and relations, even while still nursing.

Long-Term Cosleeping

Two of the main concerns that parents may have are "Will we be able to stop our child from cosleeping, once we start?" and "Will cosleeping discourage my child from becoming independent in the long term?"

It is important to remember that cosleeping, and the need for security at night, is programmed into the brain of every child as a survival instinct, as discussed previously. This explains the stubborn difficulties that we will encounter, and the extreme limits that we must go to, if we want our babies and children to sleep alone all night. Cosleeping is difficult to stop only because our children learn that their fears will be lessened, and sleeping made easier, with nighttime company.

From the perspective of evolution and safety in the wild, we could consider that our children are hardwired to comfortably sleep alone only when they can at least attempt to defend themselves from nighttime predators, which is one reason why most of us prefer company at night, including most parents.

However, cosleeping and bed sharing become more negotiable with older children, and it is almost always possible to find an arrangement that works for everyone. Solitary sleeping children may need company while falling asleep, as my children have, and appreciate easy access to a comforting adult presence during the dark hours if needed, either in their own bed (double beds work well for obvious reasons) or in a family bed. A large family bed suits some families, and a king-size bed (one of the best investments for family sleep) can be turned sideways to comfortably sleep three or even four.

Parents can also be reassured that cosleeping is much more likely to benefit than harm their children's psychological development. Several studies have surveyed cosleepers from children through adults, finding no detrimental effects and some beneficial ones. For example, one study found enhanced self-esteem among college students who had bed-shared in childhood, along with less guilt and anxiety.[47] Another study found more engagement in social activities, and better scores from teachers, among military children who had bed-shared, as well as a lower chance of requiring psychiatric care.[48] A U.S. survey of 1,400 adults from different ethnic backgrounds found more positive adult outcomes, including more satisfaction with life, among those who had bed-shared as children.[49] Another large U.S. study, which followed children to age eighteen, found no benefits or harm for offspring who had bed-shared as children.[50] These studies are well summarized in McKenna and McDade's excellent review.[10]

Parental intimacy can be another concern, but again, creativity, flexibility with timing, and double beds elsewhere are helpful. Young babies seem to have an intimacy radar and will often awake at the most inconvenient times, even when sleeping in another room.

Simple Sleep for Tired Parents

Perhaps all the fuss about babies and sleep isn't really about our babies' ability to sleep through the night but about our own perceived need for uninterrupted sleep. Research and anecdotes from other cultures show that this is not a universal expectation,[14] and that worldwide, most new mothers would not say that their baby or child had a sleep problem because he or she woke frequently at night.[14]

However, our Western expectations and activities are different. For example, most new mothers need to "operate heavy machinery" (that is, drive a car) every day, an activity that requires a high level of concentration, especially compared with the more straightforward tasks that women have traditionally combined with early mothering. Many women are also working full- or part-time outside the home in their baby's first year, which may require a degree of intellectual focus that is harder to achieve when nights are busy.

However, if we can focus more on our own need for rest, simple solutions may arise. For example, I recommend a daytime nap for all mothers of young children. At least an hour spent horizontal while the baby sleeps is ideal and can often be combined with a rest or sleep time for other children; even fifteen minutes can be helpful. This is usually a better investment in family sanity than time spent doing domestic or other work while the baby sleeps. It is important to remember (and to remind others) that this need for extra rest will pass as our babies mature.

Sharing parenting responsibilities with your spouse or another adult is also ideal, and many fathers excel at, and enjoy, a morning or evening shift with their babies and other children. Again, I recommend paring back other commitments and expectations and focusing on rest and restoration, or another replenishing activity, during this time. When nights were busy with my babies and small children, my own rule of thumb was to be in bed for twelve hours—for example, from 8 P.M. to 8 A.M.

Mothers who work full-time outside the home may find this more challenging, but may also enjoy the intimacy and extra contact that co-sleeping provides, using what Canadian obstetrician and mother of four Alison Barrett describes as "reverse cycle mothering."[51]

Concluding with a Little Rest . . .

Caring for a young baby is a huge task, day and night, and we need as much support, and rest, as possible.

Australian cartoonist Michael Leunig has inspired me to take many restful interludes during the intense years of early parenting. His mythical exchange between cartoon heroes Mr. Curly and Vasco Pyjama on the subject "What is worth doing and what is worth having"[52] ends in this way:

> I gently urge you Vasco, do as we do in Curly Flat—learn to curl up and rest—feel your noble tiredness—learn about it and make a generous place for it in your life, and enjoyment will surely follow. I repeat: it's worth doing nothing and having a rest.

Ten Tips for Safe Sleeping

Whether your baby sleeps in a nearby cot, bassinet, crib, or "side car," or shares your bed, there are some general principles that will make your baby's sleep as safe as possible. These apply to all babies under the age of one.

1. **Put your baby on his or her back to sleep**

   Babies are more at risk of sudden infant death syndrome (SIDS) when they sleep prone; that is, face down. A baby in the prone position can't get rid of body heat as efficiently and can't kick off excess bedding. Both factors can contribute to overheating, a risk factor for SIDS. "Back to sleep" campaigns in many countries have reduced the number of babies dying of SIDS by up to 70 percent.

   If you are breastfeeding and bed sharing, your baby may spend time in the side position during and following nursing. Although this position is recognized as a SIDS risk factor, we do not know if this also applies to breastfeeding, bed sharing babies, who are much less likely to roll into the prone position (see page 257). It may be safer to turn your baby onto her or his back.

2. **Keep your baby's head uncovered during sleep**

   Babies are safest without soft bedding around them. This includes pillows (no child under one needs a pillow), duvets, or comforters (blankets are safer), crib or cot bumper pads (not recommended), and soft toys, all of which can end up over the baby's head. Sheets need to be tucked in firmly, or fitted snugly, so that they can't come loose. Loose bedding can cover and suffocate.

   Babies in a crib or cot are safest tucked in firmly with their foot at the bottom. Bed sharing babies also need to be kept from slipping under the bedding.

   Water beds and beanbags are not safe places for sleeping babies, who can slip into a soft pocket of bedding. Firm mattresses are recommended wherever your baby sleeps. If one parent is very heavy, use a very firm mattress to ensure that the baby cannot roll into a depression in the mattress. If bed sharing with another adult as well as your baby, it is probably safest to sleep your baby on the outside edge, rather than between two adults.

3. **Avoid entrapment hazards**

A young baby can wriggle into a small gap and suffocate. A hazardous gap may be formed:

- Between a mattress and the side of a crib (cot): most standards allow a gap no greater than one inch (2.5 centimeters or two finger widths)
- Between the mattress of an adult bed and the wall or adjoining furniture
- Between the mattress and headboard, footboard, and railings
- Between a mattress and a bed guard rail (bed guard rails are not recommended for children under one, but I highly recommend the simple "Humanity Family Bed cosleeper" for a safe guard system)

An adult mattress used for bed sharing may be safer on the floor well away from walls, but you should always ensure that a baby who rolls off is safe from entrapment and injury.

4. **Avoid strangulation hazards**

Check your baby's sleep environment for long strings or ties. This also applies to mobiles hung over cribs (cots). It is recommended that bed sharing adults prevent entanglement or strangulation by tying up their hair if it is longer than waist length. Again, crib (cot) bumpers (with or without ties) are not recommended.

5. **Dress your baby appropriately for the room temperature**

It is important to avoid both over- and underheating. In winter, your baby does not need both very warm clothing and very warm bedding. A solitary sleeping baby can be dressed in a blanket sleeper or securely tucked into bedding appropriate to the season.

A bed sharing baby will stay warm via body contact and does not need more than one layer of clothing. A cotton singlet or T-shirt, long- or short-sleeved according to the climate, and a diaper (nappy) are usually sufficient. Natural-fiber (cotton, wool, hemp, silk) clothing and bedding is recommended.

Also ensure that the room is neither overheated nor too cool. Consider whether the heating, bedding, and clothing would add up to a comfortable sleeping temperature for you.

6. **Keep yourself smoke- and drug-free**

This means avoiding smoking during pregnancy as well as after birth. Studies show that babies born to mothers who smoked in pregnancy have an increased risk of SIDS, and it is recommended that these mothers do not bed-share with their babies.

After birth, keep cigarette smoke away from your baby at all times. For mothers who cannot quit, cutting down will reduce the risk to some extent. Babies are also generally safer from SIDS if the father does not smoke, and bed sharing with a smoking father may increase the risk of SIDS. If either parent smokes, they can still safely sleep their baby on a separate surface close by.

It is also important that bed sharing parents are not under the influence of drugs or alcohol. These can make them sleep too deeply to monitor their baby's safety overnight.

7. **Do not put your baby to sleep alone in an adult bed**
Adult beds present entrapment hazards, as noted, as well as the danger of suffocation from soft bedding. Your baby is safer sleeping alone in a crib (cot) or in a safe place on a mattress on the floor, away from pets. It is also unsafe to sleep a baby next to a sibling or young child who might roll onto them.

Cultures with low SIDS rates incorporate baby sleep time into family life; for example, having babies sleep in a family room rather than isolating them at sleep time (which may increase SIDS vulnerability). Most babies will sleep happily with a large amount of noise and activity around them. (Consider how noisy and active it was in your belly!)

8. **Ensure that older babies in cribs (cots) cannot climb or fall out**
Once your baby can sit, lower the mattress if it is adjustable. Once the baby can stand, put the mattress at the lowest level and ensure that there are no aids to escape—that is, items the baby can stand on or pull down into the crib (cot). A child who is taller than 35 inches (90 centimeters) has outgrown the crib (cot).

9. **Do not put your baby to sleep on a sofa or chair**
Not only is this dangerous in terms of falling off, but babies can become entrapped in the gaps of a sofa or chair, which are much more hazardous than a bed, crib, or cot.

Also check your baby carriage or stroller and do not leave your baby sleeping there without adult supervision. Babies can become entrapped or suffocated while sleeping in these, which are not designed for unsupervised sleep.

10. Breastfeed your baby

In some studies, breastfeeding has been shown to give added protection against SIDS, which may be greater with more frequent breastfeeding. Breast-fed babies arouse more readily from deep sleep, which may help protect from SIDS.

Breastfeeding and bed sharing are an ideal combination, because bed sharing babies nurse more frequently but with less effort on the mother's part. This extra breastfeeding provides more nourishment for the baby and benefits the mother by delaying the return of her fertility, acting as a natural birth control mechanism.

If you are formula feeding, bed sharing may be less safe: it may be prefer-able to provide a separate, close-by sleep surface for your baby.

EPILOGUE: BECOMING A PARENT

PREPARING FOR PREGNANCY; conceiving a new soul; growing a child within our bodies; releasing our babies into the world at birth; caring for our vulnerable newborns: these powerful experiences involve great joy and great responsibility, and are the beginnings of our lifelong journey as parents.

In this book I have striven to provide information and ideas for informed decision-making, so that mothers- and fathers-to-be can make the choices that are right for themselves, their babies, and their families. Sometimes those decisions will align with cultural expectations and conventional medical advice: at other times, a family's right choices may be radically different from the mainstream, and even from their previous beliefs. The overall message I hope you take away from this book is the importance of taking the time to think *and* feel: of using instinct and intelligence, heart and mind as we make the choices that will best serve our children-to-be, our families, and ourselves.

When Things Go Wrong

Events will not always turn out as we would hope, even with openhearted intentions and thoughtful decision making. Birth and parenting, like life, may involve unexpected, disappointing, or even tragic events for ourselves or our babies, and we may wonder whether different outcomes might have accompanied different choices. In other situations we may find no explanation or reasons, and may ultimately have to accept that there was no way to avoid the unexpected.

Following any unwelcome outcome, which can include birth experiences that could be defined as "normal" but where there was fear, helplessness, confusion, or horror, it is important to acknowledge our questions and disappointments, ideally with the help of a partner, husband, trusted friend, or professional. This may open to deeper emotions such as sadness, hurt, and anger. We can help resolve these important feelings with deep reflection: ongoing conversations with supportive friends, counseling, healing groups (including women's circles), and other forms of therapy. Ideally we will work with people who have experience or expertise in dealing with birth or parenting trauma.

Acknowledging the trauma and asking for help are important first steps, but our healing can be simple and primarily solitary, if we wish, using techniques such as journaling and drawing. Sometimes physical forms of healing, such as osteopathy, chiropractic, cranio-sacral therapy, homeopathy, or Chinese medicine may be beneficial, especially when we carry some bodily damage from our experiences. Online groups and resources may also be helpful—see www.sarahjbuckley.com for a current list of suggested websites.

Whatever paths to healing we choose (and we may have to trust our intuition to tell us), it is above all crucial to be kind and loving to ourselves in the midst of major events and throughout our recovery from them. We will also need to take the space and time for this healing work, as far as our family commitments allow. This may involve trying to convey the magnitude and importance of healing work to partners, family, and friends.

Remember, too, that our partners, husbands, or friends may have strong feelings in relation to birth and parenting experiences, especially if they were present, and may need safety and support to express their own fears and feelings, and seek their own healing. It is important that all involved take the necessary time to talk through events and emotions and work towards resolution.

For all of us, events at birth can trigger memories and feelings from our own birth and early times. These may be addressed with homeopathy, flower essences, cranio-sacral therapy, and other healing modalities. Some practitioners may work more directly with birth experiences using techniques such as hypnosis, rebirthing, and bodywork, either individually or in dedicated groups and workshops: see www.sarahjbuckley.com for more resources. Examining and healing our own birth experiences is also important preparation for birth, and may be initiated simply by asking our mother how we were born.

Many women have used the grief and passion from unexpected events in labor and birth, especially when there seemed to be deficits in care, to advocate for enhanced choices and better care for other women. Some of the world's most dynamic birth activists have had disappointing or traumatic births, often followed by an awakening and subsequent empowered birth, and have committed to help others have the best experience possible.

Healing for Children

We may also consider talking about these events with our children, especially if we feel that early experiences may have impacted their well-being. It can be helpful to begin by expressing our own feelings in simple ways, emphasizing our care and concern, and our regret for any suffering. Our children will have their own experiences, perhaps even conscious memories, and may deeply appreciate validation of their memories and feelings.

This simple sharing can be profoundly healing, even with young babies who do not consciously understand our words. Some parents have shared these feelings in the middle of the night, with their children deeply asleep, and experienced powerful shifts and resolutions.

We can access gentle physical healing therapies for our children. Chiropractic, osteopathy, and cranio-sacral therapy in particular can resolve subtle malfunctions from the physical effects of birth, sometimes dramatically resolving problems with breastfeeding, digestion, and sleep in newborns and older babies.

Babies and young children may also carry strong emotions, including fear and trauma, from their birth and early experiences. Here again, gentle therapies such as those already mentioned can help heal the body memories, and specialized therapists are available in some places to work with children who have experienced trauma from conception through to infancy. (See www.birthpsychology.com for more information.)

We can help our babies and young children to self-heal by supporting their emotional expression, holding them lovingly when they cry or rage. (See Aletha Solter's books in the Resources list.) With older children, we can encourage, or even participate in, games that allow replaying of difficult experiences; a sleeping bag is a wonderful start for playing birth games, or wearing a large T-shirt that children can crawl into.

Children's need to express their story through words, play and replay, questions, stories, emotional expression, and more may continue, on and off, for an extended time. This need may resurface with other triggers, such as a birthday which is a perfect time to reflect or retell the child's birth story); or the birth of a sibling, which can be a deeply healing experience.

In my experience, children's memories of birth and early life can be conscious and accessible from around two years, and asking simple questions may help to evoke these experiences. My own approach is to be respectful and silently appreciative when my children honor me by sharing these memories. Keeping in mind that these stories belong to my children, I always ask before I share them with others (including publishing their birth stories in this book).

These practices of healing, integration, and care around difficult birth experiences can help us begin our parenting journey in wisdom and strength.

The Path of Parenting

Parenting will inevitably provide its own challenges and traumas, inviting us to examine and refurbish our attitudes and expectations and to heal any trauma from our own childhood. These aspects of parenting are not often addressed, but can be among the greatest gifts that our children give us. As midwife and mother of six Jeannine Parvati Baker observed: "Our children make us a whole lot better than we ever wanted to be."

Our parenting path will be immeasurably easier and more relaxed if we follow our children's leads, even from babyhood, as described in these pages. When we allow our child to lead, we create the possibility of fully meeting their unique and individual needs, which are harder to discern and may even become invisible when we habitually impose our own ideas or expert-generated solutions. This trusting approach also imprints initiative in our children, along with the confidence that they can effect change in the world—qualities that will not only make parenting easier through the teen years, but will also equip our offspring to be leaders and change-agents for the next generation.

Following our children's lead does not mean ignoring our own needs. In fact, I strongly advocate being self-centered as a parent—attending to our own needs, so that we can care for our children from a place of nurture. Being self-centered is an essential balance to a child-centered parenting philosophy, and we can accommodate both when we look for ways that meet everyone's needs. For specific parenting techniques, see my article on Gentle Discipline at www.sarahjbuckley.com: I also recommend

Parent Effectiveness Training (PET) and Nonviolent Communication (NVC) as practical and effective parenting tools.

Perfect Parent, Imperfect Parent

Through our parenting years, there will be many times when we are off track: when we mess up, do the wrong thing, and cause some major or minor hurts and harms to others as well as ourselves. The two most useful things we can do in this situation are to recognize and own our mistakes, at least to ourselves, and to keep breathing. We can then allow our feelings of regret, sadness, and perhaps even shame to arise, focusing at the same time on loving and accepting ourselves and our children.

It is especially important in this situation to avoid blame, and to realize that we are doing the best that we can with the knowledge and resources that we have. We can also accept that parenting is an imperfect art, and that striving for parental perfection can create stress and guilt, which can erode our confidence and our self-esteem and actually impoverish our parenting.

Admitting and accepting our imperfection humbles us, and helps us to perfect the art of apology, which I also highly recommend. There is nothing as sweet as being forgiven by our children, who are usually much kinder than we are to ourselves, and their forgiveness can melt not only our hearts but also any residual harshness and guilt that we carry as part of our parenting load.

Staying real, asking for help, healing our own hurts and trauma, admitting our mistakes, extending compassion to our partners and children, being gentle on ourselves, appreciating our own efforts, and forgiving ourselves: these habits will sustain and support parents and families on the parenting path, where our imperfections can make us truly perfect.

In Conclusion

I hope this book has given you information, inspiration, nourishment, and support as you make the huge transition to parenthood—humankind's most important role.

I hope that, as you progress in your parenthood, your confidence in your own abilities flourishes as you realize you are the expert in your own child, whose unfolding is unique and who deserves your loving attention and one-of-a-kind decision-making.

I also hope that you will regard any advice and opinion, including everything in this book, with healthy skepticism, and accept it only if it works for you, your child, and your family, as judged using your most sensitive criteria.

Finally, I hope you will trust your own instincts and listen to your child's communications with all your senses and sensitivity.

Blending instinct and responsiveness, wisdom and love, may you and your family experience the happiness and fulfillment that is a birthright for parents and children alike. Through your gentle parenting, may you contribute to the global revolution that is turning us all towards peace, participation, compassion, and connection.

So be it.

RESOURCES

FOR A FULL LIST of resources, see www.sarahjbuckley.com.

Birth

Abbott, Zuki. *This Sacred Life: Transforming Our World through Birth.* Crestone, CO. Wisdom's Birth Keepers, 2006.

Arms, Suzanne. *Immaculate Deception II: Myth, Magic and Birth.* Revised ed. Berkeley CA: Celestial Arts, 1996.

Baker, Jeannine Parvati. *Prenatal Yoga and Natural Childbirth.* 3rd ed. Berkeley CA: North Atlantic Books, 2001.

Baker, Jeannine Parvati, and Frederick Baker. *Conscious Conception: Elementary Journey through the Labyrinth of Sexuality.* Third ed. Berkeley CA: North Atlantic Books, 1986.

Balaskas, Janet. *Active Birth: The New Approach to Giving Birth Naturally.* Revised ed. Boston: The Harvard Common Press, 1992.

———. *The Waterbirth Book.* London: Thorsons, 2004.

Block, Jennifer. *Pushed: The Painful Truth about Childbirth and Modern Maternity Care.* Cambridge MA: Da Capo Press, 2007.

Blyth, Jenny. *Birthwork: A Compassionate Guide to Being with Birth.* Qld Australia: www.birthwork.com, 2005.

Cassidy, Tina. *Birth: The Surprising History of How We Are Born.* New York: Atlantic Monthly Press; 2006.

Dahl, Gail J. *Pregnancy and Childbirth Secrets.* Calgary: Innovative Publishing, 2007.

Davis, Elizabeth. *Heart & Hands: A Midwife's Guide to Pregnancy & Birth.* Revised 4th ed. Berkeley CA: Celestial Arts, 2004.

Daub, Cathy. *Birthing in the Spirit.* Medford NJ: Birth Works Press, 2007.

Donna, Sylvie. *Birth: Countdown to Optimal.* Chester le Street UK: Fresh Heart, 2008.

Edwards, Nadine P. *Birthing Autonomy: Women's Experiences of Planned Home Births.* Abingdon UK: Routledge; 2005.

England, Pam, and Rob Horowitz. *Birthing from Within: An Extra-Ordinary Guide to Childbirth Preparation.* Albuquerque NM: Partera Press, 1998.

Frye, Anne. *Holistic Midwifery: A Comprehensive Textbook for Midwives in Homebirth Practice. Volume 1 Care During Pregnancy.* Portland OR: Labrys Press, 1998

———. *Holistic Midwifery: A Comprehensive Textbook for Midwives in Homebirth Practice. Volume 2 Care During Labor and Birth.* Portland OR: Labrys Press, 2004.

———. *Understanding Diagnostic Tests in the Childbearing Year.* 7th ed. Portland OR: Labrys Press, 2007.

Gaskin, Ina May. *Ina May's Guide to Childbirth.* New York: Bantam, 2003.

———. *Spiritual Midwifery.* 4th ed. Summertown TN: The Book Publishing Co, 1977.

Goer, Henci. *The Thinking Woman's Guide to a Better Birth.* New York: Perigee, 1999.

————.*Obstetric Myths Versus Research Realities.* Westport CT: Bergin & Garvey, 1995.

Gurmukh. *Beautiful, Bountiful, Blissful: Experience the Natural Power of Pregnancy and Birth with Kundalini Yoga and Meditation.* New York: St. Martin's Griffin, 2004.

Harper, Barbara. *Gentle Birth Choices.* Rochester VT: Healing Arts Press, 2005.

Houser, Patrick M. *The Fathers-to-Be Handbook: A Road Map for the Transition to Fatherhood.* Kent UK: Creative Life Systems, 2008.

Johnson, Ingrid and Paul. *The Paper Midwife: A Guide to Responsible Homebirth.* Dunedin, New Zealand: Caveman Press, 1980.

Kitzinger, Sheila. *Birth Crisis.* London: Routledge, 2006.

————. *Birth, Your Way.* London: Dorling Kindersley, 2002.

————. *The Complete Book of Pregnancy and Childbirth.* 5th ed. New York: Knopf, 2003.

————. *Rediscovering Birth.* London: Little, Brown, 2000.

Lim, Robin. *After the Baby's Birth: A Woman's Way to Wellness.* Revised ed. Berkeley CA: Ten Speed, 2001.

Minelli, Sheri L. *Journey into Motherhood: Inspirational Stories of Natural Birth.* Encinitas CA: White Heart, 2005.

Mongan, Marie F. *Hypnobirthing: The Mongan Method.* Deerfield FL: Health Communications Ltd, 2005.

Muhlhahn, Cara. *Labor of Love: A Midwife's Memoir.* New York: Kaplan, 2008.

Newman, Robert. *Calm Birth: New Method for Conscious Childbirth.* Berkeley CA: North Atlantic Books, 2005.

Noble, Elizabeth. *Essential Exercises for the Childbearing Year: A Guide to Health and Comfort before and after Your Baby Is Born.* Revised 4th ed. Harwich MA: New Life Images, 2003.

————. *Primal Connections: How our experiences from birth influence our emotions, behavior and health.* Revised 4th ed. New York: Fireside/Simon and Schuster; 1993

Noble, Elizabeth, and Leo Sorger. *Having Twins: A Parent's Guide to Multiple Pregnancy, Birth and Early Childhood.* 3rd ed. Boston MA: Houghton Mifflin, 2003.

Odent, Michel. *Birth and Breastfeeding: Rediscovering the Needs of Women in Pregnancy and Childbirth.* East Sussex UK: Clairview, 2003.

————. *Birth Reborn: What Childbirth Should Be.* 2nd ed. London: Souvenir Press, 1994.

————. *The Caesarean.* Revised ed. London: Free Association Books, 2004.

————. *Primal Health: Understanding the Critical Period between Conception and the First Birthday.* East Sussex UK: Clairview, 2002.

————. *The Scientification of Love.* Revised ed. London: Free Association Books, 2001.

O'Mara, Peggy. *Mothering Magazine's Having a Baby, Naturally: The Mothering Magazine Guide to Pregnancy and Childbirth.* New York: Atria, 2003.

Overend, Jenni, and Julie Vivas. *Welcome with Love.* La Jolla CA: Kane/Miller, 1999.

Pearce, Joseph Chilton. *Evolution's End: Claiming the Potential of Our Intelligence.* San Francisco: Harper San Francisco, 1992.

Rachana, Shivam. *Lotus Birth.* Yarra Glen Australia: Greenwood Press, 2000.

Shanley, Laura Kaplan. *Unassisted Childbirth.* Westport CT: Bergin & Garvey, 1994.

Simkin, Penny, and Phyllis Klaus. *When Survivors Give Birth: Understanding and Healing the Effects of Early Sexual Abuse on Childbearing Women.* Seattle: Classic Day Publishing, 2004.

Simkin, Penny, Janet Whalley, and Ann Keppler. *Pregnancy, Childbirth, and the Newborn: The Complete Guide.* Revised, updated ed. Minnetonka MN: Meadowbrook Press, 2001.

Sutton, J, and Pauline Scott. *Optimal Foetal Positioning.* Tauranga New Zealand: Birth-Concepts, 1996.

Wagner, Marsden. *Creating Your Birth Plan: The Definitive Guide to a Safe and Empowering Birth.* New York: Perigee, 1993.

Wagner, Marsden. *Born in the USA: How a Broken Maternity System Must Be Fixed to Put Women and Children First.* Berkeley CA: University of California Press, 2006.

Weed, Susan. *Wise Woman Herbal for the Childbearing Year.* Woodstock, NY: Ash Tree, 1985

Wesson, Nicky. *Home Birth: A Practical Guide.* Revised 4th ed. London: Pinter & Martin Ltd, 2006.

Prenatal Testing

Beck, Martha. *Expecting Adam: A True Story of Birth, Rebirth, and Everyday Magic.* New York: Berkley Books, 2001.

de Crespigny, Lachlan, and Rhonda Dredge. *Which Tests for My Unborn Baby? Ultrasound and Other Prenatal Tests.* 2nd ed. Melbourne: Oxford University Press, 1996.

de Crespigny, Lachlan, and Frank Chervenak. *Prenatal Tests: The Facts.* 2nd ed. New York: Oxford University Press, 2006.

Kuckoff, Mitchell. *Choosing Naia: A Family's Journey.* Boston: Beacon Press, 2002.

Kuebelbeck, Amy. *Waiting with Gabriel: A Story of Cherishing a Baby's Brief Life.* Chicago: Loyola Press, 2003

Rapp, Rayna. *Testing Women, Testing the Fetus: The Social Impact of Amniocentesis in America (the Anthropology of Everyday Life).* Kentucky TN: Routledge, 2000.

Reist, Melinda Tankard. *Defiant Birth: Women Who Resist Medical Eugenics.* Melbourne: Spinifex, 2006

Rothman, Barbara Katz. *The Tentative Pregnancy: How Amniocentesis Changes the Experience of Motherhood.* 2nd ed. London: W. W. Norton & Company, 1993.

Sheffield, Kylie. *Not Compatible with Life: A Diary of Keeping Daniel.* Melbourne: Best Legenz, 2008. www.trisomyoz.bounce.com.au/#/danielsbook/4528173715

Soper, Kathryn Lynard. *Gifts: Mothers Reflect on How Children with Down Syndrome Enrich Their Lives.* Bethesda MD: Woodbine House, 2007.

Breastfeeding

Bumgarner, Norma Jane. *Mothering Your Nursing Toddler*. Schaumburg IL: La Leche
   League International, 2000

Flower, Hilary. *Adventures in Tandem Nursing: Breastfeeding During Pregnancy and
   Beyond*. Schaumburg IL: La Leche League International, 2003.

Huggins, Kathleen. *The Nursing Mother's Companion*. Revised ed. Boston, MA: Harvard
   Common Press, 2005.

La Leche League International. *The Womanly Art of Breastfeeding*. New York: Plume,
   2004.

Mohrbacher, Nancy, Julie Stock, and La Leche League International. *The Breastfeeding
   Answer Book*. Revised ed. Schaumburg IL: La Leche League International, 2003.

Renfrew, Mary, Chloe Fisher and Suzanne Arms. *Bestfeeding: How to Breastfeed Your
   Baby*, 3rd Rev Ed. Berkeley CA: Celestial Arts, 2004. Published in the UK as: *Bestfeeding: Why Breastfeeding is Best for You and Your Baby*, 3rd Rev Ed.

Robinson, Veronika Sophia. *The Drinks Are on Me: Everything Your Mother Never Told
   You About Breastfeeding*. East Grinstead UK: The Art of Change, 2007.

Sears, Martha, and William Sears. *The Breastfeeding Book: Everything You Need to
   Know About Nursing Your Child from Birth through Weaning*. Boston: Little, Brown,
   2000.

Cosleeping

Jackson, Deborah. *Three in a Bed: The Benefits of Sleeping with Your Baby*. London:
   Bloomsbury, 2003.

McKenna, James. *Sleeping with Your Baby: A Parents Guide to Cosleeping*. Washington
   DC: Platypus Media, 2006.

Sears, William. *Nighttime Parenting*. Schaumburg IL: La Leche League International,
   1999.

Small, Meredith E. *Our Babies, Ourselves*. New York: Random House, 1998.

Thevenin, Tine. *The Family Bed*. New York: Perigee Trade, 2002.

Parenting

Aldort, Naomi. *Raising Our Children, Raising Ourselves*. Bothell WA: Book Publishers
   Network, 2006.

Bauer, Ingrid. *Diaper Free! The Gentle Wisdom of Natural Infant Hygiene*. New York:
   Plume, 2006.

Blythe, Sally G. *What Babies and Children Really Need: How Mothers and Fathers
   Can Nurture Children's Growth for Health and Wellbeing*. Gloucestershire, UK:
   Hawthorn Press, 2008

Brott, Armin A., and Jennifer Ash. *A Dad's Guide to the Toddler Years*. New York:
   Abbeville Press, 2004.

———. *Father Knows Best: The Expectant Father, Facts, Tips, and Advice for Dads-to-
   Be*. New York: Abbeville Press, 2004.

———. *The New Father, a Dad's Guide to the First Year*. New York: Abbeville Press,
   2004.

Buckley Sarah J. *More Gentle Mothering: Extended Breastfeeding and Raising your Baby without Nappies/Diapers* (ebook). One Moon Press, 2008. Available at: www .sarahjbuckley.com/shop.

———. *Babies and Sleep for Tired Parents plus Yoga and Motherhood* (ebook). One Moon Press, 2008. Available at: www.sarahjbuckley.com/shop

———. *Gentle Discipline* (ebook). One Moon Press, 2008. Available at: www .sarahjbuckley.com/shop.

Chamberlain, David. *The Mind of Your Newborn Baby.* Berkeley CA: North Atlantic Books, 1998.

Cohen, Lawrence J. *Playful Parenting.* New York: Ballantine Books, 2002.

Contey, Carrie, and Debby Takikawa. *CALMS: A Guide to Soothing Your Baby.* Los Olivos CA: Hana Peace Works, 2007.

Gerhardt, Sue. *Why Love Matters: How Affection Shapes Your Baby's Brain.* London: Routledge, 2004.

Gordon, Thomas. *Parent Effectiveness Training.* New York: Penguin, 1975.

Granju, Katie. *Attachment Parenting: Instinctive Care for Your Baby and Young Child.* New York: Simon and Schuster, 1999.

Grille, Robin. *Heart to Heart Parenting: Nurturing Your Child's Emotional Intelligence from Conception to School Age.* Sydney: ABC Books, 2008.

———. *Parenting for a Peaceful World.* Sydney: Longueville Books, 2005.

Hart, Sura, and Victoria Kindle. *Respectful Parents, Respectful Kids: 7 Keys to Turn Family Conflict into Cooperation.* Encinitas CA: Puddle Dancer Press, 2006.

Hunt, Jan. *The Natural Child: Parenting from the Heart.* Gabriola Island, BC, Canada: New Society Publishers, 2001.

Klaus, Marshall H., John H. Kennell, and Phyllis Klaus. *Bonding: Building the Foundations of Secure Attachment and Independence.* Cambridge MA: Da Capo Press, 1996

Klaus, Marshall H., and Phyllis Klaus. *Your Amazing Newborn.* Cambridge MA: Da Capo Press, 2000.

Kohn, Alfie. *Unconditional Parenting: Moving from Rewards and Punishments to Love and Reason.* New York: Atria, 2006.

Kabat-Zinn, Myla and Jon. *Everyday Blessings: The Inner Work of Mindful Parenting.* New York: Hyperion, 1998.

Leo, Pam. *Connection Parenting: Parenting through Connection Instead of Coercion, through Love Instead of Fear.* 2nd ed. Deadwood OR: Wyatt-MacKenzie Publishing.

Liedloff, J. *The Continuum Concept: In Search of Happiness Lost.* Reading MA: Perseus Books, 1997.

Napthali, Sarah. *Buddhism for Mothers: A Calm Approach to Caring for Yourself and Your Children.* Sydney: Allen and Unwin, 2003.

O'Mara, Peggy. *Natural Family Living: The Mothering Magazine Guide to Parenting.* New York: Pocket Books, 2000.

———. *A Quiet Place: Essays on Life and Family.* Santa Fe: Mothering Publications, 2006.

Montague, Ashley. *Touch: the Human Significance of the Skin.* New York: Harper, 1996.

Muthri, Gowra, and Karen Swan Macleod. *Gentle First Year: The Essential Guide to Mother and Baby Wellbeing in the First Twelve Months.* Glasgow: Harper Thorsons, 2004.

Palisi, Tiffany. *Loving Mama: Essays on Natural Parenting and Motherhood.* Tucson AZ: Hats Off Books, 2004.

Palmer, Linda Folden. *Baby Matters: What Your Doctor May Not Tell You About Caring for Your Baby.* Revised 2nd ed. San Diego CA: Baby Reference, 2007.

Pearce, Joseph Chilton. *Magical Child: Rediscovering Nature's Plan for Our Children.* New York: Dutton, 1977.

Rosenberg, Marshall. *Nonviolent Communication: A Language of Life.* 2nd ed. Encinitas CA: Puddle Dancer Press, 2003.

Sears, William, and Martha Sears. *The Baby Book: Birth to Two Years.* Boston: Little, Brown, 2003.

———. *The Discipline Book: Everything You Need to Know to Have a Better-Behaved Child - from Birth to Age Ten.* Boston: Little, Brown, 1995.

Small, Meredith E. *Our Babies, Ourselves.* New York: Random House, 1998.

Solter, Aletha. *The Aware Baby: A New Approach to Parenting.* Goleta CA: Shining Star Press, 2001.

———. *Helping Young Children Flourish.* Goleta CA: Shining Star Press, 1989.

———. *Tears and Tantrums.* Goleta CA: Shining Star Press, 1998.

Staton, Laura, and Sarah Perron. *Baby Om.* Villa Park IL: Newleaf, 2003.

Sunderland, Margot. *The Science of Parenting: Practical Guidance on Sleep, Crying, Play and Building Emotional Wellbeing for Life.* London: Dorling Kindersley, 2006

Films and DVDs

The Big Stretch: Insights about Birth. Director: Alieta Belle (Australia, 2006) www.birthwork.com

Birth as We Know It. Director: Elena Tonetti (United States, 2005).

Birth in the Squatting Position. Moyses and Claudio Paciornik (Brazil, 1982) www.birthworks.org

The Business of Being Born. Directors: Abby Epstein and Rikki Lake (United States, 2008).

Orgasmic Birth. Director: Debra Pascali-Bonaro (United States, 2008).

What Babies Want. Director. Debby Takikawa (United States, 2004).

ACKNOWLEDGMENTS

FIRST, I THANK my beloved parents, Nola and Tim, who loved and supported me through my rather tempestuous and precocious childhood, encouraged me through my studies, and continue to love and support me and my family.

Second, I am grateful beyond words to my own children, my best teachers: Emma, Zoe, Jacob, and Maia, who have given me such deep and rich experiences of pregnancy, birth, and mothering. Thank you, too, for the space you have given me for my writing and for the new understandings you bring to me every day.

Equally, I thank Nicholas, the love of my life, for his love, support, tolerance, and sense of humor, and for walking alongside me on this wild and wonderful path of parenting.

Thanks also to Nicholas's sister, New Zealand midwife Sue Lennox, whose wisdom and enthusiasm helped to make homebirth an easy choice for us, immeasurably enriching our family and leading, eighteen years later, to the book you hold in your hands.

I am also grateful to all the women in my "advanced women's mysteries" circle based in Melbourne, who provide such a solid foundation for my work. Thanks especially to Bachana—circle leader, teacher, wise woman, and friend—who has been a true midwife to me and to so many others. Thanks also to my many other supporters and mentors around the world, including Michel Odent, Deva Daricha, and the late Jeannine Parvati Baker, whose work on the cutting edge of consciousness continues to inspire me.

Thanks to all my woman friends, my homebirth and midwife friends, and the Brisbane Home Midwifery Association circle, who help to keep alive the spirit and love of birth and babies. Thanks especially to my faithful moon circle, Suzanne, Georgina, Susan, and Mary.

Appreciation to the people who have nurtured and supported my writing, especially Ashisha and Peggy at *Mothering*; Jan Tritten at *Midwifery Today*; Veronika Robinson at *The Mother* magazine (UK); and Kali Wendorf at *Kindred* magazine (Australia).

Thanks to Soni Stecker, whose editorial skills and support helped me to shape the original *Gentle Birth, Gentle Mothering*; to my friend John

Travis, for his advocacy for my book and his amazing networking talents; and to Celestial Arts and my editor Clancy Drake for support with this U.S. edition, which takes *Gentle Birth, Gentle Mothering* to a worldwide readership.

Thanks also to the many people who continue to support my talks and lectures around the world through invitations, organization, and attendance: your support fulfills my need for joyful contribution to mothers, babies, fathers, and families everywhere.

Appreciation also to the midwives, doulas, childbirth educators, physicians, and others whose practical support for gentle birth is so potent and important in these times: may the wisdom and support that you generously share, and the courage and passion that you bring to a culture that has lost its understanding of the primacy of birth, be returned to you one thousandfold.

A special mention to the founders and members of the Association for Prenatal and Perinatal Psychology and Health (APPPAH), who have been truly revolutionary in their understanding of, and advocacy for, the needs of unborn babies.

Thanks also to the growing global network of birth activists: women and men of incredible courage and commitment, who are all working to heal birth in our culture.

On a more personal note, thanks to those superb practitioners who have supported my health and my body, so that I can do the work of mother and writer, especially my masseuse Narelle Clark, homeopath Patricia Hatherly, shiatsu practitioner Michie Araki, and naturopath and craniosacral therapist Claire Brassard.

Finally, gratitude to all my readers—mothers, fathers, families, and professionals worldwide—for your feedback, appreciation, and patronage, and for giving me the opportunity to bring together my mothering heart, my scientific mind, and my love of writing.

Many blessings on your journey.

NOTES

Chapter 1: RECLAIMING EVERY WOMAN'S BIRTH RIGHT

1. Block J. *Pushed: the Painful Truth about Childbirth and Modern Maternity Care.* Cambridge MA: Da Capo Press; 2007.

2. Davis-Floyd R. *Birth as an American Rite of Passage.* Berkeley CA: University of California Press; 2003.

3. Organisation for Economic Cooperation and Development. *OECD Health Data 2007: a comparative analysis of 30 countries.* Paris: OECD; 2007.

4. Minino AM, Heron MP, Murphy SL, Kochanek KD. *Deaths: Final Data for 2004.* Hyattsville, MD: National Center for Health Statistics; 2007.

5. Hamilton BE, Martin JA, Ventura SJ. *Births: preliminary data for 2006.* Hyattsville, MD: National Center for Health Statistics; 2007. vol 56 no 7.

6. Canadian Institute for Health Information. *Health Indicators 2007.* Ottawa: CIHI; 2007.

7. Richardson A, Mmata C. *Statistical bulletin: NHS maternity statistics, England: 2005-6.* London: The Information Centre; 2007.

8. Morbidity and Mortality Weekly Report. *Rates of Cesarean Delivery—United States, 1993.* Atlanta GA: Center for Disease Control; April 21, 1995; 44(15).

9. World Health Organisation. Appropriate technology for birth. *Lancet.* Aug 24 1985;2(8452):436-437.

10. Declercq E, Sakala C, Corry M, Applebaum S, Risher P. *Listening to Mothers: Report of the First U.S. National Survey of Women's Childbearing Experiences.* New York: Maternity Center Association; 2002.

11. Declercq ER, Sakala C, Corry MP, Applebaum S. *Listening to Mothers II: Report of the Second National U.S. Survey of Women's Childbearing Experiences.* New York: Childbirth Connection; October 2006.

12. Fisher J, Smith A, Astbury J. Private health insurance and a healthy personality: new risk factors for obstetric intervention? *J Psychosom Obstet Gynaecol.* Mar 1995;16(1):1-9.

13. Jacobson B, Nyberg K, Gronbladh L, Eklund G, Bygdeman M, Rydberg U. Opiate addiction in adult offspring through possible imprinting after obstetric treatment. *Br Med J.* Nov 10 1990;301(6760):1067-1070.

14. Boyce PM. Risk factors for postnatal depression: a review and risk factors in Australian populations. *Arch Women Ment Health.* Aug 2003;6 Suppl 2:S43-50.

15. Lobel M, DeLuca RS. Psychosocial sequelae of cesarean delivery: review and analysis of their causes and implications. *Soc Sci Med.* Jun 2007;64(11):2272-2284.

16. Rowe-Murray HJ, Fisher JR. Operative intervention in delivery is associated with compromised early mother-infant interaction. *Br J Obstet Gynaecol.* Oct 2001;108(10):1068-1075.

17. Hodnett ED. Pain and women's satisfaction with the experience of childbirth: a systematic review. *Am J Obstet Gynecol.* May 2002;186(5 Suppl Nature):S160-172.

18. Olsen O, Jewell MD. Home versus hospital birth. *Cochrane Database Syst Rev.* 2000(2):CD000352.

19. Hodnett ED. Continuity of caregivers for care during pregnancy and childbirth. *Cochrane Database Syst Rev.* 2000(2):CD000062.

20. Enkin M, Keirse M, Neilson J, et al. *Effective Care in Pregnancy and Childbirth.* 3rd ed. Oxford: Oxford University Press; 2000.

21. Cochrane Collaborative. The Cochrane Library: John Wiley; 2005. www.thecochranelibrary.org.

22. Enkin M, Keirse M, Neilson J, et al. *Effective Care in Pregnancy and Childbirth.* 3rd ed. Oxford: Oxford University Press; 2000, p 486.

Chapter 2: VISION AND TOOLS FOR INSTINCTIVE BIRTH

1. Odent M. *Birth Reborn.* 2nd ed. London: Souvenir Press; 1994.

2. Common Knowledge Trust. *The Pink Kit; Essential preparations for your birthing body.* Nelson New Zealand: Common Knowledge Trust www.birthingbetter.com; 2001.

3. International College of Spiritual Midwifery. Melbourne: www.womenofspirit.asn.au.

4. Naish F, Roberts J. *Healthy Parents, Better Babies: A Couple's Guide to Natural Preconception.* Freedom CA: The Crossing Press; 1990.

5. Kitzinger S. Sheila Kitzinger's letter from Europe: the clock, the bed, the chair, the pool. *Birth.* Mar 2003;30(1):54-56.

6. Balaskas J. *Active Birth: the new approach to giving birth naturally.* Revised ed. Boston: The Harvard Common Press; 1992.

7. Sutton J, Scott P. *Optimal Foetal Positioning.* Tauranga New Zealand: BirthConcepts; 1996.

8. England P, Horowitz R. *Birthing from within: an extraordinary guide to childbirth preparation.* Albuquerque NM: Partera Press; 1998.

9. Gaskin IM. *Spiritual Midwifery.* 4th ed. Summertown TN: The Book Publishing Co; 2002.

10. Baker JP. *Prenatal Yoga and Natural Childbirth.* 3rd ed. Berkeley CA: North Atlantic Books; 2001 p 90.

11. Shanley LK. *Unassisted Childbirth.* Westport CT: Bergin & Garvey; 1994.

12. McCracken L. *Resexualizing Childbirth.* Coquitlam BC: Birthlove; 2000.

13. Banks M. *Breech Birth, Woman Wise.* Hamilton New Zealand: Birthspirit Books; 1998.

Chapter 3: HEALING BIRTH, HEALING THE EARTH

1. Baker JP. Hygieia College Mystery School. www.birthkeeper.com.

2. Baker JP. *Prenatal Yoga and Natural Childbirth.* 3rd ed. Berkeley CA: North Atlantic Books; 2001.

Chapter 4: YOUR BODY, YOUR BABY, YOUR CHOICE

1. Dunn PM. Wilhelm Conrad Roentgen (1845-1923), the discovery of x rays and perinatal diagnosis. *Arch Dis Child Fetal Neonatal Ed.* Mar 2001;84(2):F138-139.

2. Centers for Disease Control and Prevention. DES Update. *United States Department of Health and Human Services.* Available at: www.cdc.gov/DES.

3. American College of Obstetricians and Gynecologists. Informed Consent. *Ethics in Obstetrics and Gynecology.* Washington, DC: ACOG; 2004:9-17.

4. Royal College of Obstetricians and Gynecologists. *Obtaining valid consent* 2004. Number 6.

5. ACOG Committee on Ethics. ACOG Committee Opinion #321: Maternal decision making, ethics, and the law. *Obstet Gynecol.* 2005;106:1127-1137, p 1135.

6. American College of Obstetricians and Gynecologists. ACOG Committee Opinion No. 306. Informed refusal. *Obstet*

Gynecol. Dec 2004;104(6):1465-1466, p 1466.

7. Murphy-Lawless J. *Reading Birth and Death: A History of Obstetric Thinking.* Bloomington, IN: Indiana University Press; 1999.

8. Chamberlain D. *The Mind of Your Newborn Baby.* Berkeley CA: North Atlantic Books; 1998.

9. Odent M. *The Scientification of Love.* Revised ed. London: Free Association Books; 2001.

10. Odent M. *Primal Health Database.* http://www.birthworks.org/ primalhealth.

11. Odent M. *Primal Health: Understanding the critical period between conception and the first birthday.* East Sussex UK: Clairview; 2002.

12. Odent M. Gestational Diabetes: A diagnosis still looking for a disease. *Primal Health Research.* 1998;12(1):1-6, p 4.

13. Odent M. The Function of Joy in Pregnancy. *Journal of Prenatal and Perinatal Psychology and Health.* 2007;21(4):307-313, p 311.

14. Field T, Diego M. Cortisol: the culprit prenatal stress variable. *Int J Neurosci.* Aug 2008;118(8):1181.

15. Field T, Hernandez-Reif M, Hart S, Theakston H, Schanberg S, Kuhn C. Pregnant women benefit from massage therapy. *J Psychosom Obstet Gynaecol.* Mar 1999;20(1):31-38.

16. Field T, Diego M, Hernandez-Reif M. Prematurity and potential predictors. *Int J Neurosci.* Feb 2008;118(2):277-289.

17. Hillier TA, Vesco KK, Pedula KL, Beil TL, Whitlock EP, Pettitt DJ. Screening for gestational diabetes mellitus: a systematic review for the U.S. Preventive Services Task Force. *Ann Intern Med.* May 20 2008;148(10):759-766.

18. Alberti KG, Zimmet PZ. Definition, diagnosis and classification of diabetes mellitus and its complications. Part 1: diagnosis and classification of diabetes mellitus provisional report of a WHO consultation. *Diabet Med.* Jul 1998;15(7):539-553.

19. Berger H, Crane J, Farine D, et al. Screening for gestational diabetes mellitus. *J Obstet Gynaecol Can.* Nov 2002;24(11):894-912.

20. Sermer M, Naylor CD, Farine D, et al. The Toronto Tri-Hospital Gestational Diabetes Project. A preliminary review. *Diabetes Care.* Aug 1998;21 Suppl 2:B33-42.

21. Frye A. *Understanding Diagnostic Tests in the Childbearing Year: A Holistic Approach.* 7th ed. Portland OR: Labrys Press; 2007.

22. National Institute for Clinical Excellence. *Diabetes in pregnancy: management of diabetes and its complications from preconception to the postnatal period.* London: National Collaborating Centre for Women's and Children's Health; 2004.

23. Lain KY, Catalano PM. Metabolic Changes in Pregnancy. *Clin Obstet Gynecol.* Dec 2007;50(4):938-948.

24. U.S. Department of Health and Human Services: National Diabetes Education Program. *Type 2 Diabetes Risk After Gestational Diabetes* 2006.

25. National Heart Lung and Blood Institute: Obesity Education Initiative. Body Mass Index Calculator. Available at: http://www.nhlbisupport.com/bmi/ bmicalc.htm

26. Metzger BE. Long-term Outcomes in Mothers Diagnosed With Gestational Diabetes Mellitus and Their Offspring. *Clin Obstet Gynecol.* Dec 2007;50(4):972-979.

27. Cheng YW, Caughey AB. Gestational diabetes: diagnosis and management. *J Perinatol.* Jul 17 2008.

28. American College of Obstetricians and Gynecologists. ACOG Practice Bulletin. Clinical management guidelines for

obstetrician-gynecologists. Number 30, September 2001 (replaces Technical Bulletin Number 200, December 1994). Gestational diabetes. *Obstet Gynecol.* Sep 2001;98(3):525-538.

29. Crowther CA, Hiller JE, Moss JR, McPhee AJ, Jeffries WS, Robinson JS. Effect of treatment of gestational diabetes mellitus on pregnancy outcomes. *N Engl J Med.* Jun 16 2005;352(24):2477-2486.

30. Metzger BE, Lowe LP, Dyer AR, et al. Hyperglycemia and adverse pregnancy outcomes. *N Engl J Med.* May 8 2008;358(19):1991-2002.

31. Boney CM, Verma A, Tucker R, Vohr BR. Metabolic syndrome in childhood: association with birth weight, maternal obesity, and gestational diabetes mellitus. *Pediatrics.* Mar 2005;115(3): e290-296.

32. Gillman MW, Rifas-Shiman S, Berkey CS, Field AE, Colditz GA. Maternal gestational diabetes, birth weight, and adolescent obesity. *Pediatrics.* Mar 2003;111(3):e221-226.

33. Jarrett RJ, Castro-Soares J, Dornhorst A, Beard RW. Should we screen for gestational diabetes? *BMJ.* Sep 20 1997;315(7110):736-739.

34. U.S. Preventive Services Task Force. Screening for diabetes mellitus. *Preventive Services Task Force. Guide to clinical preventive services: report of the U.S. Preventive Services Task Force.* 2nd ed. Baltimore: Williams & Wilkins; 1996:193-208.

35. Naylor CD, Sermer M, Chen E, Farine D. Selective screening for gestational diabetes mellitus. Toronto Trihospital Gestational Diabetes Project Investigators. *N Engl J Med.* Nov 27 1997;337(22):1591-1596.

36. Jovanovic-Peterson L, Bevier W, Peterson CM. The Santa Barbara County Health Care Services program: birth weight change concomitant with

screening for and treatment of glucose-intolerance of pregnancy: a potential cost-effective intervention? *Am J Perinatol.* Apr 1997;14(4):221-228.

37. Boulvain M, Stan C, Irion O. Elective delivery in diabetic pregnant women. *Cochrane Database Syst Rev.* 2001(2):CD001997.

38. Graves CR. Antepartum fetal surveillance and timing of delivery in the pregnancy complicated by diabetes mellitus. *Clin Obstet Gynecol.* Dec 2007;50(4):1007-1013.

39. Rouse DJ, Owen J, Goldenberg RL, Cliver SP. The effectiveness and costs of elective cesarean delivery for fetal macrosomia diagnosed by ultrasound. *JAMA.* Nov 13 1996;276(18):1480-1486.

40. Lurie S, Matzkel A, Weissman A, Gotlibe Z, Friedman A. Outcome of pregnancy in class A1 and A2 gestational diabetic patients delivered beyond 40 weeks' gestation. *Am J Perinatol.* Sep-Nov 1992;9(5-6):484-488.

41. Nahum GG, Stanislaw H. Ultrasonographic prediction of term birth weight: how accurate is it? *Am J Obstet Gynecol.* Feb 2003;188(2):566-574.

42. Hillier TA, Vesco KK, Pedula KL, Beil TL, Whitlock EP, Pettitt DJ. Screening for gestational diabetes mellitus: a systematic review for the U.S. Preventive Services Task Force. *Ann Intern Med.* May 20 2008;148(10):766-775.

43. U.S. Preventive Services Task Force. Screening for gestational diabetes mellitus: U.S. Preventive Services Task Force recommendation statement. *Ann Intern Med.* May 20 2008;148(10):759-765, p 762.

44. Galtier F, Raingeard I, Renard E, Boulot P, Bringer J. Optimizing the outcome of pregnancy in obese women: from pregestational to long-term management. *Diabetes Metab.* Feb 2008;34(1):19-25.

45. Gavard JA, Artal R. Effect of exercise on pregnancy outcome. *Clin Obstet Gynecol.* Jun 2008;51(2):467-480.

46. Clapp JF. Effects of Diet and Exercise on Insulin Resistance during Pregnancy. *Metab Syndr Relat Disord.* Summer 2006;4(2):84-90.

47. University of Sydney. Glycemic Index and GI Database. Available at: www.glycemicindex.com.

48. Saldana TM, Siega-Riz AM, Adair LS. Effect of macronutrient intake on the development of glucose intolerance during pregnancy. *Am J Clin Nutr.* Mar 2004;79(3):479-486.

49. Thomas B, Ghebremeskel K, Lowy C, Crawford M, Offley-Shore B. Nutrient intake of women with and without gestational diabetes with a specific focus on fatty acids. *Nutrition.* Mar 2006;22(3):230-236.

50. A.D.A.M. Health and Age: Alternative medicine: Diabetes. Available at: http://www.healthandage.com/html/res/com/ConsConditions/DiabetesMellituscc.html#NutritionDiet.

51. Hunter DJ, Milner R. Gestational diabetes and birth trauma. *Am J Obstet Gynecol.* Aug 1 1985;152(7 Pt 1): 918-919.

52. Greenberg JA. Gestational diabetes: what's the problem? *Am J Obstet Gynecol.* Jan 2006;194(1):299; author reply 299-300.

53. Odent M. Gestational Diabetes: A diagnosis still looking for a disease. *Primal Health Research.* 1998;12(1):1-6.

54. U.S. Preventive Services Task Force. Screening for gestational diabetes mellitus: U.S. Preventive Services Task Force recommendation statement. *Ann Intern Med.* May 20 2008;148(10):759-765, p 759.

55. Centers for Disease Control and Prevention. *Prevention of Perinatal Group B Streptococcal Disease.* Atlanta, GA: Centers for Disease Control and Prevention; August 16, 2002.

56. Royal College of Obstetricians and Gynaecologists. *Prevention Of Early Onset Neonatal Group B Streptococcal Disease* 2003.

57. Thinkhamrop J, Limpongsanurak S, Festin MR, et al. Infections in international pregnancy study: performance of the optical immunoassay test for detection of group B streptococcus. *J Clin Microbiol.* Nov 2003;41(11):5288-5290.

58. Schrag SJ, Zell ER, Lynfield R, et al. A population-based comparison of strategies to prevent early-onset group B streptococcal disease in neonates. *N Engl J Med.* Jul 25 2002;347(4):233-239.

59. Money DM, Dobson S. The prevention of early-onset neonatal group B streptococcal disease. *J Obstet Gynaecol Can.* Sep 2004;26(9):826-840.

60. Campbell N, Eddy A, Darlow B, Stone P, Grimwood K. The prevention of early-onset neonatal group B streptococcus infection: technical report from the New Zealand GBS Consensus Working Party. *N Z Med J.* Aug 20 2004;117(1200):U1023.

61. National Collaborating Centre for Women's and Children's Health. *Antenatal care: routine care for the healthy pregnant woman.* London: National Institute for Health and Clinical Excellence; 2008.

62. Towers CV, Briggs GG. Antepartum use of antibiotics and early-onset neonatal sepsis: the next 4 years. *Am J Obstet Gynecol.* Aug 2002;187(2):495-500.

63. Alarcon A, Pena P, Salas S, Sancha M, Omenaca F. Neonatal early onset Escherichia coli sepsis: trends in incidence and antimicrobial resistance in the era of intrapartum antimicrobial prophylaxis. *Pediatr Infect Dis J.* Apr 2004;23(4): 295-299.

64. Glasgow TS, Young PC, Wallin J, et al. Association of intrapartum antibiotic exposure and late-onset serious bacterial

infections in infants. *Pediatrics.* Sep 2005;116(3):696-702.

65. Bedford Russell AR, Murch SH. Could peripartum antibiotics have delayed health consequences for the infant? *BJOG.* Jul 2006;113(7):758-765.

66. Sullivan A, Edlund C, Nord CE. Effect of antimicrobial agents on the ecological balance of human microflora. *Lancet Infect Dis.* Sep 2001;1(2):101-114.

67. Jaureguy F, Carton M, Panel P, Foucaud P, Butel MJ, Doucet-Populaire F. Effects of intrapartum penicillin prophylaxis on intestinal bacterial colonization in infants. *J Clin Microbiol.* Nov 2004;42(11):5184-5188.

68. Penders J, Thijs C, Vink C, et al. Factors influencing the composition of the intestinal microbiota in early infancy. *Pediatrics.* Aug 2006;118(2):511-521.

69. Bedford Russell AR, Murch SH. Could peripartum antibiotics have delayed health consequences for the infant? *BJOG.* Jul 2006;113(7):758-765, p 761.

70. Bedford Russell AR, Murch SH. Could peripartum antibiotics have delayed health consequences for the infant? *BJOG.* Jul 2006;113(7):758-765, p 763.

71. Rusconi F, Galassi C, Forastiere F, et al. Maternal complications and procedures in pregnancy and at birth and wheezing phenotypes in children. *Am J Respir Crit Care Med.* Jan 1 2007;175(1):16-21.

72. Montgomery SM, Wakefield AJ, Morris DL, Pounder RE, Murch SH. The initial care of newborn infants and subsequent hay fever. *Allergy.* Oct 2000;55(10):916-922.

73. Rowland IR, Robinson RD, Doherty RA. Effects of diet on mercury metabolism and excretion in mice given methylmercury: role of gut flora. *Arch Environ Health.* Nov-Dec 1984;39(6):401-408.

74. Adams JB, Romdalvik J, Ramanujam VM, Legator MS. Mercury, lead, and zinc in baby teeth of children with autism versus controls. *J Toxicol Environ Health A.* Jun 2007;70(12):1046-1051.

75. McKinney PA, Parslow R, Gurney KA, Law GR, Bodansky HJ, Williams R. Perinatal and neonatal determinants of childhood type 1 diabetes. A case-control study in Yorkshire, U.K. *Diabetes Care.* Jun 1999;22(6):928-932.

76. Patterson CC, Carson DJ, Hadden DR, Waugh NR, Cole SK. A case-control investigation of perinatal risk factors for childhood IDDM in Northern Ireland and Scotland. *Diabetes Care.* May 1994;17(5):376-381.

77. Dahlquist G, Kallen B. Maternal-child blood group incompatibility and other perinatal events increase the risk for early-onset type 1 (insulin-dependent) diabetes mellitus. *Diabetologia.* Jul 1992;35(7):671-675.

78. Rescigno M. The pathogenic role of intestinal flora in IBD and colon cancer. *Curr Drug Targets.* May 2008;9(5):395-403.

79. DiBaise JK, Zhang H, Crowell MD, Krajmalnik-Brown R, Decker GA, Rittmann BE. Gut microbiota and its possible relationship with obesity. *Mayo Clin Proc.* Apr 2008;83(4):460-469.

80. Natural Standard Research Collaboration. Medline Plus: Herbs and Supplements. *United States National Library of Medicine and National Institutes of Health.* Available at: http://www.nlm.nih.gov/medlineplus/druginfo/herb_All.html. Accessed 22 July 2008.

81. Stade B, Shah V, Ohlsson A. Vaginal chlorhexidine during labour to prevent early-onset neonatal group B streptococcal infection. *Cochrane Database Syst Rev.* 2004;(3):CD003520.

82. Konrad G, Katz A. Epidemiology of early-onset neonatal group B streptococcal infection: implications for screening. *Can Fam Physician.* Jun 2007;53(6):1055, 2001:e 1051-1056, 1054.

83. Martin JA, Hamilton BE, Sutton PD, et al. *Births: Final data for 2005 National vital statistics reports.* Hyattsville, MD: National Center for Health Statistics; 2007;56(6)

84. Declercq ER, Sakala C, Corry MP, Applebaum S. *Listening to Mothers II: Report of the Second National U.S. Survey of Women's Childbearing Experiences.* New York: Childbirth Connection; October 2006.

85. Gulmezoglu AM, Crowther CA, Middleton P. Induction of labour for improving birth outcomes for women at or beyond term. *Cochrane Database Syst Rev.* 2006(4):CD004945.

86. Rand L, Robinson JN, Economy KE, Norwitz ER. Post-term induction of labor revisited. *Obstet Gynecol.* Nov 2000;96(5 Pt 1):779-783.

87. Sanchez-Ramos L, Olivier F, Delke I, Kaunitz AM. Labor induction versus expectant management for postterm pregnancies: a systematic review with meta-analysis. *Obstet Gynecol.* Jun 2003;101(6):1312-1318.

88. Gardosi J, Vanner T, Francis A. Gestational age and induction of labour for prolonged pregnancy. *Br J Obstet Gynaecol.* Jul 1997;104(7):792-797.

89. Mittendorf R, Williams MA, Berkey CS, Cotter PF. The length of uncomplicated human gestation. *Obstet Gynecol.* Jun 1990;75(6):929-932.

90. Nguyen TH, Larsen T, Engholm G, Moller H. Evaluation of ultrasound-estimated date of delivery in 17,450 spontaneous singleton births: do we need to modify Naegele's rule? *Ultrasound Obstet Gynecol.* Jul 1999;14(1):23-28.

91. Bergsjo P, Denman DW, 3rd, Hoffman HJ, Meirik O. Duration of human singleton pregnancy. A population-based study. *Acta Obstet Gynecol Scand.* 1990;69(3):197-207.

92. Mittendorf R, Williams MA, Berkey CS, Lieberman E, Monson RR. Predictors of human gestational length. *Am J Obstet Gynecol.* Feb 1993;168(2):480-484.

93. Smith GC. Life-table analysis of the risk of perinatal death at term and post term in singleton pregnancies. *Am J Obstet Gynecol.* Feb 2001;184(3):489-496.

94. Smith GC, Fretts RC. Stillbirth. *Lancet.* Nov 17 2007;370(9600):1715-1725.

95. Hilder L, Costeloe K, Thilaganathan B. Prolonged pregnancy: evaluating gestation-specific risks of fetal and infant mortality. *Br J Obstet Gynaecol.* Feb 1998;105(2):169-173.

96. Hilder L, Costeloe K, Thilaganathan B. Prospective risk of stillbirth. Study's results are flawed by reliance on cumulative prospective risk. *BMJ.* Feb 12 2000;320(7232):444-445; author reply 446.

97. Hollis B. Prolonged pregnancy. *Curr Opin Obstet Gynecol.* Apr 2002;14(2):203-207.

98. Yuan H, Platt RW, Morin L, Joseph KS, Kramer MS. Fetal deaths in the United States, 1997 vs. 1991. *Am J Obstet Gynecol.* Aug 2005;193(2):489-495.

99. Divon MY, Ferber A, Sanderson M, Nisell H, Westgren M. A functional definition of prolonged pregnancy based on daily fetal and neonatal mortality rates. *Ultrasound Obstet Gynecol.* May 2004;23(5):423-426.

100. National Collaborating Centre for Women's and Children's Health. *Induction of Labour.* London: National Institute for Health and Clinical Excellence; 2008.

101. Campbell MK. Factors affecting outcome in post-term birth. *Curr Opin Obstet Gynecol.* Dec 1997;9(6):356-360.

102. Manzanares S, Carrillo MP, Gonzalez-Peran E, Puertas A, Montoya F. Isolated oligohydramnios in term pregnancy as an indication for induction of labor. *J Matern Fetal Neonatal Med.* Mar 2007;20(3):221-224.

103. Luton D, Alran S, Fourchotte V, Sibony O, Oury JF. Paris heat wave and oligohydramnios. *Am J Obstet Gynecol.* Dec 2004;191(6):2103-2105.

104. Manz F. Hydration and disease. *J Am Coll Nutr.* Oct 2007;26(5 Suppl):535S-541S.

105. Schreyer P, Sherman DJ, Ervin MG, Day L, Ross MG. Maternal dehydration: impact on ovine amniotic fluid volume and composition. *J Dev Physiol.* May 1990;13(5):283-287.

106. Ross MG. Dehydration-induced oligohydramnios. *Am J Obstet Gynecol.* Sep 1990;163(3):1091-1092.

107. Varner MW, Noble WD, Dombrowski M, et al. Is there a seasonal variation in the diagnosis of oligohydramnios? *J Matern Fetal Neonatal Med.* Mar 2005;17(3):173-177.

108. Sadeh-Mestechkin D, Walfisch A, Shachar R, Shoham-Vardi I, Vardi H, Hallak M. Suspected macrosomia? Better not tell. *Arch Gynecol Obstet.* Sep 2008;278(3):225-230.

109. Chauhan SP, Grobman WA, Gherman RA, et al. Suspicion and treatment of the macrosomic fetus: a review. *Am J Obstet Gynecol.* Aug 2005;193(2):332-346.

110. Chanrachakul B, Herabutya Y. Postterm with favorable cervix: is induction necessary? *Eur J Obstet Gynecol Reprod Biol.* Feb 10 2003;106(2):154-157.

111. Dandolu V, Lawrence L, Gaughan JP, et al. Trends in the rate of shoulder dystocia over two decades. *J Matern Fetal Neonatal Med.* Nov 2005;18(5):305-310.

112. Caughey AB, Stotland NE, Washington AE, Escobar GJ. Maternal and obstetric complications of pregnancy are associated with increasing gestational age at term. *Am J Obstet Gynecol.* Feb 2007;196(2):155 e151-156.

113. Olesen AW, Westergaard JG, Olsen J. Perinatal and maternal complications related to postterm delivery: a national register-based study, 1978-1993. *Am J Obstet Gynecol.* Jul 2003;189(1):222-227.

114. Hilder L, Sairam S, Thilaganathan B. Influence of parity on fetal mortality in prolonged pregnancy. *Eur J Obstet Gynecol Reprod Biol.* Jun 2007;132(2):167-170.

115. Gulmezoglu AM, Crowther CA, Middleton P. Induction of labour for improving birth outcomes for women at or beyond term. *Cochrane Database Syst Rev.* 2006(4):CD004945, p004941.

116. Sue-A-Quan AK, Hannah ME, Cohen MM, Foster GA, Liston RM. Effect of labour induction on rates of stillbirth and cesarean section in post-term pregnancies. *CMAJ.* Apr 20 1999;160(8):1145-1149.

117. Menticoglou SM, Hall PF. Routine induction of labour at 41 weeks gestation: nonsensus consensus. *Br J Obstet Gynaecol.* May 2002;109(5):485-491.

118. Heimstad R, Romundstad PR, Salvesen KA. Induction of labour for post-term pregnancy and risk estimates for intrauterine and perinatal death. *Acta Obstet Gynecol Scand.* 2008;87(2):247-249, p 248.

119. Heimstad R, Skogvoll E, Mattsson LA, Johansen OJ, Eik-Nes SH, Salvesen KA. Induction of labor or serial antenatal fetal monitoring in postterm pregnancy: a randomized controlled trial. *Obstet Gynecol.* Mar 2007;109(3):609-617.

120. Monarch Pharmaceuticals. Pitocin (package insert). Available at: http://www.kingpharm.com/uploads/pdf_inserts/Pitocin_PI.pdf.

121. Herbst A, Wolner-Hanssen P, Ingemarsson I. Risk factors for acidemia at birth. *Obstet Gynecol.* Jul 1997;90(1):125-130.

122. Milsom I, Ladfors L, Thiringer K, Niklasson A, Odeback A, Thornberg E. Influence of maternal, obstetric and fetal risk factors on the prevalence of birth asphyxia at term in a Swedish

urban population. *Acta Obstet Gynecol Scand.* Oct 2002;81(10):909-917.

123. Oscarsson ME, Amer-Wahlin I, Rydhstroem H, Kallen K. Outcome in obstetric care related to oxytocin use. A population-based study. *Acta Obstet Gynecol Scand.* 2006;85(9):1094-1098.

124. Cammu H, Martens G, Ruyssinck G, Amy JJ. Outcome after elective labor induction in nulliparous women: a matched cohort study. *Am J Obstet Gynecol.* Feb 2002;186(2):240-244.

125. Battista L, Chung JH, Lagrew DC, Wing DA. Complications of labor induction among multiparous women in a community-based hospital system. *Am J Obstet Gynecol.* Sep 2007;197(3):241 e241-247; discussion 322-243, e241-244.

126. Dublin S, Lydon-Rochelle M, Kaplan RC, Watts DH, Critchlow CW. Maternal and neonatal outcomes after induction of labor without an identified indication. *Am J Obstet Gynecol.* Oct 2000;183(4):986-994.

127. Heffner LJ, Elkin E, Fretts RC. Impact of labor induction, gestational age, and maternal age on cesarean delivery rates. *Obstet Gynecol.* Aug 2003;102(2):287-293.

128. Luthy DA, Malmgren JA, Zingheim RW. Cesarean delivery after elective induction in nulliparous women: the physician effect. *Am J Obstet Gynecol.* Nov 2004;191(5):1511-1515.

129. Seyb ST, Berka RJ, Socol ML, Dooley SL. Risk of cesarean delivery with elective induction of labor at term in nulliparous women. *Obstet Gynecol.* Oct 1999;94(4):600-607.

130. Yeast JD, Jones A, Poskin M. Induction of labor and the relationship to cesarean delivery: A review of 7001 consecutive inductions. *Am J Obstet Gynecol.* Mar 1999;180(3 Pt 1):628-633.

131. Parry E, Parry D, Pattison N. Induction of labour for post term pregnancy: an observational study. *Aust N Z J Obstet Gynaecol.* Aug 1998;38(3):275-280.

132. Hannah ME, Hannah WJ, Hellmann J, Hewson S, Milner R, Willan A. Induction of labor as compared with serial antenatal monitoring in post-term pregnancy. A randomized controlled trial. The Canadian Multicenter Post-term Pregnancy Trial Group. *N Engl J Med.* Jun 11 1992;326(24):1587-1592.

133. van Gemund N, Hardeman A, Scherjon SA, Kanhai HH. Intervention rates after elective induction of labor compared to labor with a spontaneous onset. A matched cohort study. *Gynecol Obstet Invest.* 2003;56(3):133-138.

134. Phillip H, Fletcher H, Reid M. The impact of induced labour on postpartum blood loss. *J Obstet Gynaecol.* Jan 2004;24(1):12-15.

135. Gilbert L, Porter W, Brown VA. Postpartum haemorrhage—a continuing problem. *Br J Obstet Gynaecol.* Jan 1987;94(1):67-71.

136. Stones RW, Paterson CM, Saunders NJ. Risk factors for major obstetric haemorrhage. *Eur J Obstet Gynecol Reprod Biol.* Jan 1993;48(1):15-18.

137. El-Mahally AA, Kharboush IF, Amer NH, Hussein M, Abdel Salam T, Youssef AA. Risk factors of puerperal sepsis in Alexandria. *J Egypt Public Health Assoc.* 2004;79(3-4):311-331.

138. Dare FO, Bako AU, Ezechi OC. Puerperal sepsis: a preventable postpartum complication. *Trop Doct.* Apr 1998;28(2):92-95.

139. Schwarcz R, Diaz AG, Belizan JM, Fescina R, Caldeyro-Barcia R. Influence of amniotomy and maternal position on labor. Paper presented at: VIII World Congress of Gynecology and Obstetrics; 17-22 October 1976, 1976; Mexico City.

140. Goffinet F, Fraser W, Marcoux S, Breart G, Moutquin JM, Daris M. Early amniotomy increases the frequency of fetal heart rate abnormalities.

Amniotomy Study Group. *Br J Obstet Gynaecol.* May 1997;104(5):548-553.

141. Garite TJ, Porto M, Carlson NJ, Rumney PJ, Reimbold PA. The influence of elective amniotomy on fetal heart rate patterns and the course of labor in term patients: a randomized study. *Am J Obstet Gynecol.* Jun 1993;168(6 Pt 1):1827-1831; discussion 1831-1822.

142. Barrett JF, Savage J, Phillips K, Lilford RJ. Randomized trial of amniotomy in labour versus the intention to leave membranes intact until the second stage. *Br J Obstet Gynaecol.* Jan 1992;99(1):5-9.

143. Schwarcz R, Althabe O, Belitzky R, et al. Fetal heart rate patterns in labors with intact and with ruptured membranes. *J Perinat Med.* 1973;1(3):153-165.

144. Looney CB, Smith JK, Merck LH, et al. Intracranial hemorrhage in asymptomatic neonates: prevalence on MR images and relationship to obstetric and neonatal risk factors. *Radiology.* Feb 2007;242(2):535-541.

145. Caldeyro-Barcia R. Some Consequences of Obstetrical Intervention. *Birth and the Family Journal.* 1977;2(2):1-2.

146. Fedrick J, Butler NR. Certain causes of neonatal death. V. Cerebral birth trauma. *Biol Neonate.* 1971;18(5):321-329.

147. Muller PF, Campbell HE, Graham WE, et al. Perinatal factors and their relationship to mental retardation and other parameters of development. *Am J Obstet Gynecol.* Apr 15 1971;109(8):1205-1210.

148. Lydon-Rochelle M, Holt VL, Easterling TR, Martin DP. Risk of uterine rupture during labor among women with a prior cesarean delivery. *N Engl J Med.* Jul 5 2001;345(1):3-8.

149. Catanzarite V, Cousins L, Dowling D, Daneshmand S. Oxytocin-associated rupture of an unscarred uterus in a primigravida. *Obstet Gynecol.* Sep 2006;108(3 Pt 2):723-725.

150. Miller DA, Goodwin TM, Gherman RB, Paul RH. Intrapartum rupture of the unscarred uterus. *Obstet Gynecol.* May 1997;89(5 Pt 1):671-673.

151. Kramer MS, Rouleau J, Baskett TF, Joseph KS. Amniotic-fluid embolism and medical induction of labour: a retrospective, population-based cohort study. *Lancet.* Oct 21 2006;368(9545):1444-1448.

152. Odent M. Is taking castor oil for inducing labor okay for both the unborn child and mother? *Mothering Magazine Expert Panel.* Available at: http://www.mothering.com/sections/experts/odent-archive.html#castoroil.

153. Adair CD. Nonpharmacologic approaches to cervical priming and labor induction. *Clin Obstet Gynecol.* Sep 2000;43(3):447-454.

154. Hill MJ, McWilliams GD, Garcia-Sur D, Chen B, Munroe M, Hoeldtke NJ. The effect of membrane sweeping on prelabor rupture of membranes: a randomized controlled trial. *Obstet Gynecol.* Jun 2008;111(6):1313-1319.

155. Boulvain M, Stan C, Irion O. Membrane sweeping for induction of labour. *Cochrane Database Syst Rev.* 2005(1):CD000451.

156. Tan PC, Jacob R, Omar SZ. Membrane sweeping at initiation of formal labor induction: a randomized controlled trial. *Obstet Gynecol.* Mar 2006;107(3):569-577.

157. Frye A. *Holistic Midwifery; A comprehensive textbook for midwives in homebirth practice. Volume 1 Care During Pregnancy.* Portland OR: Labrys Press; 1998, p 759.

158. American College of Obstetricians and Gynecologists. ACOG Practice Bulletin. Clinical management guidelines for obstetricians-gynecologists. Number 55, September 2004 (replaces practice pattern number 6, October 1997). Management of Postterm Pregnancy. *Obstet Gynecol.* Sep 2004;104(3):639-646.

Chapter 5: **ULTRASOUND SCANS**

1. Wagner M. Ultrasound: more harm than good? *Midwifery Today Int Midwife.* Summer 1999(50):28-30.

2. Woo DJ. A Short History of the Development of Ultrasound in Obstetrics and Gynecology. Available at: http://www. ob-ultrasound.net/history1.htm.

3. de Crespigny L, Dredge R. *Which Tests for my Unborn Baby? Ultrasound and other prenatal tests.* 2nd ed. Melbourne: Oxford University Press; 1996.

4. Oakley A. The history of ultrasonography in obstetrics. *Birth.* Mar 1986;13(1):8-13.

5. Martin J, Hamilton B, Sutton P, Ventura S, Menacker F, Munson M. *Births: Final data for 2002. National vital statistics reports.* Vol 52. Hyattsville MD: National Center for Health Statistics; 2003.

6. American College of Obstetricians and Gynecologists. ACOG Practice Bulletin No. 58. Ultrasonography in pregnancy. *Obstet Gynecol.* Dec 2004;104(6):1449-1458.

7. Beech BL. Ultrasound unsound? Talk at Mercy Hospital, Melbourne; April 1993.

8. Neilson JP. Ultrasound for fetal assessment in early pregnancy. *Cochrane Database Syst Rev.* 2000(2):CD000182.

9. Meire HB. The safety of diagnostic ultrasound. *Br J Obstet Gynaecol.* Dec 1987;94(12):1121-1122, p 1122.

10. American Institute of Ultrasound in Medicine. Keepsake Fetal Imaging; 2005.

11. Health Canada. Fetal Ultrasound For Keepsake Videos. Available at: http://www.hc-sc.gc.ca/iyh-vsv/med/ultrasound-echographic_e.html.

12. Canadian Society of Diagnostic Medical Sonographers. Position on the use of diagnostic ultrasound for nonmedical purposes. Available at: http://www.csdms.com/docs/02.pdf.

13. American College of Obstetricians and Gynecologists. ACOG Committee Opinion. Number 297, August 2004. Nonmedical use of obstetric ultrasonography. *Obstet Gynecol.* Aug 2004;104(2):423-424.

14. United States Food and Drug Administration. Official Statement on Ultrasonic Fetal Imaging. Available at: http://www.fda.gov/FDAC/features/2004/104_images.htm.

15. Richards DS, Cornwall G. Accuracy of Ultrasound Dating. Available at: http://www.obgyn.ufl.edu/ultrasound/MedInfoVersion/sec6/6_6.htm.

16. Kieler H, Axelsson O, Nilsson S, Waldenstrom U. Comparison of ultrasonic measurement of biparietal diameter and last menstrual period as a predictor of day of delivery in women with regular 28-day cycles. *Acta Obstet Gynecol Scand.* Jul 1993;72(5):347-349.

17. Olsen O, Aaroe Clausen J. Routine ultrasound dating has not been shown to be more accurate than the calendar method. *Br J Obstet Gynaecol.* Nov 1997;104(11):1221-1222.

18. Stefos T, Plachouras N, Sotiriadis A, et al. Routine obstetrical ultrasound at 18-22 weeks: our experience on 7,236 fetuses. *J Matern Fetal Med.* Mar-Apr 1999;8(2):64-69.

19. Saltvedt S, Almstrom H, Kublickas M, Valentin L, Grunewald C. Detection of malformations in chromosomally normal fetuses by routine ultrasound at 12 or 18 weeks of gestation-a randomised controlled trial in 39,572 pregnancies. *BJOG.* Jun 2006;113(6):664-674.

20. Grandjean H, Larroque D, Levi S. Sensitivity of routine ultrasound screening of pregnancies in the Eurofetus database. The Eurofetus Team. *Ann N Y Acad Sci.* Jun 18 1998;847:118-124.

21. Crane JP, LeFevre ML, Winborn RC, et al. A randomized trial of prenatal ultrasonographic screening: impact on the

detection, management, and outcome of anomalous fetuses. The RADIUS Study Group. *Am J Obstet Gynecol.* Aug 1994;171(2):392-399.

22. Chan F. Limitations of Ultrasound. *Perinatal Society of Australia and New Zealand 1st Annual Congress.* Freemantle, Australia; 1997.

23. Brand IR, Kaminopetros P, Cave M, Irving HC, Lilford RJ. Specificity of antenatal ultrasound in the Yorkshire Region: a prospective study of 2261 ultrasound detected anomalies. *Br J Obstet Gynaecol.* May 1994;101(5):392-397.

24. Borsellino A, Zaccara A, Nahom A, et al. False-positive rate in prenatal diagnosis of surgical anomalies. *J Pediatr Surg.* Apr 2006;41(4):826-829.

25. Martinez-Zamora MA, Borrell A, Borobio V, et al. False positives in the prenatal ultrasound screening of fetal structural anomalies. *Prenat Diagn.* Jan 2007;27(1):18-22.

26. Saari-Kemppainen A, Karjalainen O, Ylostalo P, Heinonen OP. Ultrasound screening and perinatal mortality: controlled trial of systematic one-stage screening in pregnancy. The Helsinki Ultrasound Trial. *Lancet.* Aug 18 1990;336(8712):387-391.

27. Sparling JW, Seeds JW, Farran DC. The relationship of obstetric ultrasound to parent and infant behavior. *Obstet Gynecol.* Dec 1988;72(6):902-907.

28. Whittle M. Ultrasonographic "soft markers" of fetal chromosomal defects. *Br Med J.* Mar 29 1997;314(7085):918.

29. Stewart TL. Screening for aneuploidy: the genetic sonogram. *Obstet Gynecol Clin North Am.* Mar 2004;31(1):21-33.

30. Brookes A. Women's experience of routine prenatal ultrasound. *Healthsharing Women: The Newsletter of Healthsharing Women's Health Resource Service,* Melbourne. 1994/5;5(3-4):1-5.

31. Khan AT, Stewart KS. Ultrasound placental localisation in early pregnancy. *Scott Med J.* Feb 1987;32(1):19-21.

32. Chama CM, Wanonyi IK, Usman JD. From low-lying implantation to placenta praevia: a longitudinal ultrasonic assessment. *J Obstet Gynaecol.* Aug 2004;24(5):516-518.

33. Page IJ, Wolstenhulme S. Does the ultrasound diagnosis of low-lying placenta in early pregnancy warrant a repeat scan? *J R Army Med Corps.* Jun 1991;137(2):84-87.

34. Ancona S, Chatterjee M, Rhee I, Sicurenza B. The mid-trimester placenta previa: a prospective follow-up. *Eur J Radiol.* May-Jun 1990;10(3):215-216.

35. Morris JM, Thompson K, Smithey J, et al. The usefulness of ultrasound assessment of amniotic fluid in predicting adverse outcome in prolonged pregnancy: a prospective blinded observational study. *BJOG.* Nov 2003;110(11):989-994.

36. Hofmeyr GJ, Gulmezoglu AM. Maternal hydration for increasing amniotic fluid volume in oligohydramnios and normal amniotic fluid volume. *Cochrane Database Syst Rev.* 2002(1):CD000134.

37. Iams JD, Goldenberg RL, Mercer BM, et al. The preterm prediction study: can low-risk women destined for spontaneous preterm birth be identified? *Am J Obstet Gynecol.* Mar 2001;184(4):652-655.

38. Owen J, Yost N, Berghella V, et al. Mid-trimester endovaginal sonography in women at high risk for spontaneous preterm birth. *JAMA.* Sep 19 2001;286(11):1340-1348.

39. Kreiser D, el-Sayed YY, Sorem KA, Chitkara U, Holbrook RH, Jr., Druzin ML. Decreased amniotic fluid index in low-risk pregnancy. *J Reprod Med.* Aug 2001;46(8):743-746.

40. Roberts T, Henderson J, Mugford M, Bricker L, Neilson J, Garcia J. Antenatal

ultrasound screening for fetal abnormalities: a systematic review of studies of cost and cost effectiveness. *BJOG*. Jan 2002;109(1):44-56.

41. Van den Hof MC, Wilson D. Obstetric Ultrasound: Is It Time for Informed Consent? *J Obstet Gynaecol Can*. 2005;27(6):569.

42. American Institute of Ultrasound in Medicine Bioeffects Committee. Bioeffects considerations for the safety of diagnostic ultrasound. *J Ultrasound Med*. Sep 1988;7(9 Suppl):S1-38.

43. Deane C. Safety of Diagnostic Ultrasound in Fetal Scanning. In: Kypros Nicolaides GR, Kurt Hecker and Renato Ximenes, ed. *Doppler in Obstetrics*. Centrus; 2002.

44. Barnett SB. Intracranial temperature elevation from diagnostic ultrasound. *Ultrasound Med Biol*. Jul 2001;27(7):883-888.

45. Jago JR, Henderson J, Whittingham TA, and Mitchell G. A comparison of AIUM/NEMA thermal indices with calculated temperature rises for a simple third-trimester pregnancy tissue model. *Ultrasound in Med. & Biol* 1999;25(4):623-628.

46. Barnett SB, Maulik D. Guidelines and recommendations for safe use of Doppler ultrasound in perinatal applications. *J Matern Fetal Med*. Apr 2001;10(2):75-84.

47. Church CC, Miller MW. Quantification of risk from fetal exposure to diagnostic ultrasound. *Prog Biophys Mol Biol*. Jan-Apr 2007;93(1-3):331-353, p 336.

48. Pohl EE, Rosenfeld EH, Pohl P, Millner R. Effects of ultrasound on agglutination and aggregation of human erythrocytes in vitro. *Ultrasound Med Biol*. 1995;21(5):711-719.

49. Liebeskind D, Bases R, Elequin F, et al. Diagnostic ultrasound: effects on the DNA and growth patterns of animal cells. *Radiology*. Apr 1979;131(1):177-184.

50. Ellisman MH, Palmer DE, Andre MP. Diagnostic levels of ultrasound may disrupt myelination. *Exp Neurol*. Oct 1987;98(1):78-92.

51. Stanton MT, Ettarh R, Arango D, Tonra M, Brennan PC. Diagnostic ultrasound induces change within numbers of cryptal mitotic and apoptotic cells in small intestine. *Life Sci*. Feb 16 2001;68(13):1471-1475.

52. Dalecki D, Child SZ, Raeman CH, Cox C. Hemorrhage in murine fetuses exposed to pulsed ultrasound. *Ultrasound Med Biol*. Sep 1999;25(7):1139-1144.

53. Suresh R, Uma Devi P, Ovchinnikov N, McRae A. Long-term effects of diagnostic ultrasound during fetal period on postnatal development and adult behavior of mouse. *Life Sci*. Jun 7 2002;71(3):339-350.

54. Ang ES, Jr., Gluncic V, Duque A, Schafer ME, Rakic P. Prenatal exposure to ultrasound waves impacts neuronal migration in mice. *Proc Natl Acad Sci U S A*. Aug 22 2006;103(34):12903 12910.

55. Arulkumaran S, Talbert DG, Nyman M, Westgren M, Su HT, Ratnam SS. Audible in utero sound caused by the ultrasonic radiation force from a real-time scanner. *J Obstet Gynaecol Res*. Dec 1996;22(6):523-527.

56. Fatemi M, Ogburn PL, Jr, Greenleaf JF. Fetal stimulation by pulsed diagnostic ultrasound. *J Ultrasound Med*. Aug 2001;20(8):883-889.

57. Crum LA, Walton AJ, Mortimer A, Dyson M, Crawford DC, Gaitan DF. Free radical production in amniotic fluid and blood plasma by medical ultrasound. *J Ultrasound Med*. Nov 1987;6(11):643-647.

58. Tarantal AF, O'Brien WD, Hendrickx AG. Evaluation of the bioeffects of prenatal ultrasound exposure in the cynomolgus macaque (*Macaca fascicularis*):

III. Developmental and hematologic studies. *Teratology.* Feb 1993;47(2):159-170.

59. Tarantal AF, Gargosky SE, Ellis DS, O'Brien WD, Jr., Hendrickx AG. Hematologic and growth-related effects of frequent prenatal ultrasound exposure in the long-tailed macaque (*Macaca fascicularis*). *Ultrasound Med Biol.* 1995;21(8):1073-1081.

60. American Institute of Ultrasound in Medicine. Section 4—bioeffects in tissues with gas bodies. American Institute of Ultrasound in Medicine. *J Ultrasound Med.* Feb 2000;19(2):97-108, 154-168, p 107.

61. Testart J, Thebault A, Souderes E, Frydman R. Premature ovulation after ovarian ultrasonography. *Br J Obstet Gynaecol.* Sep 1982;89(9):694-700.

62. Lorenz RP, Comstock CH, Bottoms SF, Marx SR. Randomized prospective trial comparing ultrasonography and pelvic examination for preterm labor surveillance. *Am J Obstet Gynecol.* Jun 1990;162(6):1603-1607; discussion 1607-1610.

63. Geerts LT, Brand EJ, Theron GB. Routine obstetric ultrasound examinations in South Africa: cost and effect on perinatal outcome—a prospective randomised controlled trial. *Br J Obstet Gynaecol.* Jun 1996;103(6):501-507.

64. Newnham JP, Evans SF, Michael CA, Stanley FJ, Landau LI. Effects of frequent ultrasound during pregnancy: a randomised controlled trial. *Lancet.* Oct 9 1993;342(8876):887-891.

65. Newnham JP, O'Dea MR, Reid KP, Diepeveen DA. Doppler flow velocity waveform analysis in high risk pregnancies: a randomized controlled trial. *Br J Obstet Gynaecol.* Oct 1991;98(10): 956-963.

66. Davies JA, Gallivan S, Spencer JA. Randomised controlled trial of Doppler ultrasound screening of placental perfusion during pregnancy. *Lancet.* Nov 28 1992;340(8831):1299-1303.

67. Stark CR, Orleans M, Haverkamp AD, Murphy J. Short- and long-term risks after exposure to diagnostic ultrasound in utero. *Obstet Gynecol.* Feb 1984;63(2):194-200.

68. Campbell JD, Elford RW, Brant RF. Case-control study of prenatal ultrasonography exposure in children with delayed speech. *Can Med Assoc J.* Nov 15 1993;149(10):1435-1440.

69. Kieler H, Axelsson O, Haglund B, Nilsson S, Salvesen KA. Routine ultrasound screening in pregnancy and the children's subsequent handedness. *Early Hum Dev.* Jan 9 1998;50(2):233-245.

70. Kieler H, Cnattingius S, Haglund B, Palmgren J, Axelsson O. Sinistrality—a side-effect of prenatal sonography: a comparative study of young men. *Epidemiology.* Nov 2001;12(6):618-623.

71. Salvesen KA, Eik-Nes SH. Ultrasound during pregnancy and subsequent childhood non-right handedness: a meta-analysis. *Ultrasound Obstet Gynecol.* Apr 1999;13(4):241-246.

72. Salvesen KA, Vatten LJ, Eik-Nes SH, Hugdahl K, Bakketeig LS. Routine ultrasonography in utero and subsequent handedness and neurological development. *Br Med J.* Jul 17 1993;307(6897):159-164.

73. Odent M. Where does handedness come from? Handedness from a primal health research perspective. *Primal Health Research.* 1998;6(1):1-6.

74. Salvesen KA. Epidemiological prenatal ultrasound studies. *Prog Biophys Mol Biol.* Jan-Apr 2007;93(1-3):295-300.

75. Kieler H, Ahlsten G, Haglund B, Salvesen K, Axelsson O. Routine ultrasound screening in pregnancy and the children's subsequent neurologic development. *Obstet Gynecol.* May 1998;91(5 Pt 1):750-756.

76. Kieler H, Haglund B, Waldenstrom U, Axelsson O. Routine ultrasound screening in pregnancy and the children's subsequent growth, vision and hearing. *Br J Obstet Gynaecol.* Nov 1997;104(11):1267-1272.

77. Salvesen KA, Jacobsen G, Vatten LJ, Eik-Nes SH, Bakketeig LS. Routine ultrasonography in utero and subsequent growth during childhood. *Ultrasound Obstet Gynecol.* Jan 1 1993;3(1):6-10.

78. Salvesen KA, Vatten LJ, Bakketeig LS, Eik-Nes SH. Routine ultrasonography in utero and speech development. *Ultrasound Obstet Gynecol.* Mar 1 1994;4(2):101-103.

79. Salvesen KA, Vatten LJ, Jacobsen G, et al. Routine ultrasonography in utero and subsequent vision and hearing at primary school age. *Ultrasound Obstet Gynecol.* Jul 1 1992;2(4):243-244, 245-247.

80. Salvesen KA, Bakketeig LS, Eik-nes SH, Undheim JO, Okland O. Routine ultrasonography in utero and school performance at age 8-9 years. *Lancet.* Jan 11 1992;339(8785):85-89.

81. Kieler H, Cnattingius S, Palmgren J, Haglund B, Axelsson O. First trimester ultrasound scans and left-handedness. *Epidemiology.* May 2002;13(3):370.

82. Henderson J, Willson K, Jago J, Whittingham T. A survey of the acoustic outputs of diagnostic ultrasound equipment in current clinical use. *Ultrasound Med Biol.* 1995;21(5):699-705.

83. Newnham JP, Doherty DA, Kendall GE, Zubrick SR, Landau LL, Stanley FJ. Effects of repeated prenatal ultrasound examinations on childhood outcome up to 8 years of age: follow-up of a randomised controlled trial. *Lancet.* Dec 4 2004;364(9450):2038-2044.

84. Newnham JP, Doherty DA, Kendall GE, Zubrick SR, Landau LL, Stanley FJ. Effects of repeated prenatal ultrasound examinations on childhood outcome

up to 8 years of age: follow-up of a randomised controlled trial. *Lancet.* Dec 4 2004;364(9450):2038-2044, p 2043.

85. Salvesen KA. Epidemiological prenatal ultrasound studies. *Prog Biophys Mol Biol.* Jan-Apr 2007;93(1-3):295-300, p 301.

86. Marinac-Dabic D, Krulewitch CJ, Moore RM, Jr. The safety of prenatal ultrasound exposure in human studies. *Epidemiology.* May 2002;13(3 Suppl):S19-22., p S19.

87. Marinac-Dabic D, Krulewitch CJ, Moore RM, Jr. The safety of prenatal ultrasound exposure in human studies. *Epidemiology.* May 2002;13(3 Suppl):S19-22., p S22.

88. Meire HB. The safety of diagnostic ultrasound. *Br J Obstet Gynaecol.* Dec 1987;94(12):1121-1122.

89. American Institute of Ultrasound in Medicine. Section 7—discussion of the mechanical index and other exposure parameters. *J Ultrasound Med.* Feb 2000;19(2):143-148, 154-168.

90. Fowlkes JB, Holland CK. Mechanical bioeffects from diagnostic ultrasound: AIUM consensus statements. American Institute of Ultrasound in Medicine. *J Ultrasound Med.* Feb 2000;19(2):69-72, p 70.

91. Lumley J. Through a glass darkly: ultrasound and prenatal bonding. *Birth.* Dec 1990;17(4):214-217.

92. Sedgmen B, McMahon C, Cairns D, Benzie RJ, Woodfield RL. The impact of two-dimensional versus three-dimensional ultrasound exposure on maternal-fetal attachment and maternal health behavior in pregnancy. *Ultrasound Obstet Gynecol.* Mar 2006;27(3):245-251.

93. Garcia J, Bricker L, Henderson J, et al. Women's views of pregnancy ultrasound: a systematic review. *Birth.* Dec 2002;29(4):225-250.

94. Nicol M. Vulnerability of first-time expectant mothers during ultrasound scans: an evaluation of the external pressures that influence the process of informed choice. *Health Care Women Int.* Jul 2007;28(6):525-533.

95. Greer G. The Goddess or The Birth Machine (talk). Paper presented at: Homebirth Austalia National Conference; Sept 1993; Byron Bay, Australia.

96. Lalor JG, Devane D. Information, knowledge and expectations of the routine ultrasound scan. *Midwifery.* Mar 2007;23(1):13-22.

97. Lalor JG, Devane D. Information, knowledge and expectations of the routine ultrasound scan. *Midwifery.* Mar 2007;23(1):13-22, p 21.

98. Reist MT. *Defiant Birth: Women who Resist Medical Eugenics.* Melbourne: Spinifex; 2006.

99. Kuebelbeck A. *Waiting with Gabriel: A Story of Cherishing a Baby's Brief Life.* Chicago: Loyola Press; 2003.

100. Sheffield K. *Not Compatible with Life: A diary of keeping Daniel.* Melbourne: Best Legenz; 2008. Free at www.trisomyoz.bounce.com.au.

101. Loach E. The hardest thing I have ever done. *Sunday Herald Sun.* August 3 2004; Sunday magazine: 8-12.

102. Mulder EJ, Robles de Medina PG, Huizink AC, Van den Bergh BR, Buitelaar JK, Visser GH. Prenatal maternal stress: effects on pregnancy and the (unborn) child. *Early Hum Dev.* Dec 2002;70(1-2):3-14.

103. Rothman BK. *The Tentative Pregnancy. How Amniocentesis Changes the Experience of Motherhood.* 2nd ed. London: W. W. Norton & Company; 1993.

Chapter 6: UNDISTURBED BIRTH

1. Pearce JC. *Evolution's End: Claiming the Potential of Our Intelligence.* San Francisco: Harper San Francisco; 1992.

2. Rosenberg KR, Trevathan WR. The evolution of human birth. *Sci Am.* Nov 2001;285(5):72-77.

3. Goland RS, Wardlaw SL, Blum M, Tropper PJ, Stark RI. Biologically active corticotropin-releasing hormone in maternal and fetal plasma during pregnancy. *Am J Obstet Gynecol.* Oct 1988;159(4):884-890.

4. Weiss G. Endocrinology of parturition. *J Clin Endocrinol Metab.* Dec 2000;85(12):4421-4425.

5. Snegovskikh V, Park JS, Norwitz ER. Endocrinology of parturition. *Endocrinol Metab Clin North Am.* Mar 2006;35(1):173-191, viii.

6. Jenkin G, Young IR. Mechanisms responsible for parturition; the use of experimental models. *Anim Reprod Sci.* Jul 2004;82-83:567-581.

7. Smith R. Parturition. *N Engl J Med.* Jan 18 2007;356(3):271-283.

8. Mendelson CR, Condon JC. New insights into the molecular endocrinology of parturition. *J Steroid Biochem Mol Biol.* Feb 2005;93(2-5):113-119.

9. Buckley SJ. Sexuality in Labour and Birth. In: Walsh D, Downe S, eds. *Essential Midwifery Practice: Intrapartum Care.* London: Elsevier Science; 2009.

10. Russell JA, Douglas AJ, Ingram CD. Brain preparations for maternity—adaptive changes in behavioral and neuroendocrine systems during pregnancy and lactation. An overview. *Prog Brain Res.* 2001;133:1-38.

11. Jackson M, Dudley DJ. Endocrine assays to predict preterm delivery. *Clin Perinatol.* Dec 1998;25(4):837-857, vi.

12. Petrocelli T, Lye SJ. Regulation of transcripts encoding the myometrial gap junction protein, connexin-43, by estrogen and progesterone. *Endocrinology.* Jul 1993;133(1):284-290.

13. Newton N. Trebly Sensuous Woman. *Psychology Today*. July 1971:68-71; 98-99.

14. Verbalis JG, McCann MJ, McHale CM, Stricker EM. Oxytocin secretion in response to cholecystokinin and food: differentiation of nausea from satiety. *Science*. Jun 13 1986;232(4756):1417-1419.

15. Odent M. *The Scientification of Love*. Revised ed. London: Free Association Books; 2001.

16. Russell JA, Leng G, Douglas AJ. The magnocellular oxytocin system, the fount of maternity: adaptations in pregnancy. *Front Neuroendocrinol*. Jan 2003;24(1):27-61.

17. Fuchs AR, Romero R, Keefe D, Parra M, Oyarzun E, Behnke E. Oxytocin secretion and human parturition: pulse frequency and duration increase during spontaneous labor in women *Am J Obstet Gynecol*. Nov 1991;165(5 Pt 1):1515-1523.

18. Fuchs AR, Fuchs F. Endocrinology of human parturition: a review. *Br J Obstet Gynaecol*. Oct 1984;91(10):948-967.

19. Arias F. Pharmacology of oxytocin and prostaglandins. *Clin Obstet Gynecol*. Sep 2000;43(3):455-468.

20. Gonser M. Labor induction and augmentation with oxytocin: pharmacokinetic considerations. *Arch Gynecol Obstet*. 1995;256(2):63-66.

21. Steer PJ. The endocrinology of parturition in the human. *Baillieres Clin Endocrinol Metab*. Jun 1990;4(2):333-349.

22. Young WS, 3rd, Shepard E, Amico J, et al. Deficiency in mouse oxytocin prevents milk ejection, but not fertility or parturition. *J Neuroendocrinol*. Nov 1996;8(11):847-853.

23. Lundeberg T, Uvnas-Moberg K, Agren G, Bruzelius G. Anti-nociceptive effects of oxytocin in rats and mice. *Neurosci Lett*. Mar 28 1994;170(1):153-157.

24. Malek A, Blann E, Mattison DR. Human placental transport of oxytocin. *J Matern Fetal Med*. Sep-Oct 1996;5(5):245-255.

25. Chard T. Fetal and maternal oxytocin in human parturition. *Am J Perinatol*. Apr 1989;6(2):145-152.

26. Dawood MY, Raghavan KS, Pociask C, Fuchs F. Oxytocin in human pregnancy and parturition. *Obstet Gynecol*. Feb 1978;51(2):138-143.

27. Odent M. The foetus ejection reflex. *Birth and Breastfeeding*. East Sussex, UK: Clairview; 2007:34-49.

28. Matthiesen AS, Ransjo-Arvidson AB, Nissen E, Uvnas-Moberg K. Postpartum maternal oxytocin release by newborns: effects of infant hand massage and sucking. *Birth*. Mar 2001;28(1):13-19.

29. Uvnas-Moberg K. *The Oxytocin Factor*. Cambridge MA: Da Capo Press; 2003.

30. Nissen E, Lilja G, Widstrom AM, Uvnas-Moberg K. Elevation of oxytocin levels early post partum in women. *Acta Obstet Gynecol Scand*. Aug 1995;74(7):530-533.

31. Gimpl G, Fahrenholz F. The oxytocin receptor system: structure, function, and regulation. *Physiol Rev*. Apr 2001;81(2):629-683.

32. Leake RD, Weitzman RE, Fisher DA. Oxytocin concentrations during the neonatal period. *Biol Neonate*. 1981;39(3-4):127-131.

33. Takeda S, Kuwabara Y, Mizuno M. Concentrations and origin of oxytocin in breastmilk. *Endocrinol Jpn*. Dec 1986;33(6):821-826.

34. Levy F, Keller M, Poindron P. Olfactory regulation of maternal behavior in mammals. *Horm Behav*. Sep 2004;46(3):284-302.

35. Lundblad EG, Hodgen GD. Induction of maternal-infant bonding in rhesus and cynomolgus monkeys after cesarean delivery. *Lab Anim Sci*. Oct 1980;30(5):913.

36. Varendi H, Christensson K, Porter RH, Winberg J. Soothing effect of amniotic fluid smell in newborn infants. *Early Hum Dev.* Apr 17 1998;51(1):47-55.

37. Marlier L, Schaal B, Soussignan R. Neonatal responsiveness to the odor of amniotic and lacteal fluids: a test of perinatal chemosensory continuity. *Child Dev.* Jun 1998;69(3):611-623.

38. Axel R. The molecular logic of smell. *Sci Am.* Oct 1995;273(4):154-159.

39. Chapman M. Oxytocin has big role in maternal behaviour: interview with Professor K Uvnas-Moberg. *Australian Doctor.* August 7 1998:38.

40. Agren G, Olsson C, Uvnas-Moberg K, Lundeberg T. Olfactory cues from an oxytocin-injected male rat can reduce energy loss in its cagemates. *Neuroreport.* Jul 28 1997;8(11):2551-2555.

41. Agren G, Uvnas-Moberg K, Lundeberg T. Olfactory cues from an oxytocin-injected male rat can induce anti-nociception in its cagemates. *Neuroreport.* Sep 29 1997;8(14):3073-3076.

42. Giovenardi M, Padoin MJ, Cadore LP, Lucion AB. Hypothalamic paraventricular nucleus modulates maternal aggression in rats: effects of ibotenic acid lesion and oxytocin antisense. *Physiol Behav.* Feb 1 1998;63(3):351-359.

43. Kinsley CH, Bridges RS. Opiate involvement in postpartum aggression in rats. *Pharmacol Biochem Behav.* Nov 1986;25(5):1007-1011.

44. Gutkowska J, Jankowski M, Mukaddam-Daher S, McCann SM. Oxytocin is a cardiovascular hormone. *Braz J Med Biol Res.* Jun 2000;33(6):625-633.

45. Uvnas-Moberg K. Oxytocin linked antistress effects—the relaxation and growth response. *Acta Physiol Scand Suppl.* 1997;640:38-42.

46. Taylor SE, Klein LC, Lewis BP, Gruenewald TL, Gurung RA, Updegraff JA. Biobehavioral responses to stress in females: tend-and-befriend, not fight-or-flight. *Psychol Rev.* Jul 2000;107(3):411-429.

47. Feifel D, Reza T. Oxytocin modulates psychotomimetic-induced deficits in sensorimotor gating. *Psychopharmacology (Berl).* Jan 1999;141(1):93-98.

48. Insel TR, O'Brien DJ, Leckman JF. Oxytocin, vasopressin, and autism: is there a connection? *Biol Psychiatry.* Jan 15 1999;45(2):145-157.

49. Knox SS, Uvnas-Moberg K. Social isolation and cardiovascular disease: an atherosclerotic pathway? *Psychoneuroendocrinology.* Nov 1998;23(8):877-890.

50. Sarnyai Z, Kovacs GL. Role of oxytocin in the neuroadaptation to drugs of abuse. *Psychoneuroendocrinology.* 1994;19(1):85-117.

51. Uvnas-Moberg K, Bjokstrand E, Hillegaart V, Ahlenius S. Oxytocin as a possible mediator of SSRI-induced antidepressant effects. *Psychopharmacology (Berl)* . Feb 1999;142(1):95-101.

52. Laatikainen TJ. Corticotropin-releasing hormone and opioid peptides in reproduction and stress. *Ann Med.* 1991;23(5):489-496.

53. Brinsmead M, Smith R, Singh B, Lewin T, Owens P. Peripartum concentrations of beta endorphin and cortisol and maternal mood states. *Aust N Z J Obstet Gynaecol.* Aug 1985;25(3):194-197.

54. Bacigalupo G, Riese S, Rosendahl H, Saling E. Quantitative relationships between pain intensities during labor and beta-endorphin and cortisol concentrations in plasma. Decline of the hormone concentrations in the early postpartum period. *J Perinat Med.* 1990;18(4):289-296.

55. Foley KM, Kourides IA, Inturrisi CE, et al. Beta-Endorphin: analgesic and hormonal effects in humans. *Proc Natl Acad Sci USA.* Oct 1979;76(10):5377-5381.

56. Facchinetti F, Lanzani A, Genazzani AR. Fetal intermediate lobe is stimulated by parturition. *Am J Obstet Gynecol.* Nov 1989;161(5):1267-1270.

57. Facchinetti F, Garuti G, Petraglia F, Mercantini F, Genazzani AR. Changes in beta-endorphin in fetal membranes and placenta in normal and pathological pregnancies. *Acta Obstet Gynecol Scand.* 1990;69(7-8):603-607.

58. Jevremovic M, Terzic M, Kartaljevic G, Filipovic B, Filipovic S, Rostic B. [The opioid peptide, beta-endorphin, in spontaneous vaginal delivery and cesarean section]. *Srp Arh Celok Lek.* Sep-Oct 1991;119(9-10):271-274.

59. Kimball CD. Do endorphin residues of beta lipotropin in hormone reinforce reproductive functions? *Am J Obstet Gynecol.* May 15 1979;134(2):127-132, p 128.

60. Jowitt M. Beta-endorphin and stress in pregnancy and labour. *Midwifery Matters.* 1995;56:3-4.

61. Douglas AJ, Bicknell RJ, Russell JA. Pathways to parturition. *Adv Exp Med Biol.* 1995;395:381-394.

62. Rivier C, Vale W, Ling N, Brown M, Guillemin R. Stimulation in vivo of the secretion of prolactin and growth hormone by beta-endorphin. *Endocrinology.* Jan 1977;100(1):238-241.

63. Voogt JL, Lee Y, Yang S, Arbogast L. Regulation of prolactin secretion during pregnancy and lactation. *Prog Brain Res.* 2001;133:173-185.

64. Mendelson CR, Boggaram V. Hormonal and developmental regulation of pulmonary surfactant synthesis in fetal lung. *Baillieres Clin Endocrinol Metab.* Jun 1990;4(2):351-378.

65. Franceschini R, Venturini PL, Cataldi A, Barreca T, Ragni N, Rolandi E. Plasma beta-endorphin concentrations during suckling in lactating women. *Br J Obstet Gynaecol.* Jun 1989;96(6):711-713.

66. Zanardo V, Nicolussi S, Carlo G, et al. Beta endorphin concentrations in human milk. *J Pediatr Gastroenterol Nutr.* Aug 2001;33(2):160-164.

67. Zanardo V, Nicolussi S, Giacomin C, Faggian D, Favaro F, Plebani M. Labor pain effects on colostral milk beta-endorphin concentrations of lactating mothers. *Biol Neonate.* Feb 2001;79(2):87-90.

68. Alehagen S, Wijma B, Lundberg U, Wijma K. Fear, pain and stress hormones during childbirth. *J Psychosom Obstet Gynaecol.* Sep 2005;26(3):153-165.

69. Segal S, Csavoy AN, Datta S. The tocolytic effect of catecholamines in the gravid rat uterus. *Anesth Analg.* Oct 1998;87(4):864-869.

70. Segal S, Wang SY. The effect of maternal catecholamines on the caliber of gravid uterine microvessels. *Anesth Analg.* Mar 2008;106(3):888-892

71. Lederman RP, Lederman E, Work B, Jr., McCann DS. Anxiety and epinephrine in multiparous women in labor: relationship to duration of labor and fetal heart rate pattern. *Am J Obstet Gynecol.* Dec 15 1985;153(8):870-877.

72. Saito M, Sano T, Satohisa E. Plasma catecholamines and microvibration as labour progresses. *Shinshin-Thaku.* 1991;31:381-389.

73. Thomas SA, Palmiter RD. Impaired maternal behavior in mice lacking norepinephrine and epinephrine. *Cell.* Nov 28 1997;91(5):583-592.

74. Phillippe M. Fetal catecholamines. *Am J Obstet Gynecol.* Aug 1 1983;146(7):840-855.

75. Irestedt L, Lagercrantz H, Belfrage P. Causes and consequences of maternal and fetal sympathoadrenal activation during parturition. *Acta Obstet Gynecol Scand Suppl.* 1984;118:111-115.

76. Lagercrantz H, Slotkin TA. The "stress" of being born. *Sci Am*. Apr 1986;254(4):100-107.

77. Hagnevik K, Faxelius G, Irestedt L, Lagercrantz H, Lundell B, Persson B. Catecholamine surge and metabolic adaptation in the newborn after vaginal delivery and caesarean section. *Acta Paediatr Scand*. Sep 1984;73(5):602-609.

78. Colson S. Womb to world: a metabolic perspective. *Midwifery Today Int Midwife*. Spring 2002(61):12-17.

79. Lowe NK, Reiss R. Parturition and fetal adaptation. *J Obstet Gynecol Neonatal Nurs*. May 1996;25(4):339-349.

80. Eliot RJ, Lam R, Leake RD, Hobel CJ, Fisher DA. Plasma catecholamine concentrations in infants at birth and during the first 48 hours of life. *J Pediatr*. Feb 1980;96(2):311-315.

81. Varendi H, Porter RH, Winberg J. The effect of labor on olfactory exposure learning within the first postnatal hour. *Behav Neurosci*. Apr 2002;116(2): 206-211.

82. Grattan DR. The actions of prolactin in the brain during pregnancy and lactation. *Prog Brain Res*. 2001;133:153-171.

83. Harris J, Stanford PM, Oakes SR, Ormandy CJ. Prolactin and the prolactin receptor: new targets of an old hormone. *Ann Med*. 2004;36(6):414-425.

84. Fernandes PA, Szelazek JT, Reid GJ, Wodzicki AM, Allardice JG, McCoshen JA. Phasic maternal prolactin secretion during spontaneous labor is associated with cervical dilatation and second-stage uterine activity. *J Soc Gynecol Investig*. Jul-Aug 1995;2(4):597-601.

85. Fernandes PA, Boroditsky RS, Roberts GK, Wodzicki AM, McCoshen JA. The acute release of maternal prolactin by instrumental cervical dilatation simulates the second stage of labor. *J Soc Gynecol Investig*. Jan-Feb 1999;6(1): 22-26.

86. Stefos T, Sotiriadis A, Tsirkas P, Messinis I, Lolis D. Maternal prolactin secretion during labor. The role of dopamine. *Acta Obstet Gynecol Scand*. Jan 2001;80(1): 34-38.

87. Volpe A, Mazza V, Di Renzo GC. Prolactin and certain obstetric stress conditions. *Int J Biol Res Pregnancy*. 1982;3(4):161-166.

88. Rigg LA, Yen SS. Multiphasic prolactin secretion during parturition in human subjects. *Am J Obstet Gynecol*. May 15 1977;128(2):215-218.

89. Stern JM, Reichlin S. Prolactin circadian rhythm persists throughout lactation in women. *Neuroendocrinology*. Jan 1990;51(1):31-37.

90. Heinrichs M, Meinlschmidt G, Neumann I, et al. Effects of suckling on hypothalamic-pituitary-adrenal axis responses to psychosocial stress in postpartum lactating women. *J Clin Endocrinol Metab*. Oct 2001;86(10):4798-4804.

91. Berczi I. The role of the growth and lactogenic hormone family in immune function. *Neuroimmunomodulation*. Jul-Aug 1994;1(4):201-216.

92. Sobrinho LG, Almeida-Costa JM. Hyperprolactinaemia as a result of immaturity or regression: the concept of maternal subroutine. A new model of psychoendocrine interactions. *Psychother Psychosom*. 1992;57(3):128-132.

93. Sobrinho LG. Emotional aspects of hyperprolactinemia. *Psychother Psychosom*. 1998;67(3):133-139.

94. Keverne EB. Sexual and aggressive behaviour in social groups of talapoin monkeys. *Ciba Found Symp*. Mar 14-16 1978(62):271-297.

95. Roberts RL, Jenkins KT, Lawler T, et al. Prolactin levels are elevated after infant carrying in parentally inexperienced common marmosets. *Physiol Behav*. Apr 2001;72(5):713-720.

96. Soltis J, Wegner FH, Newman JD. Urinary prolactin is correlated with mothering and allo-mothering in squirrel monkeys. *Physiol Behav.* Feb 15 2005;84(2):295-301.

97. Ziegler TE. Hormones associated with non-maternal infant care: a review of mammalian and avian studies. *Folia Primatol (Basel)* . Jan-Apr 2000;71 (1-2):6-21.

98. Storey AE, Walsh CJ, Quinton RL, Wynne-Edwards KE. Hormonal correlates of paternal responsiveness in new and expectant fathers. *Evol Hum Behav.* Mar 1 2000;21(2):79-95.

99. Schradin C, Anzenberger G. Prolactin, the Hormone of Paternity. *News Physiol Sci.* Dec 1999;14:223-231.

100. Fleming AS, Corter C, Stallings J, Steiner M. Testosterone and prolactin are associated with emotional responses to infant cries in new fathers. *Horm Behav.* Dec 2002;42(4):399-413.

101. Grosvenor CE, Whitworth NS. Accumulation of prolactin by maternal milk and its transfer to circulation of neonatal rat—a review. *Endocrinol Exp.* Oct 1983;17(3-4):271-282.

102. Grattan DR. The actions of prolactin in the brain during pregnancy and lactation. *Prog Brain Res.* 2001;133:153-171, p 165.

103. Horwood LJ, Fergusson DM. Breastfeeding and later cognitive and academic outcomes. *Pediatrics.* Jan 1998;101(1):E9.

104. Kramer MS, Aboud F, Mironova E, et al. Breastfeeding and child cognitive development: new evidence from a large randomized trial. *Arch Gen Psychiatry.* May 2008;65(5):578-584.

105. Declercq ER, Sakala C, Corry MP, Applebaum S. *Listening to Mothers II: Report of the Second National U.S. Survey of Women's Childbearing Experiences.* New York: Childbirth Connection; October 2006. 2006.

106. Martin JA, Hamilton BE, Sutton PD, et al. *Births: Final data for 2005.* Hyattsville, MD: National Center for Health Statistics; 2007. Vol 56 no 6.

107. Laws P, Abeywardana S, Walker J, Sullivan E. *Australia's mothers and babies 2005.* Vol Cat. no. PER 40. Sydney: Australian Institute of Health and Welfare National Perinatal Statistics Unit; 2007.

108. The Information Centre Community Health Statistics. *NHS Maternity Statistics, England: 2005-06.* 2007.

109. Canadian Institute for Health Information. *Giving Birth in Canada.* Ontario: CIHA; 2004.

110. Dawood MY. Novel approach to oxytocin induction-augmentation of labor. Application of oxytocin physiology during pregnancy. *Adv Exp Med Biol.* 1995;395:585-594.

111. Stubbs TM. Oxytocin for labor induction. *Clin Obstet Gynecol.* Sep 2000;43(3):489-494.

112. Haire D. FDA Approved Obstetric Drugs: Their Effects on Mother and Baby Available at: www.aimsusa.org/ obstetricdrugs.htm.

113. Bakker PC, Kurver PH, Kuik DJ, Van Geijn HP. Elevated uterine activity increases the risk of fetal acidosis at birth. *Am J Obstet Gynecol.* Apr 2007;196(4):313 e311-316.

114. Herbst A, Wolner-Hanssen P, Ingemarsson I. Risk factors for acidemia at birth. *Obstet Gynecol.* Jul 1997;90(1):125-130.

115. Cammu H, Martens G, Ruyssinck G, Amy JJ. Outcome after elective labor induction in nulliparous women: a matched cohort study. *Am J Obstet Gynecol.* Feb 2002;186(2):240-244.

116. Monarch Pharmaceuticals. Pitocin (package insert). Available at: http:// www.kingpharm.com/uploads/pdf_ inserts/Pitocin_PI.pdf.

117. Satin AJ, Leveno KJ, Sherman ML, Brewster DS, Cunningham FG. High- versus low-dose oxytocin for labor stimulation. *Obstet Gynecol*. Jul 1992;80(1):111-116.

118. Milsom I, Ladfors L, Thiringer K, Niklasson A, Odeback A, Thornberg E. Influence of maternal, obstetric and fetal risk factors on the prevalence of birth asphyxia at term in a Swedish urban population. *Acta Obstet Gynecol Scand*. Oct 2002;81(10):909-917.

119. Ellis M, Manandhar N, Manandhar DS, Costello AM. Risk factors for neonatal encephalopathy in Kathmandu, Nepal, a developing country: unmatched case-control study. *Br Med J*. May 6 2000;320(7244):1229-1236.

120. Bidgood KA, Steer PJ. A randomized control study of oxytocin augmentation of labour. 2. Uterine activity. *Br J Obstet Gynaecol*. Jun 1987;94(6):518-522.

121. Phillip H, Fletcher H, Reid M. The impact of induced labour on postpartum blood loss. *J Obstet Gynaecol*. Jan 2004;24(1):12-15.

122. Gilbert L, Porter W, Brown VA. Postpartum haemorrhage—a continuing problem. *Br J Obstet Gynaecol*. Jan 1987;94(1):67-71.

123. Stones RW, Paterson CM, Saunders NJ. Risk factors for major obstetric haemorrhage. *Eur J Obstet Gynecol Reprod Biol*. Jan 1993;48(1):15-18.

124. Phaneuf S, Rodriguez Linares B, TambyRaja RL, MacKenzie IZ, Lopez Bernal A. Loss of myometrial oxytocin receptors during oxytocin-induced and oxytocin-augmented labour. *J Reprod Fertil*. Sep 2000;120(1):91-97.

125. Genazzani AR, Petraglia F, Facchinetti F, Galli PA, Volpe A. Lack of beta-endorphin plasma level rise in oxytocin-induced labor. *Gynecol Obstet Invest*. 1985;19(3):130-134.

126. Palmer SR, Avery A, Taylor R. The influence of obstetric procedures and social and cultural factors on breast-feeding rates at discharge from hospital. *J Epidemiol Community Health*. Dec 1979;33(4):248-252.

127. Zuppa AA, Vignetti M, Romagnoli C, Tortorolo G. [Assistance procedures in the perinatal period that condition breast feeding at the time of discharge from the hospital]. *Pediatr Med Chir*. May-Jun 1984;6(3):367-372.

128. Out JJ, Vierhout ME, Wallenburg HC. Breast-feeding following spontaneous and induced labour. *Eur J Obstet Gynecol Reprod Biol*. Dec 1988;29(4):275-279.

129. Dewey KG. Maternal and fetal stress are associated with impaired lactogenesis in humans. *J Nutr*. Nov 2001;131(11):3012S-3015S.

130. Dawood MY, Wang CF, Gupta R, Fuchs F. Fetal contribution to oxytocin in human labor. *Obstet Gynecol*. Aug 1978;52(2):205-209.

131. Tyzio R, Cossart R, Khalilov I, et al. Maternal oxytocin triggers a transient inhibitory switch in GABA signaling in the fetal brain during delivery. *Science*. Dec 15 2006;314(5806):1788-1792.

132. Crowell DH, Sharma SD, Philip AG, Kapuniai LE, Waxman SH, Hale RW. Effects of induction of labor on the neurophysiologic functioning of newborn infants. *Am J Obstet Gynecol*. Jan 1 1980;136(1):48-53.

133. Ounsted MK, Hendrick AM, Mutch LM, Calder AA, Good FJ. Induction of labour by different methods in primiparous women. I. Some perinatal and postnatal problems. *Early Hum Dev*. Sep 1978;2(3):227-239.

134. De Coster W, Goethals A, Vandierendonck A, Thiery M, Derom R. Labor induction with prostaglandin F2alpha. Influence on psychomotor evolution of the child in the first 30 months. *Prostaglandins*. Oct 1976;12(4):559-564.

135. McBride WG, Lyle JG, Black B, Brown C, Thomas DB. A study of five

year old children born after elective induction of labour. *Med J Aust*. Oct 1 1977;2(14):456-459.

136. Winstone CL. *The relationship between artificial oxytocin (Pitocin) use at birth for labor induction or augmentation and the psychosocial functioning of three-year-olds.* Unpublished doctoral dissertation, Santa Barbara Graduate Institute; 2008.

137. Jonas W, Wiklund I, Nissen E, Ransjo-Arvidson AB, Uvnas-Moberg K. Newborn skin temperature two days postpartum during breastfeeding related to different labour ward practices. *Early Hum Dev*. Jan 2007;83(1):55-62.

138. Carter CS. Developmental consequences of oxytocin. *Physiol Behav*. Aug 2003;79(3):383-397.

139. Wahl RU. Could oxytocin administration during labor contribute to autism and related behavioral disorders? A look at the literature. *Med Hypotheses*. 2004;63(3):456-460.

140. Odent M. New reasons and new ways to study birth physiology. *Int J Gynaecol Obstet*. Nov 2001;75 Suppl 1:S39-45.

141. Winslow JT, Insel TR. The social deficits of the oxytocin knockout mouse. *Neuropeptides*. Apr-Jun 2002;36(2-3):221-229.

142. Young LJ, Pitkow LJ, Ferguson JN. Neuropeptides and social behavior: animal models relevant to autism. *Mol Psychiatry*. 2002;7 Suppl 2:S38-39.

143. Lim MM, Bielsky IF, Young LJ. Neuropeptides and the social brain: potential rodent models of autism. *Int J Dev Neurosci*. Apr-May 2005;23(2-3):235-243.

144. Hollander E, Novotny S, Hanratty M, et al. Oxytocin infusion reduces repetitive behaviors in adults with autistic and Asperger's disorders. *Neuropsychopharmacology*. Jan 2003;28(1):193-198.

145. Green L, Fein D, Modahl C, Feinstein C, Waterhouse L, Morris M. Oxytocin and autistic disorder: alterations in peptide forms. *Biol Psychiatry*. Oct 15 2001;50(8):609-613.

146. Modahl C, Green L, Fein D, et al. Plasma oxytocin levels in autistic children. *Biol Psychiatry*. Feb 15 1998;43(4):270-277.

147. Glasson EJ, Bower C, Petterson B, de Klerk N, Chaney G, Hallmayer JF. Perinatal factors and the development of autism: a population study. *Arch Gen Psychiatry*. Jun 2004;61(6):618-627.

148. Gale S, Ozonoff S, Lainhart J. Brief report: pitocin induction in autistic and nonautistic individuals. *J Autism Dev Disord*. Apr 2003;33(2):205-208.

149. Fein D, Allen D, Dunn M, et al. Pitocin induction and autism. *Am J Psychiatry*. Mar 1997;154(3):438-439.

150. Gottesman II, Hanson DR. Human development: biological and genetic processes. *Annu Rev Psychol*. 2005;56:263-286.

151. Olofsson C, Ekblom A, Ekman-Ordeberg G, Hjelm A, Irestedt L. Lack of analgesic effect of systemically administered morphine or pethidine on labour pain. *Br J Obstet Gynaecol*. Oct 1996;103(10):968-972.

152. Tsui MH, Ngan Kee WD, Ng FF, Lau TK. A double blinded randomised placebo controlled study of intramuscular pethidine for pain relief in the first stage of labour. *Br J Obstet Gynaecol*. Jul 2004;111(7):648-655.

153. Soontrapa S, Somboonporn W, Komwilaisak R, Sookpanya S. Effectiveness of intravenous meperidine for pain relief in the first stage of labour. *J Med Assoc Thai*. Nov 2002;85(11):1169-1175.

154. American College of Obstetricians and Gynecologists. Obstetric Analgesia and Anesthesia. *ACOG Technical Bulletin*. 1996;225(July).

155. Thomas TA, Fletcher JE, Hill RG. Influence of medication, pain and progress in labour on plasma beta-endorphin-like

immunoreactivity. *Br J Anaesth.* Apr 1982;54(4):401-408.

156. Thomson AM, Hillier VF. A re-evaluation of the effect of pethidine on the length of labour. *J Adv Nurs.* Mar 1994;19(3):448-456.

157. Lindow SW, van der Spuy ZM, Hendricks MS, Rosselli AP, Lombard C, Leng G. The effect of morphine and naloxone administration on plasma oxytocin concentrations in the first stage of labour. *Clin Endocrinol (Oxf).* Oct 1992;37(4):349-353.

158. Russell JA, Gosden RG, Humphreys EM, et al. Interruption of parturition in rats by morphine: a result of inhibition of oxytocin secretion. *J Endocrinol. Jun 1989;121(3):521-536.*

159. Kinsley CH, Morse AC, Zoumas C, Corl S, Billack B. Intracerebroventricular infusions of morphine, and blockade with naloxone, modify the olfactory preferences for pup odors in lactating rats. *Brain Res Bull.* 1995;37(1):103-107.

160. Misiti A, Turillazzi PG, Zapponi GA, Loizzo A. Heroin induces changes in mother-infant monkey communication and subsequent disruption of their dyadic interaction. *Pharmacol Res.* Jul 1991;24(1):93-104.

161. Bridges RS, Grimm CT. Reversal of morphine disruption of maternal behavior by concurrent treatment with the opiate antagonist naloxone. *Science.* Oct 8 1982;218(4568):166-168.

162. Stafisso-Sandoz G, Polley D, Holt E, Lambert KG, Kinsley CH. Opiate disruption of maternal behavior: morphine reduces, and naloxone restores, c-fos activity in the medial preoptic area of lactating rats. *Brain Res Bull.* 1998;45(3):307-313.

163. Kimball CD. Do endorphin residues of beta lipotropin in hormone reinforce reproductive functions? *Am J Obstet Gynecol.* May 15 1979;134(2):127-132.

164. Jacobson B, Nyberg K, Gronbladh L, Eklund G, Bygdeman M, Rydberg U. Opiate addiction in adult offspring through possible imprinting after obstetric treatment. *Br Med J.* Nov 10 1990;301(6760):1067-1070.

165. Nyberg K. Long-term effects of labor analgesia. *J Obstet Gynecol Neonatal Nurs.* May-Jun 2000;29(3):226.

166. Csaba G, Tekes K. Is the brain hormonally imprintable? *Brain Dev.* Oct 2005;27(7):465-471.

167. Kellogg CK. Sex differences in long-term consequences of prenatal diazepam exposure: possible underlying mechanisms. *Pharmacol Biochem Behav.* Dec 1999;64(4):673-680.

168. Kellogg CK, Primus RJ, Bitran D. Sexually dimorphic influence of prenatal exposure to diazepam on behavioral responses to environmental challenge and on gamma-aminobutyric acid (GABA)-stimulated chloride uptake in the brain. *J Pharmacol Exp Ther.* Jan 1991;256(1):259-265.

169. Livezey GT, Rayburn WF, Smith CV. Prenatal exposure to phenobarbital and quantifiable alterations in the electroencephalogram of adult rat offspring. *Am J Obstet Gynecol.* Dec 1992;167(6):1611-1615.

170. Mirmiran M, Swaab D. Effects of perinatal medication on the developing brain. In: Nijhuis J, ed. *Fetal behaviour.* Oxford: Oxford University Press; 1992.

171. Meyerson BJ. Neonatal beta-endorphin and sexual behavior. *Acta Physiol Scand.* May 1982;115(1):159-160.

172. Csaba G, Knippel B, Karabelyos C, Inczefi-Gonda A, Hantos M, Tekes K. Endorphin excess at weaning durably influences sexual activity, uterine estrogen receptor's binding capacity and brain serotonin level of female rats. *Horm Metab Res.* Jan 2004;36(1):39-43.

173. Meyerson BJ. Socio-sexual behaviours in rats after neonatal and adult beta-

endorphin treatment. *Scand J Psychol.* 1982;Suppl 1:85-89.

174. Csaba G, Knippel B, Karabelyos C, et al. Effect of neonatal beta-endorphin imprinting on sexual behavior and brain serotonin level in adult rats. *Life Sci.* May 23 2003;73(1):103-114.

175. Csaba G, Knippel B, Karabelyos C, Inczefi-Gonda A, Hantos M, Tekes K. Impact of single neonatal serotonin treatment (hormonal imprinting) on the brain serotonin content and sexual behavior of adult rats. *Life Sci.* Oct 10 2003;73(21):2703-2711.

176. Csaba G, Kovacs P, Pallinger E. Single treatment (hormonal imprinting) of newborn rats with serotonin increases the serotonin content of cells in adults. *Cell Biol Int.* 2002;26(8):663-668.

177. Csaba G, Karabelyos C, Inczefi Gonda A, Pallinger E. Three-generation investigation on serotonin content in rat immune cells long after beta-endorphin exposure in late pregnancy. *Horm Metab Res.* Mar 2005;37(3):172-177.

178. Csaba G, Karabelyos CS. Influence of a single treatment with vitamin E or K (hormonal imprinting) of neonatal rats on the sexual behavior of adults. *Acta Physiol Hung.* 2000;87(1):25-30.

179. Csaba G, Inczefi-Gonda A. Effect of single neonatal vitamin K1 treatment (imprinting) on the binding capacity of thymic glucocorticoid and uterine estrogen receptors of adolescent and adult rats. *Life Sci.* 1999;65(1):PL1-5.

180. Livezey GT, Rayburn WF, Smith CV. Prenatal exposure to phenobarbital and quantifiable alterations in the electroencephalogram of adult rat offspring. *Am J Obstet Gynecol.* Dec 1992;167(6):1611-1615, p 1614.

181. Scull TJ, Hemmings GT, Carli F, Weeks SK, Mazza L, Zingg HH. Epidural analgesia in early labour blocks the stress response but uterine contractions remain unchanged. *Can J Anaesth.* Jul 1998;45(7):626-630.

182. Stocche RM, Klamt JG, Antunes-Rodrigues J, Garcia LV, Moreira AC. Effects of intrathecal sufentanil on plasma oxytocin and cortisol concentrations in women during the first stage of labor. *Reg Anesth Pain Med.* Nov-Dec 2001;26(6):545-550.

183. Abboud TK, Sarkis F, Hung TT, et al. Effects of epidural anesthesia during labor on maternal plasma beta-endorphin levels. *Anesthesiology.* Jul 1983;59(1):1-5.

184. Abboud TK, Goebelsmann U, Raya J, et al. Effect of intrathecal morphine during labor on maternal plasma beta-endorphin levels. *Am J Obstet Gynecol.* Aug 1 1984;149(7):709-710.

185. Rahm VA, Hallgren A, Hogberg H, Hurtig I, Odlind V. Plasma oxytocin levels in women during labor with or without epidural analgesia: a prospective study. *Acta Obstet Gynecol Scand.* Nov 2002;81(11):1033-1039.

186. Behrens O, Goeschen K, Luck HJ, Fuchs AR. Effects of lumbar epidural analgesia on prostaglandin F2 alpha release and oxytocin secretion during labor. *Prostaglandins.* Mar 1993;45(3):285-296.

187. Goodfellow CF, Hull MG, Swaab DF, Dogterom J, Buijs RM. Oxytocin deficiency at delivery with epidural analgesia. *Br J Obstet Gynaecol.* Mar 1983;90(3):214-219.

188. Lieberman E, O'Donoghue C. Unintended effects of epidural analgesia during labor: a systematic review. *Am J Obstet Gynecol.* May 2002;186(5 Suppl Nature):S31-68.

189. Jones CM, 3rd, Greiss FC, Jr. The effect of labor on maternal and fetal circulating catecholamines. *Am J Obstet Gynecol.* Sep 15 1982;144(2):149-153.

190. Jouppila R, Puolakka J, Kauppila A, Vuori J. Maternal and umbilical cord plasma noradrenaline concentrations

during labour with and without segmental extradural analgesia, and during
caesarean section. *Br J Anaesth.* Mar
1984;56(3):251-255.

191. Vogl SE, Worda C, Egarter C, et al. Mode
of delivery is associated with maternal
and fetal endocrine stress response.
BJOG. Apr 2006;113(4):441-445.

192. Swanstrom S, Bratteby LE. Metabolic
effects of obstetric regional analgesia and of asphyxia in the newborn
infant during the first two hours after
birth. I. Arterial blood glucose concentrations. *Acta Paediatr Scand.* Nov
1981;70(6):791-800.

193. Swanstrom S, Bratteby LE. Metabolic
effects of obstetric regional analgesia
and of asphyxia in the newborn infant
during the first two hours after birth.
II. Arterial plasma concentrations of
glycerol, free fatty acids and beta-
hydroxybutyrate. *Acta Paediatr Scand.*
Nov 1981;70(6):801-809.

194. Leighton BL, Halpern SH. The effects
of epidural analgesia on labor, maternal,
and neonatal outcomes: a systematic
review. *Am J Obstet Gynecol.* May
2002;186(5 Suppl Nature):S69-77.

195. Howell CJ. Epidural versus nonepidural analgesia for pain relief in
labour. *Cochrane Database Syst Rev.*
2000(2):CD000331.

196. Brinsmead M. Fetal and neonatal effects
of drugs administered in labour. *Med J
Aust.* May 4 1987;146(9):481-486.

197. Fernando R, Bonello E, Gill P, Urquhart
J, Reynolds F, Morgan B. Neonatal welfare and placental transfer of fentanyl
and bupivacaine during ambulatory
combined spinal epidural analgesia for
labour. *Anaesthesia.* Jun 1997;52(6):517-
524.

198. Hale T. *Medications and Mother's Milk.*
Amarillo TX: Pharmasoft; 1997.

199. Mueller MD, Bruhwiler H, Schupfer
GK, Luscher KP. Higher rate of fetal
acidemia after regional anesthesia for

elective cesarean delivery. *Obstet Gynecol.* Jul 1997;90(1):131-134.

200. Roberts SW, Leveno KJ, Sidawi JE,
Lucas MJ, Kelly MA. Fetal acidemia
associated with regional anesthesia for
elective cesarean delivery. *Obstet Gynecol.* Jan 1995;85(1):79-83.

201. Krehbiel D, Poindron P, Levy F,
Prud'Homme MJ. Peridural anesthesia
disturbs maternal behavior in primiparous and multiparous parturient ewes.
Physiol Behav. 1987;40(4):463-472.

202. Sepkoski CM, Lester BM, Ostheimer
GW, Brazelton TB. The effects of
maternal epidural anesthesia on
neonatal behavior during the first
month. *Dev Med Child Neurol.* Dec
1992;34(12):1072-1080.

203. Murray AD, Dolby RM, Nation RL,
Thomas DB. Effects of epidural anes-
thesia on newborns and their mothers.
Child Dev. Mar 1981;52(1):71-82.

204. Harper MA, Byington RP, Espeland
MA, Naughton M, Meyer R, Lane K.
Pregnancy-related death and health
care services. *Obstet Gynecol.* Aug
2003;102(2):273-278.

205. Enkin M, Keirse M, Neilson J, et al.
*Effective Care in Pregnancy and Child-
birth.* 3rd ed. Oxford: Oxford University
Press; 2000.

206. Deneux-Tharaux C, Carmona E,
Bouvier-Colle MH, Breart G. Postpartum maternal mortality and cesarean
delivery. *Obstet Gynecol.* Sep 2006;108(3
Pt 1):541-548.

207. Bewley S, Cockburn J. II. The unfacts of
'request' caesarean section. *Br J Obstet
Gynaecol.* Jun 2002;109(6):597-605.

208. Villar J, Carroli G, Zavaleta N, et al.
Maternal and neonatal individual risks
and benefits associated with caesarean
delivery: multicentre prospective study.
BMJ. Nov 17 2007;335(7628):1025.

209. MacDorman MF, Declercq E, Menacker
F, Malloy MH. Infant and neonatal mor-

tality for primary cesarean and vaginal births to women with "no indicated risk," United States, 1998-2001 birth cohorts. *Birth.* Sep 2006;33(3):175-182.

210. Marchini G, Lagercrantz H, Winberg J, Uvnas-Moberg K. Fetal and maternal plasma levels of gastrin, somatostatin and oxytocin after vaginal delivery and elective cesarean section. *Early Hum Dev.* Nov 1988;18(1):73-79.

211. Jones CR, McCullouch J, Butters L, Hamilton CA, Rubin PC, Reid JL. Plasma catecholamines and modes of delivery: the relation between catecholamine levels and in-vitro platelet aggregation and adrenoreceptor radioligand binding characteristics. *Br J Obstet Gynaecol.* Jun 1985;92(6):593-599.

212. Heasman L, Spencer JA, Symonds ME. Plasma prolactin concentrations after caesarean section or vaginal delivery. *Arch Dis Child Fetal Neonatal Ed.* Nov 1997;77(5):F237-238.

213. Faxelus G, Hagnevik K, Lagercrantz H, Lundell B, Irestedt L. Catecholamine surge and lung function after delivery. *Arch Dis Child.* Apr 1983;58(4):262-266.

214. Zanardo V, Simbi AK, Franzoi M, Solda G, Salvadori A, Trevisanuto D. Neonatal respiratory morbidity risk and mode of delivery at term: influence of timing of elective caesarean delivery. *Acta Paediatr.* May 2004;93(5):643-647.

215. Levine EM, Ghai V, Barton JJ, Strom CM. Mode of delivery and risk of respiratory diseases in newborns. *Obstet Gynecol.* Mar 2001;97(3):439-442.

216. Kolas T, Saugstad OD, Daltveit AK, Nilsen ST, Oian P. Planned cesarean versus planned vaginal delivery at term: comparison of newborn infant outcomes. *Am J Obstet Gynecol.* Dec 2006;195(6):1538-1543.

217. Richardson BS, Czikk MJ, daSilva O, Natale R. The impact of labor at term on measures of neonatal outcome. *Am J Obstet Gynecol.* Jan 2005;192(1):219-226.

218. Christensson K, Siles C, Cabrera T, et al. Lower body temperatures in infants delivered by caesarean section than in vaginally delivered infants. *Acta Paediatr.* Feb 1993;82(2):128-131.

219. Isobe K, Kusaka T, Fujikawa Y, et al. Measurement of cerebral oxygenation in neonates after vaginal delivery and cesarean section using full-spectrum near infrared spectroscopy. *Comp Biochem Physiol A Mol Integr Physiol.* May 2002;132(1):133-138.

220. Buckley SJ. Leaving well alone: A natural approach to third stage. *Medical Veritas.* 2005;2(2):492-499.

221. Otamiri G, Berg G, Ledin T, Leijon I, Lagercrantz H. Delayed neurological adaptation in infants delivered by elective cesarean section and the relation to catecholamine levels. *Early Hum Dev.* Jul 1991;26(1):51-60.

222. Kim HR, Jung KY, Kim SY, Ko KO, Lee YM, Kim JM. Delivery modes and neonatal EEG: spatial pattern analysis. *Early Hum Dev.* Dec 2003;75(1-2):35-53.

223. Vladimirova E, Smirnova EE. [The CNS status of newborn infants delivered by cesarean section (based on EEG data)]. *Zh Nevropatol Psikhiatr Im S S Korsakova.* 1994;94(3):16-18.

224. Freudigman KA, Thoman EB. Infants' earliest sleep/wake organization differs as a function of delivery mode. *Dev Psychobiol.* May 1998;32(4):293-303.

225. Bagnoli F, Bruchi S, Garosi G, Pecciarini L, Bracci R. Relationship between mode of delivery and neonatal calcium homeostasis. *Eur J Pediatr.* Aug 1990;149(11):800-803.

226. Broughton Pipkin F, Symonds EM. Factors affecting angiotensin II concentrations in the human infant at birth. *Clin Sci Mol Med.* May 1977;52(5):449-456.

227. Fujimura A, Morimoto S, Uchida K, Takeda R, Ohshita M, Ebihara A. The influence of delivery mode on

biological inactive renin level in umbilical cord blood. *Am J Hypertens.* Jan 1990;3(1):23-26.

228. Tetlow HJ, Broughton Pipkin F. Studies on the effect of mode of delivery on the renin-angiotensin system in mother and fetus at term. *Br J Obstet Gynaecol.* Mar 1983;90(3):220-226.

229. Okamoto E, Otsuki Y, Iwata I, et al. Plasma concentrations of human atrial natriuretic peptide at vaginal delivery and elective cesarean section. *Asia Oceania J Obstet Gynaecol.* Jun 1989;15(2):199-202.

230. Aisien AO, Towobola OA, Otubu JA, Imade GE. Umbilical cord venous progesterone at term delivery in relation to mode of delivery. *Int J Gynaecol Obstet.* Oct 1994;47(1):27-31.

231. Malamitsi-Puchner A, Minaretzis D, Martzeli L, Papas C. Serum levels of creatine kinase and its isoenzymes during the 1st postpartum day in healthy newborns delivered vaginally or by cesarean section. *Gynecol Obstet Invest.* 1993;36(1):25-28.

232. Boksa P, El-Khodor BF. Birth insult interacts with stress at adulthood to alter dopaminergic function in animal models: possible implications for schizophrenia and other disorders. *Neurosci Biobehav Rev.* Jan-Mar 2003;27(1-2):91-101.

233. Endo A, Izumi H, Ayusawa M, Minato M, Takahashi S, Harada K. Spontaneous labor increases nitric oxide synthesis during the early neonatal period. *Pediatr Int.* Aug 2001;43(4):340-342.

234. Endo A, Ayusawa M, Minato M, Takada M, Takahashi S, Harada K. Physiologic significance of nitric oxide and endothelin-1 in circulatory adaptation. *Pediatr Int.* Feb 2000;42(1):26-30.

235. Hills FA, Gunn LK, Hardiman P, Thamaratnam S, Chard T. IGFBP-1 in the placenta, membranes and fetal circulation: levels at term and pre-

term delivery. *Early Hum Dev.* Jan 5 1996;44(1):71-76.

236. Mitchell MD, Bibby JG, Sayers L, Anderson AB, Turnbull AC. Melatonin in the maternal and umbilical circulations during human parturition. *Br J Obstet Gynaecol.* Jan 1979;86(1):29-31.

237. Bird JA, Spencer JA, Mould T, Symonds ME. Endocrine and metabolic adaptation following caesarean section or vaginal delivery. *Arch Dis Child Fetal Neonatal Ed.* Mar 1996;74(2):F132-134.

238. Mongelli M, Kwan Y, Kay LL, Hjelm M, Rogers MS. Effect of labour and delivery on plasma hepatic enzymes in the newborn. *J Obstet Gynaecol Res.* Feb 2000;26(1):61-63.

239. Banasik M, Zeman K, Pasnik J, Malinowski A, Lewkowicz P, Tchorzewski H. [Effect of maternal labor and mode of delivery on function of neonatal cord blood neutrophils]. *Ginekol Pol.* Jun 2000;71(6):559-565.

240. Molloy EJ, O'Neill AJ, Grantham JJ, et al. Labor promotes neonatal neutrophil survival and lipopolysaccharide responsiveness. *Pediatr Res.* Jul 2004;56(1):99-103.

241. Thilaganathan B, Meher-Homji N, Nicolaides KH. Labor: an immunologically beneficial process for the neonate. *Am J Obstet Gynecol.* Nov 1994;171(5):1271-1272.

242. Agrawal S, Agrawal BM, Khurana K, Gupta K, Ansari KH. Comparative study of immunoglobulin G and immunoglobulin M among neonates in caesarean section and vaginal delivery. *J Indian Med Assoc.* Feb 1996;94(2):43-44.

243. Gronlund MM, Nuutila J, Pelto L, et al. Mode of delivery directs the phagocyte functions of infants for the first 6 months of life. *Clin Exp Immunol.* Jun 1999;116(3):521-526.

244. Lubetzky R, Ben-Shachar S, Mimouni FB, Dollberg S. Mode of delivery and

neonatal hematocrit. *Am J Perinatol.* 2000;17(3):163-165.

245. Stevenson DK, Bucalo LR, Cohen RS, Vreman HJ, Ferguson JE, 2nd, Schwartz HC. Increased immunoreactive erythropoietin in cord plasma and neonatal bilirubin production in normal term infants after labor. *Obstet Gynecol.* Jan 1986;67(1):69-73.

246. Bujko M, Sulovic V, Sbutega-Milosevic G, Zivanovic V. Mode of delivery and level of passive immunity against herpes simplex virus. *Clin Exp Obstet Gynecol.* 1989;16(1):6-8.

247. Steinborn A, Sohn C, Sayehli C, et al. Spontaneous labour at term is associated with fetal monocyte activation. *Clin Exp Immunol.* Jul 1999;117(1):147-152.

248. Brown MA, Rad PY, Halonen MJ. Method of birth alters interferon-gamma and interleukin-12 production by cord blood mononuclear cells. *Pediatr Allergy Immunol.* Apr 2003;14(2):106-111.

249. Santala M. Mode of delivery and lymphocyte beta 2-adrenoceptor density in parturients and newborns. *Gynecol Obstet Invest.* 1989;28(4):174-177.

250. Franzoi M, Simioni P, Luni S, Zerbinati P, Girolami A, Zanardo V. Effect of delivery modalities on the physiologic inhibition system of coagulation of the neonate. *Thromb Res.* Jan 1 2002;105(1):15-18.

251. Pasetto N, Piccione E, Ticconi C, Pontieri G, Lenti L, Zicari A. Leukotrienes in human umbilical plasma at birth. *Br J Obstet Gynaecol.* Jan 1989;96(1):88-91.

252. Miclat NN, Hodgkinson R, Marx GF. Neonatal gastric pH. *Anesth Analg.* Jan-Feb 1978;57(1):98-101.

253. Sangild PT, Hilsted L, Nexo E, Fowden AL, Silver M. Vaginal birth versus elective caesarean section: effects on gastric function in the neonate. *Exp Physiol.* Jan 1995;80(1):147-157.

254. Gronlund MM, Lehtonen OP, Eerola E, Kero P. Fecal microflora in healthy infants born by different methods of delivery: permanent changes in intestinal flora after cesarean delivery. *J Pediatr Gastroenterol Nutr.* Jan 1999;28(1):19-25.

255. Hallstrom M, Eerola E, Vuento R, Janas M, Tammela O. Effects of mode of delivery and necrotising enterocolitis on the intestinal microflora in preterm infants. *Eur J Clin Microbiol Infect Dis.* Jun 2004;23(6):463-470.

256. Kero J, Gissler M, Gronlund MM, et al. Mode of delivery and asthma—is there a connection? *Pediatr Res.* Jul 2002;52(1):6-11.

257. Hakansson S, Kallen K. Caesarean section increases the risk of hospital care in childhood for asthma and gastroenteritis. *Clin Exp Allergy.* Jun 2003;33(6):757-764.

258. Laubereau B, Filipiak-Pittroff B, von Berg A, et al. Caesarean section and gastrointestinal symptoms, atopic dermatitis, and sensitisation during the first year of life. *Arch Dis Child.* Nov 2004;89(11):993-997.

259. Rogers MS, Mongelli JM, Tsang KH, Wang CC, Law KP. Lipid peroxidation in cord blood at birth: the effect of labour. *Br J Obstet Gynaecol.* Jul 1998;105(7):739-744.

260. Buhimschi IA, Buhimschi CS, Pupkin M, Weiner CP. Beneficial impact of term labor: nonenzymatic antioxidant reserve in the human fetus. *Am J Obstet Gynecol.* Jul 2003;189(1):181-188.

261. Kazda H, Taylor N, Healy D, Walker D. Maternal, umbilical, and amniotic fluid concentrations of tryptophan and kynurenine after labor or cesarean section. *Pediatr Res.* Sep 1998;44(3):368-373.

262. Pohjavuori M, Fyhrquist F. Vasopressin, ACTH and neonatal haemodynamics.

Acta Paediatr Scand Suppl. 1983;305: 79-83.

263. Pohjavuori M, Rovamo L, Laatikainen T. Plasma immunoreactive beta-endorphin and cortisol in the newborn infant after elective caesarean section and after spontaneous labour. *Eur J Obstet Gynecol Reprod Biol.* Feb 1985;19(2):67-74.

264. Fisher J, Astbury J, Smith A. Adverse psychological impact of operative obstetric interventions: a prospective longitudinal study. *Aust N Z J Psychiatry.* Oct 1997;31(5):728-738.

265. Nissen E, Uvnas-Moberg K, Svensson K, Stock S, Widstrom AM, Winberg J. Different patterns of oxytocin, prolactin but not cortisol release during breastfeeding in women delivered by caesarean section or by the vaginal route. *Early Hum Dev.* Jul 5 1996;45(1-2):103-118, p 116.

266. Evans KC, Evans RG, Royal R, Esterman AJ, James SL. Effect of caesarean section on breastmilk transfer to the normal term newborn over the first week of life. *Arch Dis Child Fetal Neonatal Ed.* Sep 2003;88(5):F380-382.

267. Salariya EM, Easton PM, Cater JI. Duration of breast-feeding after early initiation and frequent feeding. *Lancet.* Nov 25 1978;2(8100):1141-1143.

268. de Chateau P, Wiberg B. Long-term effect on mother-infant behaviour of extra contact during the first hour post partum. II. A follow-up at three months. *Acta Paediatr Scand.* Mar 1977;66(2):145-151.

269. DiMatteo MR, Morton SC, Lepper HS, et al. Cesarean childbirth and psychosocial outcomes: a meta-analysis. *Health Psychol.* Jul 1996;15(4):303-314.

270. Dewey KG, Nommsen-Rivers LA, Heinig MJ, Cohen RJ. Risk factors for suboptimal infant breastfeeding behavior, delayed onset of lactation, and excess neonatal weight loss. *Pediatrics.* Sep 2003;112(3 Pt 1):607-619.

271. Lobel M, DeLuca RS. Psychosocial sequelae of cesarean delivery: review and analysis of their causes and implications. *Soc Sci Med.* Jun 2007;64(11): 2272-2284.

272. Odent M. *Primal Health Database.* Birthworks; 2003 http://www.birthworks.org/primalhealth/.

273. Widstrom AM, Wahlberg V, Matthiesen AS, et al. Short-term effects of early suckling and touch of the nipple on maternal behaviour. *Early Hum Dev.* Mar 1990;21(3):153-163.

274. Uvnas-Moberg K. The gastrointestinal tract in growth and reproduction. *Sci Am.* Jul 1989;261(1):78-83.

275. Klaus M. Mother and infant: early emotional ties. *Pediatrics.* Nov 1998;102(5 Suppl E):1244-1246, p 1246.

276. Christensson K, Siles C, Moreno L, et al. Temperature, metabolic adaptation and crying in healthy full-term newborns cared for skin-to-skin or in a cot. *Acta Paediatr.* Jun-Jul 1992;81(6-7):488-493.

277. Ferber SG, Makhoul IR. The effect of skin-to-skin contact (kangaroo care) shortly after birth on the neurobehavioral responses of the term newborn: a randomized, controlled trial. *Pediatrics.* Apr 2004;113(4):858-865.

278. Bystrova K, Matthiesen AS, Widstrom AM, et al. The effect of Russian Maternity Home routines on breastfeeding and neonatal weight loss with special reference to swaddling. *Early Hum Dev.* May 19 2006.

279. Christensson K, Cabrera T, Christensson E, Uvnas-Moberg K, Winberg J. Separation distress call in the human neonate in the absence of maternal body contact. *Acta Paediatr.* May 1995;84(5):468-473, p 468.

280. Biagini G, Pich EM, Carani C, Marrama P, Agnati LF. Postnatal maternal separation during the stress hyporesponsive period enhances the adrenocortical response to novelty in adult rats by

affecting feedback regulation in the CA1 hippocampal field. *Int J Dev Neurosci.* Jun-Jul 1998;16(3-4):187-197.

281. Bergman NJ. Skin-to-Skin Contact and Perinatal Neuroscience. Paper presented at: Capers Breastfeeding Seminar: Breastfeeding, A Lifelong Investment; May 13 2006; Brisbane, Australia.

282. Klaus M. Mother and infant: early emotional ties. *Pediatrics.* Nov 1998;102(5 Suppl E):1244-1246.

283. Buranasin B. The effects of rooming-in on the success of breastfeeding and the decline in abandonment of children. *Asia Pac J Public Health.* 1991;5(3):217-220.

284. O'Connor S, Vietze PM, Sherrod KB, Sandler HM, Altemeier WA, 3rd. Reduced incidence of parenting inadequacy following rooming-in. *Pediatrics.* Aug 1980;66(2):176-182.

285. Ringler NM, Kennell JH, Jarvella R, Navojosky BJ, Klaus MH. Mother-to-child speech at 2 years—effects of early postnatal contact. *J Pediatr.* Jan 1975;86(1):141-144.

286. Pearce JC. *Evolution's End: Claiming the Potential of Our Intelligence.* San Francisco: Harper San Francisco; 1992 p 114-5.

287. Pearce JC. *Evolution's End· Claiming the Potential of Our Intelligence.* San Francisco: Harper San Francisco; 1992 p 115.

288. Lin SH, Kiyohara T, Sun B. Maternal behavior: activation of the central oxytocin receptor system in parturient rats? *Neuroreport.* Aug 6 2003;14(11):1439-1444, p 1444.

289. Luckman SM. Fos expression within regions of the preoptic area, hypothalamus and brainstem during pregnancy and parturition. *Brain Res.* Jan 9 1995;669(1):115-124.

290. Bridges RS. Long-term effects of pregnancy and parturition upon maternal

responsiveness in the rat. *Physiol Behav.* Mar 1975;14(3):245-249.

291. Brown T. Back to Basics: Regressive Therapy Could Give You and Baby a Fresh Start. Available at: http://breast-feed.com/resources/articles/btob.htm; n.d.

292. Righard L, Alade MO. Effect of delivery room routines on success of first breast-feed. *Lancet.* Nov 3 1990;336(8723):1105-1107.

293. Baker JP. *Prenatal Yoga and Natural Childbirth.* 3rd ed. Berkley: North Atlantic Books; 2001 p 90.

294. Kloosterman G. The universal aspects of childbirth: Human birth as a socio-psychosomatic paradigm. *J Psychosom Obstet Gynaecol.* 1982;1(1):35-41, p 40.

Chapter 7: **EPIDURALS**

1. Hamilton GR, Baskett TF. In the arms of Morpheus: the development of morphine for postoperative pain relief. *Can J Anaesth.* Apr 2000;47(4):367-374.

2. Declercq ER, Sakala C, Corry MP, Applebaum S. *Listening to Mothers II: Report of the Second National U.S. Survey of Women's Childbearing Experiences.* New York: Childbirth Connection; October 2006.

3. Canadian Institute for Health Information. *Giving Birth in Canada: Regional Trends From 2001-2002 to 2005-2006.* Toronto: CIHI; 2007.

4. The Information Centre CHS. *NHS Maternity Statistics, England: 2004-05.* 2006.

5. Hodnett ED. Pain and women's satisfaction with the experience of childbirth: a systematic review. *Am J Obstet Gynecol.* May 2002;186(5 Suppl Nature):S160-172.

6. World Health Organization. *Care in Normal Birth: a Practical Guide. Report of a Technical Working Group.* Geneva: World Health Organization; 1996, p 16.

7. Rahm VA, Hallgren A, Hogberg H, Hurtig I, Odlind V. Plasma oxytocin levels in women during labor with or without epidural analgesia: a prospective study. *Acta Obstet Gynecol Scand.* Nov 2002;81(11):1033-1039.

8. Stocche RM, Klamt JG, Antunes-Rodrigues J, Garcia LV, Moreira AC. Effects of intrathecal sufentanil on plasma oxytocin and cortisol concentrations in women during the first stage of labor. *Reg Anesth Pain Med.* Nov-Dec 2001;26(6):545-550.

9. Goodfellow CF, Hull MG, Swaab DF, Dogterom J, Buijs RM. Oxytocin deficiency at delivery with epidural analgesia. *Br J Obstet Gynaecol.* Mar 1983;90(3):214-219.

10. Levy F, Kendrick KM, Keverne EB, Piketty V, Poindron P. Intracerebral oxytocin is important for the onset of maternal behavior in inexperienced ewes delivered under peridural anesthesia. *Behav Neurosci.* Apr 1992;106(2):427-432.

11. Behrens O, Goeschen K, Luck HJ, Fuchs AR. Effects of lumbar epidural analgesia on prostaglandin F2 alpha release and oxytocin secretion during labor. *Prostaglandins.* Mar 1993;45(3):285-296.

12. Jouppila R, Jouppila P, Karlqvist K, Kaukoranta P, Leppaluoto J, Vuolteenaho O. Maternal and umbilical venous plasma immunoreactive beta-endorphin levels during labor with and without epidural analgesia. *Am J Obstet Gynecol.* Dec 1 1983;147(7):799-802.

13. Scull TJ, Hemmings GT, Carli F, Weeks SK, Mazza L, Zingg HH. Epidural analgesia in early labour blocks the stress response but uterine contractions remain unchanged. *Can J Anaesth.* Jul 1998;45(7):626-630.

14. Browning AJ, Butt WR, Lynch SS, Shakespear RA, Crawford JS. Maternal and cord plasma concentrations of beta-lipotrophin, beta-endorphin and gamma-lipotrophin at delivery; effect

of analgesia. *Br J Obstet Gynaecol.* Dec 1983;90(12):1152-1156.

15. Costa A, De Filippis V, Voglino M, et al. Adrenocorticotropic hormone and catecholamines in maternal, umbilical and neonatal plasma in relation to vaginal delivery. *J Endocrinol Invest.* Nov 1988;11(10):703-709.

16. Lederman RP, Lederman E, Work B, Jr., McCann DS. Anxiety and epinephrine in multiparous women in labor: relationship to duration of labor and fetal heart rate pattern. *Am J Obstet Gynecol.* Dec 15 1985;153(8):870-877.

17. Neumark J, Hammerle AF, Biegelmayer C. Effects of epidural analgesia on plasma catecholamines and cortisol in parturition. *Acta Anaesthesiol Scand.* Aug 1985;29(6):555-559.

18. Jouppila R, Puolakka J, Kauppila A, Vuori J. Maternal and umbilical cord plasma noradrenaline concentrations during labour with and without segmental extradural analgesia, and during caesarean section. *Br J Anaesth.* Mar 1984;56(3):251-255.

19. Jones CR, McCullouch J, Butters L, Hamilton CA, Rubin PC, Reid JL. Plasma catecholamines and modes of delivery: the relation between catecholamine levels and in-vitro platelet aggregation and adrenoreceptor radioligand binding characteristics. *Br J Obstet Gynaecol.* Jun 1985;92(6):593-599.

20. Arici G, Karsli B, Kayacan N, Akar M. The effects of bupivacaine, ropivacaine and mepivacaine on the contractility of rat myometrium. *Int J Obstet Anesth.* Apr 2004;13(2):95-98.

21. Cheek TG, Samuels P, Miller F, Tobin M, Gutsche BB. Normal saline i.v. fluid load decreases uterine activity in active labour. *Br J Anaesth.* Nov 1996;77(5):632-635.

22. Leighton BL, Halpern SH. The effects of epidural analgesia on labor, maternal, and neonatal outcomes: a systematic

review. *Am J Obstet Gynecol.* May 2002;186(5 Suppl Nature):S69-77.

23. Lieberman E, Davidson K, Lee-Parritz A, Shearer E. Changes in fetal position during labor and their association with epidural analgesia. *Obstet Gynecol.* May 2005;105(5):974-982.

24. Ponkey SE, Cohen AP, Heffner LJ, Lieberman E. Persistent fetal occiput posterior position: obstetric outcomes. *Obstet Gynecol.* May 2003;101(5 Pt 1):915-920.

25. Fitzpatrick M, McQuillan K, O'Herlihy C. Influence of persistent occiput posterior position on delivery outcome. *Obstet Gynecol.* Dec 2001;98(6):1027-1031.

26. COMET Study Group UK. Effect of low-dose mobile versus traditional epidural techniques on mode of delivery: a randomised controlled trial. *Lancet.* Jul 7 2001;358(9275):19-23.

27. Torvaldsen S, Roberts CL, Bell JC, Raynes-Greenow CH. Discontinuation of epidural analgesia late in labour for reducing the adverse delivery outcomes associated with epidural analgesia. *Cochrane Database Syst Rev.* 2004(4):CD004457.

28. Carroll TG, Engelken M, Mosier MC, Nazir N. Epidural analgesia and severe perineal laceration in a community-based obstetric practice. *J Am Board Fam Pract.* Jan-Feb 2003;16(1):1-6.

29. Robinson JN, Norwitz ER, Cohen AP, McElrath TF, Lieberman ES. Epidural analgesia and third- or fourth-degree lacerations in nulliparas. *Obstet Gynecol.* Aug 1999;94(2):259-262.

30. Thompson JF, Roberts CL, Currie M, Ellwood DA. Prevalence and persistence of health problems after childbirth: associations with parity and method of birth. *Birth.* Jun 2002;29(2):83-94.

31. Brown S, Lumley J. Maternal health after childbirth: results of an Australian population based survey. *Br J Obstet Gynaecol.* Feb 1998;105(2):156-161.

32. Johanson RB, Heycock E, Carter J, Sultan AH, Walklate K, Jones PW. Maternal and child health after assisted vaginal delivery: five-year follow up of a randomised controlled study comparing forceps and ventouse. *Br J Obstet Gynaecol.* Jun 1999;106(6):544-549.

33. Johnson JH, Figueroa R, Garry D, Elimian A, Maulik D. Immediate maternal and neonatal effects of forceps and vacuum-assisted deliveries. *Obstet Gynecol.* Mar 2004;103(3):513-518.

34. Jhawar BS, Ranger A, Steven D, Del Maestro RF. Risk factors for intracranial hemorrhage among full-term infants: a case-control study. *Neurosurgery.* Mar 2003;52(3):581-590; discussion 588-590.

35. McBride WG, Black BP, Brown CJ, Dolby RM, Murray AD, Thomas DB. Method of delivery and developmental outcome at five years of age. *Med J Aust.* Apr 21 1979;1(8):301-304.

36. Wesley BD, van den Berg BJ, Reece EA. The effect of forceps delivery on cognitive development. *Am J Obstet Gynecol.* Nov 1993;169(5):1091-1095.

37. Poggi SH, Allen RH, Patel C, et al. Effect of epidural anaesthesia on clinician-applied force during vaginal delivery. *Am J Obstet Gynecol.* Sep 2004;191(3):903-906.

38. Roberts CL, Tracy S, Peat B. Rates for obstetric intervention among private and public patients in Australia: population based descriptive study. *Br Med J.* Jul 15 2000;321(7254):137-141.

39. Serati M, Salvatore S, Khullar V, et al. Prospective study to assess risk factors for pelvic floor dysfunction after delivery. *Acta Obstet Gynecol Scand.* 2008;87(3):313-318.

40. Casey BM, Schaffer JI, Bloom SL, Heartwell SF, McIntire DD, Leveno KJ. Obstetric antecedents for postpartum pelvic floor dysfunction. *Am J Obstet Gynecol.* May 2005;192(5):1655-1662.

41. Snooks SJ, Swash M, Henry MM, Setchell M. Risk factors in childbirth causing damage to the pelvic floor innervation. *Int J Colorectal Dis.* Jan 1986;1(1):20-24.

42. Schaffer JI, Bloom SL, Casey BM, McIntire DD, Nihira MA, Leveno KJ. A randomized trial of the effects of coached vs uncoached maternal pushing during the second stage of labor on postpartum pelvic floor structure and function. *Am J Obstet Gynecol.* May 2005;192(5):1692-1696.

43. Lieberman E, O'Donoghue C. Unintended effects of epidural analgesia during labor: a systematic review. *Am J Obstet Gynecol.* May 2002;186(5 Suppl Nature):S31-68.

44. Kotaska AJ, Klein MC, Liston RM. Epidural analgesia associated with low-dose oxytocin augmentation increases cesarean births: a critical look at the external validity of randomized trials. *Am J Obstet Gynecol.* Mar 2006;194(3):809-814.

45. Thorp JA, Parisi VM, Boylan PC, Johnston DA. The effect of continuous epidural analgesia on cesarean section for dystocia in nulliparous women. *Am J Obstet Gynecol.* Sep 1989;161(3):670-675.

46. Golub MS. Labor analgesia and infant brain development. *Pharmacol Biochem Behav.* Dec 1996;55(4):619-628, p 619.

47. DeBalli P, Breen TW. Intrathecal opioids for combined spinal-epidural analgesia during labour. *CNS Drugs.* 2003;17(12):889-904.

48. Buggy D, Hughes N, Gardiner J. Posterior column sensory impairment during ambulatory extradural analgesia in labour. *Br J Anaesth.* Oct 1994;73(4):540-542.

49. Shennan A, Cooke V, Lloyd-Jones F, Morgan B, de Swiet M. Blood pressure changes during labour and whilst ambulating with combined spinal epidural analgesia. *Br J Obstet Gynaecol.* Mar 1995;102(3):192-197.

50. Goetzl LM. ACOG Practice Bulletin. Clinical Management Guidelines for Obstetrician-Gynecologists Number 36, July 2002. Obstetric analgesial and anesthesia. *Obstet Gynecol.* Jul 2002;100(1):177-191.

51. Mayberry LJ, Clemmens D, De A. Epidural analgesia side effects, co-interventions, and care of women during childbirth: a systematic review. *Am J Obstet Gynecol.* May 2002;186(5 Suppl Nature):S81-93.

52. Scott DB, Hibbard BM. Serious non-fatal complications associated with extradural block in obstetric practice. *Br J Anaesth.* May 1990;64(5):537-541.

53. Buggy D, Gardiner J. The space blanket and shivering during extradural analgesia in labour. *Acta Anaesthesiol Scand.* May 1995;39(4):551-553.

54. Goetzl L, Rivers J, Zighelboim I, Wali A, Badell M, Suresh MS. Intrapartum epidural analgesia and maternal temperature regulation. *Obstet Gynecol.* Mar 2007;109(3):687-690.

55. Lieberman E, Lang JM, Frigoletto F, Jr., Richardson DK, Ringer SA, Cohen A. Epidural analgesia, intrapartum fever, and neonatal sepsis evaluation. *Pediatrics.* Mar 1997;99(3):415-419.

56. Gaiser R. Neonatal effects of labor analgesia. *Int Anesthesiol Clin.* Fall 2002;40(4):49-65.

57. DeBalli P, Breen TW. Intrathecal opioids for combined spinal-epidural analgesia during labour. *CNS Drugs.* 2003;17(12):889-904, p 892-883.

58. Saunders NS, Paterson CM, Wadsworth J. Neonatal and maternal morbidity in relation to the length of the second stage of labour. *Br J Obstet Gynaecol.* May 1992;99(5):381-385.

59. St George L, Crandon AJ. Immediate postpartum complications. *Aust N Z J Obstet Gynaecol.* Feb 1990;30(1):52-56.

60. Magann EF, Evans S, Hutchinson M, Collins R, Howard BC, Morrison JC. Postpartum hemorrhage after vaginal birth: an analysis of risk factors. *South Med J.* Apr 2005;98(4):419-422.

61. Eggebo TM, Gjessing LK. [Hemorrhage after vaginal delivery]. *Tidsskr Nor Laegeforen.* Oct 10 2000;120(24):2860-2863.

62. Ploeckinger B, Ulm MR, Chalubinski K, Gruber W. Epidural anaesthesia in labour: influence on surgical delivery rates, intrapartum fever and blood loss. *Gynecol Obstet Invest.* 1995;39(1):24-27.

63. Gilbert L, Porter W, Brown VA. Postpartum haemorrhage—a continuing problem. *Br J Obstet Gynaecol.* Jan 1987;94(1):67-71.

64. Paech MJ, Godkin R, Webster S. Complications of obstetric epidural analgesia and anaesthesia: a prospective analysis of 10,995 cases. *Int J Obstet Anesth.* Jan 1998;7(1):5-11.

65. Stride PC, Cooper GM. Dural taps revisited. A 20-year survey from Birmingham Maternity Hospital. *Anaesthesia.* Mar 1993;48(3):247-255.

66. Costigan SN, Sprigge JS. Dural puncture: the patients' perspective. A patient survey of cases at a DGH maternity unit 1983-1993. *Acta Anaesthesiol Scand.* Jul 1996;40(6):710-714.

67. Scott DB, Tunstall ME. Serious complications associated with epidural/spinal blockade in obstetrics: a two-year prospective study. *Int J Obstet Anesth.* Jul 1995;4(3):133-139.

68. Crawford JS. Some maternal complications of epidural analgesia for labour. *Anaesthesia.* Dec 1985;40(12):1219-1225.

69. Reynolds F. Epidural analgesia in obstetrics. *Br Med J.* Sep 23 1989;299(6702):751-752.

70. MIDIRS and The NHS Centre for Reviews and Dissemination. *Epidural pain relief during labour.* Informed choice for profesionals. Bristol: MIDIRS; 1999.

71. Fernando R, Bonello E, Gill P, Urquhart J, Reynolds F, Morgan B. Neonatal welfare and placental transfer of fentanyl and bupivacaine during ambulatory combined spinal epidural analgesia for labour. *Anaesthesia.* Jun 1997;52(6): 517-524.

72. Capogna G. Effect of epidural analgesia on the fetal heart rate. *Eur J Obstet Gynecol Reprod Biol.* Oct 2001;98(2):160-164.

73. Nicolet J, Miller A, Kaufman I, Guertin MC, Deschamps A. Maternal factors implicated in fetal bradycardia after combined spinal epidural for labour pain. *Eur J Anaesthesiol.* Apr 10 2008: 1-5.

74. Van de Velde M, Teunkens A, Hanssens M, Vandermeersch E, Verhaeghe J. Intrathecal sufentanil and fetal heart rate abnormalities: a double-blind, double placebo-controlled trial comparing two forms of combined spinal epidural analgesia with epidural analgesia in labor. *Anesth Analg.* Apr 2004;98(4):1153-1159, table of contents.

75. Hill JB, Alexander JM, Sharma SK, McIntire DD, Leveno KJ. A comparison of the effects of epidural and meperidine analgesia during labor on fetal heart rate. *Obstet Gynecol.* Aug 2003;102(2):333-337.

76. Mardirosoff C, Dumont L, Boulvain M, Tramer MR. Fetal bradycardia due to intrathecal opioids for labour analgesia: a systematic review. *Br J Obstet Gynaecol.* Mar 2002;109(3):274-281.

77. Littleford J. Effects on the fetus and newborn of maternal analgesia and anesthesia: a review. *Can J Anaesth.* Jun-Jul 2004;51(6):586-609.

78. Aldrich CJ, D'Antona D, Spencer JA, et al. The effect of maternal posture on fetal cerebral oxygenation during labour. *Br J Obstet Gynaecol.* Jan 1995;102(1):14-19.

79. Lieberman E, Lang J, Richardson DK, Frigoletto FD, Heffner LJ, Cohen A. Intrapartum maternal fever and neonatal outcome. *Pediatrics.* Jan 2000;105(1 Pt 1):8-13.

80. Morishima HO, Glaser B, Niemann WH, James LS. Increased uterine activity and fetal deterioration during maternal hyperthermia. *Am J Obstet Gynecol.* Feb 15 1975;121(4):531-538.

81. Perlman JM. Hyperthermia in the delivery: potential impact on neonatal mortality and morbidity. *Clin Perinatol.* Mar 2006;33(1):55-63, vi, p 57.

82. Impey L, Greenwood C, MacQuillan K, Reynolds M, Sheil O. Fever in labour and neonatal encephalopathy: a prospective cohort study. *Br J Obstet Gynaecol.* Jun 2001;108(6):594-597.

83. Petrova A, Demissie K, Rhoads GG, Smulian JC, Marcella S, Ananth CV. Association of maternal fever during labor with neonatal and infant morbidity and mortality. *Obstet Gynecol.* Jul 2001;98(1):20-27.

84. Vroman S, Yo Le Sian A, Thiery M, et al. Elective induction of labor conducted under lumbar epidural block. I. Labor induction by amniotomy and intravenous oxytocin. *Eur J Obstet Gynecol Reprod Biol.* 1977;7(3):159-180.

85. Thiery M, Vroman S, de Hemptinne D, et al. Elective induction of labor conducted under lumbar epidural block. II. Labor induction by amniotomy and intravenous prostaglandin. *Eur J Obstet Gynecol Reprod Biol.* 1977;7(3):181-200.

86. Thorngren-Jerneck K, Herbst A. Low 5-minute Apgar score: a population-based register study of 1 million term births. *Obstet Gynecol.* Jul 2001;98(1): 65-70.

87. Kumar M, Paes B. Epidural opioid analgesia and neonatal respiratory depression. *J Perinatol.* Jul-Aug 2003;23(5):425-427.

88. Hale T. *Medications and Mother's Milk.* Amarillo TX: Pharmasoft; 1997.

89. Kuhnert BR, Zuspan KJ, Kuhnert PM, Syracuse CD, Brown DE. Bupivacaine disposition in mother, fetus, and neonate after spinal anesthesia for cesarean section. *Anesth Analg.* May 1987;66(5):407-412.

90. Hale T. The effects on breastfeeding women of anaesthetic medications used during labour. Paper presented at: The Passage to Motherhood, 1998; Brisbane Australia.

91. De Amici D, Gasparoni A, Chirico G, et al. Natural killer cell activity and delivery: possible influence of cortisol and anesthetic agents. A study on newborn cord blood. *Biol Neonate.* Dec 1999;76(6):348-354.

92. Camann W, Brazelton TB. Use and abuse of neonatal neurobehavioral testing. *Anesthesiology.* Jan 2000;92(1):3-5.

93. Halpern SH, Littleford JA, Brockhurst NJ, Youngs PJ, Malik N, Owen HC. The neurologic and adaptive capacity score is not a reliable method of newborn evaluation. *Anesthesiology.* Jun 2001;94(6):958-962.

94. Torvaldsen S, Roberts CL, Simpson JM, Thompson JF, Ellwood DA. Intrapartum epidural analgesia and breastfeeding: a prospective cohort study. *Int Breastfeed J.* 2006;1:24.

95. Brockhurst NJ, Littleford JA, Halpern SH. The Neurologic and Adaptive Capacity Score: a systematic review of its use in obstetric anesthesia research. *Anesthesiology.* Jan 2000;92(1):237-246.

96. Murray AD, Dolby RM, Nation RL, Thomas DB. Effects of epidural anesthesia on newborns and their mothers. *Child Dev.* Mar 1981;52(1):71-82, p 78.

97. Murray AD, Dolby RM, Nation RL, Thomas DB. Effects of epidural anesthesia on newborns and their mothers. *Child Dev.* Mar 1981;52(1):71-82.

98. Sepkoski CM, Lester BM, Ostheimer GW, Brazelton TB. The effects of maternal epidural anesthesia on neonatal behavior during the first month. *Dev Med Child Neurol.* Dec 1992;34(12):1072-1080.

99. Rosenblatt DB, Belsey EM, Lieberman BA, et al. The influence of maternal analgesia on neonatal behaviour: II. Epidural bupivacaine. *Br J Obstet Gynaecol.* Apr 1981;88(4):407-413.

100. Loftus JR, Hill H, Cohen SE. Placental transfer and neonatal effects of epidural sufentanil and fentanyl administered with bupivacaine during labor. *Anesthesiology.* Aug 1995;83(2):300-308.

101. Murray AD, Dolby RM, Nation RL, Thomas DB. Effects of epidural anesthesia on newborns and their mothers. *Child Dev.* Mar 1981;52(1):71-82, p 81.

102. Murray AD, Dolby RM, Nation RL, Thomas DB. Effects of epidural anesthesia on newborns and their mothers. *Child Dev.* Mar 1981;52(1):71-82, p 71.

103. Radzyminski S. Neurobehavioral functioning and breastfeeding behavior in the newborn. *J Obstet Gynecol Neonatal Nurs.* May-Jun 2005;34(3):335-341.

104. Jonas W, Wiklund I, Nissen E, Ransjo-Arvidson AB, Uvnas Moberg K. Newborn skin temperature two days postpartum during breastfeeding related to different labour ward practices. *Early Hum Dev.* Jan 2007;83(1):55-62.

105. Uvnas-Moberg K. *The Oxytocin Factor.* Cambridge MA: Da Capo Press; 2003.

106. Jonas W, Wiklund I, Nissen E, Ransjo-Arvidson AB, Uvnas-Moberg K. Newborn skin temperature two days postpartum during breastfeeding related to different labour ward practices. *Early Hum Dev.* Jan 2007;83(1):55-62, p 57.

107. Brackbill Y. Long-term effects of obstetrical anesthesia on infant autonomic function. *Dev Psychobiol.* Nov 1977;10(6):529-535.

108. Krehbiel D, Poindron P, Levy F, Prud'Homme MJ. Peridural anesthesia disturbs maternal behavior in primiparous and multiparous parturient ewes. *Physiol Behav.* 1987;40(4):463-472.

109. Golub MS, Germann SL. Perinatal bupivacaine and infant behavior in rhesus monkeys. *Neurotoxicol Teratol.* Jan-Feb 1998;20(1):29-41.

110. Righard L, Alade MO. Effect of delivery room routines on success of first breast-feed. *Lancet.* Nov 3 1990;336(8723):1105-1107.

111. Matthews MK. The relationship between maternal labour analgesia and delay in the initiation of breastfeeding in healthy neonates in the early neonatal period. *Midwifery.* Mar 1989;5(1):3-10.

112. Ransjo-Arvidson AB, Matthiesen AS, Lilja G, Nissen E, Widstrom AM, Uvnas-Moberg K. Maternal analgesia during labor disturbs newborn behavior: effects on breastfeeding, temperature, and crying. *Birth.* Mar 2001;28(1):5-12.

113. Nissen E, Lilja G, Matthiesen AS, Ransjo-Arvidsson AB, Uvnas-Moberg K, Widstrom AM. Effects of maternal pethidine on infants' developing breast feeding behaviour. *Acta Paediatr.* Feb 1995;84(2):140-145.

114. Rajan L. The impact of obstetric procedures and analgesia/anaesthesia during labour and delivery on breast feeding. *Midwifery.* Jun 1994;10(2):87-103.

115. Riordan J, Gross A, Angeron J, Krumwiede B, Melin J. The effect of labor pain relief medication on neonatal suckling and breastfeeding duration. *J Hum Lact.* Feb 2000;16(1):7-12.

116. Dewey KG, Nommsen-Rivers LA, Heinig MJ, Cohen RJ. Risk factors for suboptimal infant breastfeeding behavior, delayed onset of lactation, and excess

neonatal weight loss. *Pediatrics.* Sep 2003;112(3 Pt 1):607-619.

117. Radzyminski S. The effect of ultra low dose epidural analgesia on newborn breastfeeding behaviors. *J Obstet Gynecol Neonatal Nurs.* May-Jun 2003;32(3):322-331.

118. Moore ER, Anderson GC, Bergman N. Early skin-to-skin contact for mothers and their healthy newborn infants. *Cochrane Database Syst Rev.* 2007(3):CD003519.

119. Jordan S, Emery S, Bradshaw C, Watkins A, Friswell W. The impact of intrapartum analgesia on infant feeding. *BJOG.* Jul 2005;112(7):927-934.

120. Beilin Y, Bodian CA, Weiser J, et al. Effect of labor epidural analgesia with and without fentanyl on infant breastfeeding: a prospective, randomized, double-blind study. *Anesthesiology.* Dec 2005;103(6):1211-1217.

121. Baumgarder DJ, Muehl P, Fischer M, Pribbenow B. Effect of labor epidural anesthesia on breast-feeding of healthy full-term newborns delivered vaginally. *J Am Board Fam Pract.* Jan-Feb 2003;16(1):7-13.

122. Volmanen P, Valanne J, Alahuhta S. Breast-feeding problems after epidural analgesia for labour: a retrospective cohort study of pain, obstetrical procedures and breast-feeding practices. *Int J Obstet Anesth.* Jan 2004;13(1):25-29.

123. Henderson JJ, Dickinson JE, Evans SF, McDonald SJ, Paech MJ. Impact of intrapartum epidural analgesia on breast-feeding duration. *Aust N Z J Obstet Gynaecol.* Oct 2003;43(5):372-377.

124. Kiehl EM, Anderson GC, Wilson ME, Fosson L. Social status, mother-infant time together, and breastfeeding duration. *J Hum Lact.* Sep 1996;12(3):201-206.

125. Halpern SH, Levine T, Wilson DB, MacDonell J, Katsiris SE, Leighton BL.

Effect of labor analgesia on breastfeeding success. *Birth.* Jun 1999;26(2):83-88.

126. Chang ZM, Heaman MI. Epidural analgesia during labor and delivery: effects on the initiation and continuation of effective breastfeeding. *J Hum Lact.* Aug 2005;21(3):305-314; quiz 315-309, 326.

127. UNICEF. The Baby-Friendly Hospital Initiative. Available at: http://www.unicef.org/programme/breastfeeding/baby.htm.

128. Kannan S, Jamison RN, Datta S. Maternal satisfaction and pain control in women electing natural childbirth. *Reg Anesth Pain Med.* Sep-Oct 2001;26(5):468-472.

129. Green JM, Coupland VA, Kitzinger JV. Expectations, experiences, and psychological outcomes of childbirth: a prospective study of 825 women. *Birth.* Mar 1990;17(1):15-24.

130. Morgan BM, Bulpitt CJ, Clifton P, Lewis PJ. Analgesia and satisfaction in childbirth (the Queen Charlotte's 1000 Mother Survey). *Lancet.* Oct 9 1982;2(8302):808-810.

131. Morgan BM, Bulpitt CJ, Clifton P, Lewis PJ. Analgesia and satisfaction in childbirth (the Queen Charlotte's 1000 Mother Survey). *Lancet.* Oct 9 1982;2(8302):808-810, p 809.

132. Klein MC, Grzybowski S, Harris S, et al. Epidural analgesia use as a marker for physician approach to birth: implications for maternal and newborn outcomes. *Birth.* Dec 2001;28(4):243-248.

Chapter 8: LEAVING WELL ENOUGH ALONE

1. Matthiesen AS, Ransjo-Arvidson AB, Nissen E, Uvnas-Moberg K. Postpartum maternal oxytocin release by newborns: effects of infant hand massage and sucking. *Birth.* Mar 2001;28(1):13-19.

2. Segal S, Csavoy AN, Datta S. The tocolytic effect of catecholamines in

the gravid rat uterus. *Anesth Analg.* Oct 1998;87(4):864-869.

3. Odent M. The foetus ejection reflex. *Birth.* Jun 1987;14(2):104-105.

4. Westgren M, Lindahl SG, Norden NE. Maternal and fetal endocrine stress response at vaginal delivery with and without an epidural block. *J Perinat Med.* 1986;14(4):235-241.

5. Saito M, Sano T, Satohisa E. Plasma catecholamines and microvibration as labour progresses. *Shinshin-Thaku.* 1991;31:381-389.

6. Odent M. Don't manage the third stage of labour! *Pract Midwife.* Sep 1998;1(9):31-33.

7. Thornton S, Davison JM, Baylis PH. Plasma oxytocin during third stage of labour: comparison of natural and active management. *Br Med J.* Jul 16 1988;297(6642):167-169.

8. Leff M. The role of adrenalin (epinephrine) in labor and the use of an adrenolytic drug to prevent postpartum hemorrhage; observations based on 3,500 cases. *Am J Obstet Gynecol.* Feb 1953;65(2):278-281.

9. Grattan DR. The actions of prolactin in the brain during pregnancy and lactation. *Prog Brain Res.* 2001;133:153-171.

10. Stefos T, Sotiriadis A, Tsirkas P, Messinis I, Lolis D. Maternal prolactin secretion during labor: The role of dopamine. *Acta Obstet Gynecol Scand.* Jan 2001;80(1):34-38.

11. Christensson K, Siles C, Moreno L, et al. Temperature, metabolic adaptation and crying in healthy full-term newborns cared for skin-to-skin or in a cot. *Acta Paediatr.* Jun-Jul 1992;81(6-7):488-493.

12. Bystrova K, Widstrom AM, Matthiesen AS, et al. Skin-to-skin contact may reduce negative consequences of "the stress of being born": a study on temperature in newborn infants, subjected to different ward routines in St. Petersburg. *Acta Paediatr.* 2003;92(3):320-326.

13. Bergman NJ. Skin-to-Skin Contact and Perinatal Neuroscience. Paper presented at: Capers Breastfeeding Seminar: Breastfeeding A Lifelong Investment; May 13 2006, Brisbane, Australia.

14. Schore AN. The effects of early relational trauma on right brain development, affect regulation, and infant mental health. *Infant Mental Health Journal.* 2001;221(1-2):201-269.

15. Dettling AC, Feldon J, Pryce CR. Repeated parental deprivation in the infant common marmoset (*Callithrix jacchus,* primates) and analysis of its effects on early development. *Biol Psychiatry.* Dec 1 2002;52(11):1037-1046.

16. Kalinichev M, Easterling KW, Plotsky PM, Holtzman SG. Long-lasting changes in stress-induced corticosterone response and anxiety-like behaviors as a consequence of neonatal maternal separation in Long-Evans rats. *Pharmacol Biochem Behav.* Aug 2002;73(1):131-140.

17. Daniels WM, Pietersen CY, Carstens ME, Stein DJ. Maternal separation in rats leads to anxiety-like behavior and a blunted ACTH response and altered neurotransmitter levels in response to a subsequent stressor. *Metab Brain Dis.* Jun 2004;19(1-2):3-14.

18. Bergman NJ. Reducing NICU Stays by 40% with Skin to Skin Mothering. Paper presented at: Gentle Birth World Congress, 2007; Portland OR.

19. Carter CS. Developmental consequences of oxytocin. *Physiol Behav.* Aug 2003;79(3):383-397, p 386.

20. Jacobson B, Eklund G, Hamberger L, Linnarsson D, Sedvall G, Valverius M. Perinatal origin of adult self-destructive behavior. *Acta Psychiatr Scand.* Oct 1987;76(4):364-371.

21. Jacobson B, Nyberg K, Gronbladh L, Eklund G, Bygdeman M, Rydberg U. Opiate addiction in adult offspring

through possible imprinting after obstetric treatment. *Br Med J.* Nov 10 1990;301(6760):1067-1070.

22. Jacobson B, Bygdeman M. Obstetric care and proneness of offspring to suicide as adults: case-control study. *Br Med J.* Nov 14 1998;317(7169):1346-1349.

23. Raine A, Brennan P, Mednick SA. Birth complications combined with early maternal rejection at age 1 year predispose to violent crime at age 18 years. *Arch Gen Psychiatry.* Dec 1994;51(12):984-988.

24. Pearce JC. *Evolution's End: Claiming the Potential of Our Intelligence.* San Francisco: HarperSanFrancisco; 1995.

25. Odent M. *The Scientification of Love.* Revised ed. London: Free Association Books; 2001.

26. Brady-Fryer B, Wiebe N, Lander JA. Pain relief for neonatal circumcision. *Cochrane Database Syst Rev.* 2004(4):CD004217.

27. Olson TL, Downey VW. Infant physiological responses to noxious stimuli of circumcision with anesthesia and analgesia. *Pediatr Nurs.* Jul-Aug 1998;24(4):385-389.

28. Williamson PS, Evans ND. Neonatal cortisol response to circumcision with anesthesia. *Clin Pediatr (Phila).* Aug 1986;25(8):412-415.

29. Redmond A, Isana S, Ingall D. Relation of Onset of Respiration to Placental Transfusion. *Lancet.* Feb 6 1965;17:283-285.

30. Dunn P. Alterations in the distribution of blood between the fetus and placenta during and after delivery. Paper presented at: Canadian Pediatric Society Centennial Commonwealth Meeting, 1967; Toronto, Sept 3-9.

31. Diaz-Rossello JL. Early umbilical cord clamping and cord-blood banking. *Lancet.* Sep 2 2006;368(9538):840.

32. Gunther M. The transfer of blood between baby and placenta in the minutes after birth. *Lancet.* Jun 22 1957;272(6982):1277-1280.

33. Linderkamp O. Placental transfusion: determinants and effects. *Clin Perinatol.* Oct 1982;9(3):559-592.

34. Yao AC, Hirvensalo M, Lind J. Placental transfusion-rate and uterine contraction. *Lancet.* Feb 24 1968;1(7539):380-383.

35. Yao AC, Lind J. Effect of gravity on placental transfusion. *Lancet.* Sep 6 1969;2(7619):505-508.

36. Hutton EK, Hassan ES. Late vs early clamping of the umbilical cord in full-term neonates: systematic review and meta-analysis of controlled trials. *JAMA.* Mar 21 2007;297(11):1241-1252.

37. Dunn PM. The placental venous pressure during and after the third stage of labour following early cord ligation. *J Obstet Gynaecol Br Commonw.* Oct 1966;73(5):747-756.

38. McDonald SJ, Middleton P. Effect of timing of umbilical cord clamping of term infants on maternal and neonatal outcomes. *Cochrane Database Syst Rev.* 2008(2):CD004074.

39. International Confederation of Midwives and International Federation of Gynaecologists and Obstetricians. Joint statement: management of the third stage of labour to prevent post-partum haemorrhage. *J Midwifery Womens Health.* Jan-Feb 2004;49(1):76-77.

40. Pisacane A. Neonatal prevention of iron deficiency. *Br Med J.* Jan 20 1996;312(7024):136-137, p 136.

41. Usher R, Shephard M, Lind J. The Blood Volume of the Newborn Infant and Placental Transfusion. *Acta Paediatr.* Sep 1963;52:497-512.

42. Morley GM. Cord Closure: Can Hasty Clamping Injure the Newborn? *OBG Management.* July 1998;29-36, p 33.

43. Peltonen T. Placental transfusion—advantage and disadvantage. *Eur J Pediatr*. Oct 1981;137(2):141-146.

44. Ibid., p 142.

45. Diaz-Rossello JL. International Perspectives: Cord Clamping for Stem Cell Donation: Medical Facts and Ethics. *Neoreviews*. 2006;7:557-563, p 561.

46. Wiberg N, Kallen K, Olofsson P. Delayed umbilical cord clamping at birth has effects on arterial and venous blood gases and lactate concentrations. *BJOG*. May 2008;115(6):697-703.

47. Weeks A. Umbilical cord clamping after birth. *BMJ*. Aug 18 2007;335(7615):312-313.

48. Mercer JS, Skovgaard RL, Peareara-Eaves J, Bowman TA. Nuchal cord management and nurse-midwifery practice. *J Midwifery Womens Health*. Sep-Oct 2005;50(5):373-379.

49. Itty L, Varadi V. Cerebral palsy following cutting of the nuchal cord before delivery. *Med Law*. 1994;13(3-4):323-330.

50. Iffy L, Varadi V, Papp E. Untoward neonatal sequelae deriving from cutting of the umbilical cord before delivery. *Med Law*. 2001;20(4):627-634.

51. Kleinberg F, Dong L, Phibbs RH. Cesarean section prevents placenta-to-infant transfusion despite delayed cord clamping. *Am J Obstet Gynecol*. Jan 1 1975;121(1):66-70

52. Landau DB. Hyaline membrane formation in the newborn; hematogenic shock as a possible etiologic factor. *Mo Med*. Mar 1953;50(3):183-185.

53. Dunn P. Caesarean section and the prevention of respiratory distress syndrome of the newborn. Paper presented at: Third European Congress of Perinatal Medicine, 1972; Lausanne.

54. Morley G. To Clamp or Not to Clamp: This Is the Answer. 2002 http://www.cordclamping.com/clamp.htm.

55. Philip AG, Teng SS. Role of respiration in effecting transfusion at cesarean section. *Biol Neonate*. 1977;31(3-4):219-224.

56. Zlotkin S. Current issues for the prevention and treatment of iron deficiency anemia. *Indian Pediatr*. Feb 2002;39(2):125-129.

57. van Rheenen P, Brabin BJ. Late umbilical cord-clamping as an intervention for reducing iron deficiency anaemia in term infants in developing and industrialised countries: a systematic review. *Ann Trop Paediatr*. Mar 2004;24(1):3-16.

58. Chaparro CM, Fornes R, Neufeld LM, Tena Alavez G, Eguia-Liz Cedillo R, Dewey KG. Early umbilical cord clamping contributes to elevated blood lead levels among infants with higher lead exposure. *J Pediatr*. Nov 2007;151(5):506-512.

59. Lozoff B, Georgieff MK. Iron deficiency and brain development. *Semin Pediatr Neurol*. Sep 2006;13(3):158-165

60. Darwin E. *Zoonomia or The Laws of Organic Life*. Second ed. London: J Johnson; 1796.

61. Kinmond S, Aitchison TC, Holland BM, Jones JG, Turner TL, Wardrop CA. Umbilical cord clamping and preterm infants: a randomised trial. *Br Med J*. Jan 16 1993;306(6871):172-175.

62. Rabe H, Reynolds G, Diaz-Rossello J. Early versus delayed umbilical cord clamping in preterm infants. *Cochrane Database Syst Rev*. 2004(4):CD003248.

63. Hofmeyr GJ, Bex PJ, Skapinker R, Delahunt T. Hasty clamping of the umbilical cord may initiate neonatal intraventricular hemorrhage. *Med Hypotheses*. May 1989;29(1):5-6.

64. Meek JH, Tyszczuk L, Elwell CE, Wyatt JS. Low cerebral blood flow is a risk factor for severe intraventricular haemorrhage. *Arch Dis Child Fetal Neonatal Ed*. Jul 1999;81(1):F15-18.

65. Morley G. Neonatal encephalopathy, Hypoxic Ischemic Encephalopathy, and Subsequent Cerebral Palsy: Etiology, Pathology and Prevention. 2003 www.cordclamping.com/Lancet2003analysis.htm.

66. Morley G. Autism, ADD/ADHD, and related disorders: Is a common childbirth practice to blame? *Red Flags Weekly enewsletter.* 2002 http://redflagsweekly.com/features/Morley.html.

67. Simon E. Developmental Language Disability: One consequence of ischemic brainstem injury? 31st Annual Meeting of the Fetal and Neonatal Physiological Society, Tuscany, 2004. Available at: www.cordclamping.com/poster1.doc.

68. Simon E. *The History of Cord Clamping.* 2004 www.cordclamping.com/History.htm.

69. Jaykka S, Peltonen T, Hirvonen L. Capillary erection in the living lung. *Acta Paediatr Suppl.* Sep 1959;48(Suppl 118):41-42.

70. Jaykka S. Capillary erection and the structural appearance of fetal and neonatal lungs. *Acta Paediatr.* Sep 1958;47(5):484-500.

71. Jaykka S. Capillary erection and lung expansion; an experimental study of the effect of liquid pressure applied to the capillary network of excised fetal lungs. *Acta Paediatr Suppl.* Jan 1957;46(suppl 112):1-91.

72. Jaykka S. A new theory concerning the mechanism of the initiation of respiration in the newborn; a preliminary report. *Acta Paediatr.* Sep 1954;43(5):399-410.

73. Mercer JS, Skovgaard RL. Neonatal transitional physiology: a new paradigm. *J Perinat Neonatal Nurs.* Mar 2002;15(4):56-75.

74. Yao AC, Moinian M, Lind J. Distribution of blood between infant and placenta after birth. *Lancet.* Oct 25 1969;2(7626):871-873.

75. Saigal S, Usher RH. Symptomatic neonatal plethora. *Biol Neonate.* 1977;32(1-2):62-72.

76 Ceriani Cernadas JM, Carroli G, Pellegrini L, et al. The effect of timing of cord clamping on neonatal venous hematocrit values and clinical outcome at term: a randomized, controlled trial. *Pediatrics.* Apr 2006;117(4):e779-786.

77. Mercer JS. Current best evidence: a review of the literature on umbilical cord clamping. *J Midwifery Womens Health.* Nov-Dec 2001;46(6):402-414.

78. Morley GM. Cord Closure: Can Hasty Clamping Injure the Newborn? *OBG Management.* July 1998;29-36.

79. McDonagh A. Bilirubin the beneficent. *Pediatrics.* Dec 2004;114(6):1741-1742; author reply 1742-1743.

80. Sedlak TW, Snyder SH. Bilirubin benefits: cellular protection by a biliverdin reductase antioxidant cycle. *Pediatrics.* Jun 2004;113(6):1776-1782.

81. Shekeeb Shahab M, Kumar P, Sharma N, Narang A, Prasad R. Evaluation of oxidant and antioxidant status in term neonates: a plausible protective role of bilirubin. *Mol Cell Biochem.* Jun 17 2008.

82. Najib-Farah. Defensive role of bilirubinemia in pneumococcal infection. *Lancet.* 1937;1:505-506.

83. Weeks A. Umbilical cord clamping after birth. *BMJ.* Aug 18 2007;335(7615):312-313, p 313.

84. Garrison L. www.gentlebirth.org/archives/cordIssues.html; 1999.

85. Marquis L, Ackerman BD. Placental respiration in the immediate neonatal period. *Am J Obstet Gynecol.* Oct 1 1973;117(3):358-363.

86. Carter CS. Developmental consequences of oxytocin. *Physiol Behav.* Aug 2003;79(3):383-397.

87. Ibid., p 392.

88. Edwards NP. *Delivering Your Placenta: The Third Stage.* AIMS for British Maternity Trust; 1999.

89. Hoff DS, Maynard RC. Accidental administration of oxytocin to a premature infant. *Neonatal Netw.* Feb 2002;21(1):27-29.

90. Brereteon-Stiles GG, Winship WS, Goodwin NM, Roos RF. Accidental administration of syntometrine to a neonate. *S Afr Med J.* Dec 30 1972;46(52):2052.

91. Sullivan MJ. Banking on cord blood stem cells. *Nat Rev Cancer.* Jul 2008;8(7):555-563.

92. Steinbrook R. The cord-blood-bank controversies. *N Engl J Med.* Nov 25 2004;351(22):2255-2257.

93. Fisk NM, Roberts IA, Markwald R, Mironov V. Can routine commercial cord blood banking be scientifically and ethically justified? *PLoS Med.* Feb 2005;2(2):e44.

94. Laughlin MJ, Eapen M, Rubinstein P, et al. Outcomes After Transplantation of Cord Blood or Bone Marrow from Unrelated Donors in Adults with Leukemia. *Obstet Gynecol Surv.* May 2005;60(5):295-296.

95. Sullivan MJ. Banking on cord blood stem cells. *Nat Rev Cancer.* Jul 2008;8(7):555-563, p 561.

96. European Group on Ethics in Science and New Technologies, Gunning J. *Opinion No 19—Opinion on the ethical aspects of umbilical cord blood banking.* Luxembourg: Office for Official Publications of the European Communities; 2004.

97. Cord blood banking for potential future transplantation: subject review. American Academy of Pediatrics. Work Group on Cord Blood Banking. *Pediatrics.* Jul 1999;104(1 Pt 1):116-118.

98. Lubin BH, Shearer WT. Cord blood banking for potential future transplantation. *Pediatrics.* Jan 2007;119(1):165-170.

99. American College of Obstetricians and Gynecologists. ACOG committee opinion number 399, February 2008: umbilical cord blood banking. *Obstet Gynecol.* Feb 2008;111(2 Pt 1):475-477, p 475.

100. Agovino T. As business grows, umbilical cord blood storage prompts debate. *Boston Globe.* 4/10/2004, 2004: A4.

101. Woodhouse D. Cord blood banking movement grows. *O&G: the Royal Australian and New Zealand College of Obstetricians and Gynaecologists.* February 1999;1(1).

102. McGregor JA, Rogo LJ. Breastmilk: an unappreciated source of stem cells. *J Hum Lact.* Aug 2006;22(3):270-271.

103. Donaldson C, Armitage WJ, Laundy V, et al. Impact of obstetric factors on cord blood donation for transplantation. *Br J Haematol.* Jul 1999;106(1):128-132.

104. Smith FO, Thomson BG. Umbilical cord blood collection, banking, and transplantation: current status and issues relevant to perinatal caregivers. *Birth.* Jun 2000;27(2):127-135.

105. Lasky LC, Lane TA, Miller JP, et al. In utero or ex utero cord blood collection: which is better? *Transfusion.* Oct 2002;42(10):1261-1267.

106. Wardrop CA, Holland BM. The roles and vital importance of placental blood to the newborn infant. *J Perinat Med.* 1995;23(1-2):139-143.

107. Levy T, Blickstein I. Timing of cord clamping revisited. J Perinat Med. 2006;34(4):293-297, p 293.

108. Chouthai NS, Sampers J, Desai N, Smith GM. Changes in neurotrophin levels in umbilical cord blood from infants with different gestational ages and clinical conditions. *Pediatr Res.* Jun 2003;53(6):965-969.

109. Bracci-Laudiero L, Celestino D, Starace G, et al. CD34-positive cells in

human umbilical cord blood express nerve growth factor and its specific receptor TrkA. *J Neuroimmunol.* Mar 2003;136(1-2):130-139.

110. Kim SY, Park SY, Kim JM, et al. Differentiation of endothelial cells from human umbilical cord blood AC133-CD14+ cells. *Ann Hematol.* Jul 2005;84(7):417-422.

111. Gora-Kupilas K, Josko J. The neuroprotective function of vascular endothelial growth factor (VEGF). *Folia Neuropathol.* 2005;43(1):31-39.

112. Hao HN, Zhao J, Thomas RL, Parker GC, Lyman WD. Fetal human hematopoietic stem cells can differentiate sequentially into neural stem cells and then astrocytes in vitro. *J Hematother Stem Cell Res.* Feb 2003;12(1): 23-32.

113. Steenblock D. Umbilical Stem Cell Therapy for Autism (Microsoft Power-Point presentation). *Steenblock Research Institute.* Available at: http://www .autismone.org/uploads/2006.

114. Kiatpongsan S. Business on hope: a case study on private cord blood stem cell banking. *J Med Assoc Thai.* Apr 2008;91(4):577-580.

115. European Group on Ethics in Science and New Technologies, Gunning J. *Opinion No 19—Opinion on the ethical aspects of umbilical cord blood banking.* Luxembourg: Office for Official Publications of the European Communities; 2004.

116. Royal College of Obstetricians and Gynaecologists. *Cord blood banking: information for parents.* 2006.

117. Royal College of Obstetricians and Gynaecologists. *Umbilical Cord Blood Banking.* 2006.

118. International Federation of Gynaecologists and Obstetricians (FIGO) Committee for the Ethical Aspects of Human Reproduction. Ethical guidelines regarding the procedure of collection of cord blood (1998). *Recommendations on Ethical Issues in Obstetrics and Gynecology.* London: FIGO; 2000:42-43.

119. Diaz-Rossello JL. International Perspectives: Cord Clamping for Stem Cell Donation: Medical Facts and Ethics. *Neoreviews.* 2006;7:557-563, p 562.

120. Inch S. *Birth Rights: What Every Parent Should Know About Childbirth in Hospital.* New York: Random House; 1984.

121. Jordan S. *Pharmacology for Midwives.* Hampshire UK: Palgrave; 2002.

122. de Groot AN, van Dongen PW, Vree TB, Hekster YA, van Roosmalen J. Ergot alkaloids. Current status and review of clinical pharmacology and therapeutic use compared with other oxytocics in obstetrics and gynaecology. *Drugs.* Oct 1998;56(4):523-535.

123. Begley CM. The effect of ergometrine on breast feeding (author reply). *Midwifery. Dec 1990;6(4):231-232.*

124. Carroli G, Grant A. The effect of ergometrine on breast feeding. *Midwifery.* Dec 1990;6(4):231-232.

125. Begley CM. The effect of ergometrine on breast feeding. *Midwifery.* Jun 1990;6(2):60-72.

126. Hale T. *Medications and Mother's Milk.* 4th ed. Amarillo TX: Pharmasoft; 2006.

127. Weiss G, Klein S, Shenkman L, Kataoka K, Hollander CS. Effect of methylergonovine on puerperal prolactin secretion. *Obstet Gynecol.* Aug 1975;46(2):209-210

128. Arabin B, Ruttgers H, Kubli F. [Effects of routine administration of methylergometrin during puerperium on involution, maternal morbidity and lactation]. *Geburtshilfe Frauenheilkd.* Apr 1986;46(4):215-220.

129. Liabsuetrakul T, Choobun T, Peeyananjarassri K, Islam QM. Prophylactic use of ergot alkaloids in the third stage of labour. *Cochrane Database Syst Rev.* 2007(2):CD005456.

130. McDonald S, Abbott JM, Higgins SP. Prophylactic ergometrine-oxytocin versus oxytocin for the third stage of labour. *Cochrane Database Syst Rev.* 2004(1):CD000201.

131. McDonald S, Prendiville WJ, Elbourne D. Prophylactic syntometrine versus oxytocin for delivery of the placenta. *Cochrane Database Syst Rev.* 2000(2):CD000201.

132. Sorbe B. Active pharmacologic management of the third stage of labor. A comparison of oxytocin and ergometrine. *Obstet Gynecol.* Dec 1978;52(6):694-697.

133. Gulmezoglu AM, Forna F, Villar J, Hofmeyr GJ. Prostaglandins for prevention of postpartum haemorrhage. *Cochrane Database Syst Rev.* 2004(1):CD000494.

134. Vogel D, Burkhardt T, Rentsch K, et al. Misoprostol versus methylergometrine: pharmacokinetics in human milk. *Am J Obstet Gynecol.* Dec 2004;191(6):2168-2173.

135. Prendiville WJ, Elbourne D, McDonald S. Active versus expectant management in the third stage of labour. *Cochrane Database Syst Rev.* 2000(3):CD000007.

136. Rogers J, Wood J, McCandlish R, Ayers S, Truesdale A, Elbourne D. Active versus expectant management of third stage of labour: the Hinchingbrooke randomised controlled trial. *Lancet.* Mar 7 1998;351(9104):693-699.

137. Ibid., p 698.

138. Botha M. Management of the Umbilical Cord During Labour. *South African Journal of Obstetrics and Gynecology.* 1968;6:30-33, p 30.

139. Walsh SZ. Maternal effects of early and late clamping of the umbilical cord. *Lancet.* May 11 1968;1(7550):996-997.

140. Soltani H, F D, I S. Placental cord drainage after spontaneous vaginal delivery as part of the management of the third stage of labour. *The Cochrane Database of Systematic Reviews.* 2004;(1):CD004665.

141. Phillip H, Fletcher H, Reid M. The impact of induced labour on postpartum blood loss. *J Obstet Gynaecol.* Jan 2004;24(1):12-15.

142. Stones RW, Paterson CM, Saunders NJ. Risk factors for major obstetric haemorrhage. *Eur J Obstet Gynecol Reprod Biol.* Jan 1993;48(1):15-18.

143. MacKenzie IZ. Induction of labour and postpartum haemorrhage. *Br Med J.* Mar 17 1979;1(6165):750.

144. Brinsden PR, Clark AD. Postpartum haemorrhage after induced and spontaneous labour. *Br Med J.* Sep 23 1978;2(6141):855-856.

145. St George L, Crandon AJ. Immediate postpartum complications. *Aust N Z J Obstet Gynaecol.* Feb 1990;30(1):52-56.

146. Magann EF, Evans S, Hutchinson M, Collins R, Howard BC, Morrison JC, Postpartum hemorrhage after vaginal birth: an analysis of risk factors. *South Med J.* Apr 2005;98(4):419-422.

147. Ploeckinger B, Ulm MR, Chalubinski K, Gruber W. Epidural anaesthesia in labour: influence on surgical delivery rates, intrapartum fever and blood loss. *Gynecol Obstet Invest.* 1995;39(1):24-27.

148. Gilbert L, Porter W, Brown VA. Postpartum haemorrhage—a continuing problem. *Br J Obstet Gynaecol.* Jan 1987;94(1):67-71.

149. Chattopadhyay SK, Kharit H, Sherbeeni MM. Placenta praevia and accreta after previous caesarean section. *Eur J Obstet Gynecol Reprod Biol.* Dec 30 1993;52(3):151-156.

150. Hemminki E, Merilainen J. Long-term effects of cesarean sections: ectopic pregnancies and placental problems. *Am J Obstet Gynecol.* May 1996;174(5):1569-1574.

151. Lydon-Rochelle M, Holt VL, Easterling TR, Martin DP. First-birth cesarean and

placental abruption or previa at second birth. *Obstet Gynecol.* May 2001;97(5 1):765-769.

152. Goodfellow CF, Hull MG, Swaab DF, Dogterom J, Buijs RM. Oxytocin deficiency at delivery with epidural analgesia. *Br J Obstet Gynaecol.* Mar 1983;90(3):214-219.

153. Phaneuf S, Rodriguez Linares B, TambyRaja RL, MacKenzie IZ, Lopez Bernal A. Loss of myometrial oxytocin receptors during oxytocin-induced and oxytocin-augmented labour. *J Reprod Fertil.* Sep 2000;120(1):91-97.

154. Kennell JH, McGrath S. What babies teach us: the essential link between baby's behavior and mother's biology. *Birth.* Mar 2001;28(1):20-21, p 20.

155. Logue M. The management of the third stage of labour: a midwife's view. *J Obstet Gynaecol.* 1990;10(Suppl 2):10-12.

156. Ladipo OA. Management of third stage of labour, with particular reference to reduction of feto-maternal transfusion. *Br Med J.* Mar 18 1972;1(5802):721-723.

157. Doolittle JE, Moritz CR. Prevention of erythroblastosis by an obstetric technic. *Obstet Gynecol.* Apr 1966;27(4):529-531.

158. Beer AE. Fetal erythrocytes in maternal circulation of 155 Rh-negative women. *Obstet Gynecol.* Aug 1969;34(2):143-150.

159. Weinstein L, Farabow WS, Gusdon JP, Jr. Third stage of labor and transplacental hemorrhage. *Obstet Gynecol.* Jan 1971;37(1):90-93.

160. Bakas P, Liapis A, Giner M, Paterakis G, Creatsas G. Massive fetomaternal hemorrhage and oxytocin contraction test: case report and review. *Arch Gynecol Obstet.* Jan 2004;269(2):149-151.

161. Valdes V, Goldrey M, Hamon I, Hascoet JM. [Massive fetomaternal transfusion after induction of labor by oxytocin]. *Arch Pediatr.* Aug 2002;9(8):818-821.

162. Leavitt BG, Huff DL, Bell LA, Thurnau GR. Placental drainage of fetal

blood at cesarean delivery and feto maternal transfusion: a randomized controlled trial. *Obstet Gynecol.* Sep 2007;110(3):608-611.

163. Doolittle JE. Placental Vascular Integrity Related to Third-Stage Management. *Obstet Gynecol.* Oct 1963;22:468-472.

164. David M, Smidt J, Chen FC, Stein U, Dudenhausen JW. Risk factors for fetal-to-maternal transfusion in Rh D-negative women—results of a prospective study on 942 pregnant women. *J Perinat Med.* 2004;32(3):254-257.

165. Wickham S. *Anti-D in Midwifery: Panacea or Paradox?* Oxford: Books for Midwives; 2001.

166. Wickham S. Anti-D: Exploring midwifery knowledge. *MIDIRS Midwifery Digest.* 2000; 9(4):450-455 http://www.withwoman.co.uk/contents/info/antid.html.

167. World Health Organisation. *Care in Normal Birth: a Practical Guide. Report of a Technical Working Group.* Geneva: World Health Organisation; 1996, p 31.

168. World Health Organisation. *Care in Normal Birth: a Practical Guide. Report of a Technical Working Group.* Geneva: World Health Organisation; 1996, p 32.

169. Oxford Midwives Research Group. A study of the relationship between the delivery to cord clamping interval and the time of cord separation. *Midwifery.* Dec 1991;7(4):167-176.

170. Fetus and Newborn Committee Canadian Paediatric Society. Red blood cell transfusions in newborn infants: Revised guidelines. *Paediatrics & Child Health.* 2002;7(8):553-558.

171. Lemay G. Leaving the umbilical cord to pulse. *Online birth centre news.* 1999(14.8).

172. Rachana S. *Lotus Birth.* Yarra Glen Australia: Greenwood Press; 2000.

Jacob's Placenta

1. Profet M. *Pregnancy Sickness: Using Your Body's Natural Defenses to Protect Your Baby-To-Be.* Cambridge MA: Da Capo; 1997.

2. Morgan E. *The Descent of the Child: Human Evolution from a New Paradigm.* London: Souvenir Press; 1994.

3. DuBose TJ. *Fetal Sonography.* Philadelphia: W. B. Saunders Co; 1996.

4. Odent M. Gestational Diabetes: A diagnosis still looking for a disease. *Primal Health Research.* 1998;12(1):1-6.

5. Odent M. *The Scientification of Love.* Revised ed. London: Free Association Books; 2001.

6. Falcao R. Locating Placenta Using a Hand held Doppler. Available at: www .gentlebirth.org/archives/placprev.html.

7. Buckley SJ. Lotus Birth: a ritual for our times. In: *Gentle Birth, Gentle Mothering: The wisdom and science of gentle choices in pregnancy, birth and parenting.* Brisbane Australia: One Moon Press; 2005, pp. 40-43. Also at www .sarahjbuckley.com

8. Fox H. A contemporary view of the human placenta. *Midwifery.* Mar 1991;7(1):31 39.

9. Ochedalski T, Zylinska K, Laudanski T, Lachowicz A. Corticotrophin-releasing hormone and ACTH levels in maternal and fetal blood during spontaneous and oxytocin-induced labour. *Eur J Endocrinol.* Feb 2001;144(2);117-121.

10. Morley G. Autism, ADD/ADHD, and related disorders: Is a common childbirth practice to blame? Red Flags Weekly enewsletter. 2002. http://www .whale.to/a/morley5.html.

11. Gilbert E. *Eat, Pray, Love: One Woman's Search for Everything Across Italy, India and Indonesia.* New York: Penguin; 2006.

12. Blythe J. Traditional Midwifery and Childbirth Practices in Zimbabwe. Paper presented at: Traditional Midwifery, 29 August 1998; Brisbane, Australia.

13. Frazer SJ. *The Golden Bough.* New York: Macmillan; 1922, p 40.

14. Baker JP. Freestone Innerprizes Newsletter. Spring; 2000.

15. Baker JP. *Prenatal Yoga and Natural Childbirth.* 3rd ed. Berkeley CA: North Atlantic Books; 2001.

16. Rachana S. *Lotus Birth.* Yarra Glen Australia: Greenwood Press; 2000.

Chapter 9: CESAREAN SURGERY

1. de Costa CM. "Ript from the womb": a short history of caesarean section. *Med J Aust.* Jan 15 2001;174(2):97-100.

2. Lurie S. The changing motives of cesarean section: from the ancient world to the twenty-first century. *Arch Gynecol Obstet.* Apr 2005;271(4):281-285.

3. Solomon B, Falkner N, *Tweedy's Practical Obstetrics.* Oxford: Oxford University Press p 582 4; 1937.

4. Kerr JMM. The technique of cesarean section, with special reference to the lower uterine segment incision *Am J Obstet Gynecol.* 1926;12:729-734.

5. Morbidity and Mortality Weekly Report. *Rates of Cesarean Delivery—United States, 1993.* Atlanta GA: Center for Disease Control; April 21, 1995; 44(15).

6. Hamilton BE, Martin JA, Ventura SJ. *Births: Preliminary data for 2006.* Hyattsville, MD: National Center for Health Statistics, 2007. vol 56 no 7.

7. Canadian Institute for Health Information. *Health Indicators 2007.* Ottawa: CIHI; 2007.

8. Richardson A, Mmata C. *Statistical bulletin: NHS maternity statistics, England: 2005 6.* London: The Information Centre; 2007.

9. Declercq E, Barger M, Cabral HJ, et al. Maternal outcomes associated with planned primary cesarean births

compared with planned vaginal births. *Obstet Gynecol.* Mar 2007;109(3):669-677.

10. National Institute for Clinical Excellence. *Caesarean Section: Clinical Guideline.* London: National Collaborating Centre for Women's and Children's Health; 2004.

11. Petrou S, Glazener C. The economic costs of alternative modes of delivery during the first two months postpartum: results from a Scottish observational study. *BJOG.* Feb 2002;109(2):214-217

12. Althabe F, Sosa C, Belizan JM, Gibbons L, Jacquerioz F, Bergel E. Cesarean section rates and maternal and neonatal mortality in low-, medium-, and high-income countries: an ecological study. *Birth.* Dec 2006;33(4):270-277.

13. Sreevidya S, Sathiyasekaran BW. High caesarean rates in Madras (India): a population-based cross sectional study. *BJOG.* Feb 2003;110(2):106-111.

14. Laws P, Abeywardana S, Walker J, Sullivan E. *Australia's mothers and babies 2005.* Vol Cat. no. PER 40. Sydney: Australian Institute of Health and Welfare National Perinatal Statistics Unit; 2007.

15. Barros FC, Victora CG, Barros AJ, et al. The challenge of reducing neonatal mortality in middle-income countries: findings from three Brazilian birth cohorts in 1982, 1993, and 2004. *Lancet.* Mar 5-11 2005;365(9462):847-854.

16. World Health Organization. Appropriate technology for birth. *Lancet.* Aug 24 1985;2(8452):436-437.

17. Harper MA, Byington RP, Espeland MA, Naughton M, Meyer R, Lane K. Pregnancy-related death and health care services. *Obstet Gynecol.* Aug 2003;102(2):273-278.

18. Enkin M, Keirse M, Neilson J, et al. *Effective Care in Pregnancy and Childbirth.* 3rd ed. Oxford: Oxford University Press; 2000.

19. Deneux-Tharaux C, Carmona E, Bouvier-Colle MH, Breart G. Postpartum maternal mortality and cesarean delivery. *Obstet Gynecol.* Sep 2006;108(3 Pt 1):541-548.

20. Allen VM, O'Connell CM, Liston RM, Baskett TF. Maternal morbidity associated with cesarean delivery without labor compared with spontaneous onset of labor at term. *Obstet Gynecol.* Sep 2003;102(3):477-482.

21. Hager RM, Daltveit AK, Hofoss D, et al. Complications of cesarean deliveries: rates and risk factors. *Am J Obstet Gynecol.* Feb 2004;190(2):428-434.

22. Henderson E, Love EJ. Incidence of hospital-acquired infections associated with caesarean section. *J Hosp Infect.* Apr 1995;29(4):245-255.

23. van Ham MA, van Dongen PW, Mulder J. Maternal consequences of caesarean section. A retrospective study of intraoperative and postoperative maternal complications of caesarean section during a 10-year period. *Eur J Obstet Gynecol Reprod Biol.* Jul 1997;74(1):1-6.

24. Villar J, Carroli G, Zavaleta N, et al. Maternal and neonatal individual risks and benefits associated with caesarean delivery: multicentre prospective study. *BMJ.* Nov 17 2007;335(7628):1025.

25. Liu S, Liston RM, Joseph KS, Heaman M, Sauve R, Kramer MS. Maternal mortality and severe morbidity associated with low-risk planned cesarean delivery versus planned vaginal delivery at term. *CMAJ.* Feb 13 2007;176(4):455-460.

26. Lin SY, Hu CJ, Lin HC. Increased risk of stroke in patients who undergo cesarean section delivery: a nationwide population-based study. *Am J Obstet Gynecol.* Apr 2008;198(4):391 e391-397.

27. Lobel M, DeLuca RS. Psychosocial sequelae of cesarean delivery: review and analysis of their causes and implications. *Soc Sci Med.* Jun 2007;64(11):2272-2284.

28. Thompson JF, Roberts CL, Currie M, Ellwood DA. Prevalence and persistence of health problems after childbirth: associations with parity and method of birth. *Birth*. Jun 2002;29(2):83-94.

29. DiMatteo MR, Morton SC, Lepper HS, et al. Cesarean childbirth and psychosocial outcomes: a meta-analysis. *Health Psychol*. Jul 1996;15(4):303-314.

30. Boyce PM, Todd AL. Increased risk of postnatal depression after emergency caesarean section. *Med J Aust*. Aug 3 1992;157(3):172-174.

31. Johnstone SJ, Boyce PM, Hickey AR, Morris-Yatees AD, Harris MG. Obstetric risk factors for postnatal depression in urban and rural community samples. *Aust N Z J Psychiatry*. Feb 2001;35(1):69-74.

32. Patel RR, Murphy DJ, Peters TJ. Operative delivery and postnatal depression: a cohort study. *BMJ*. Apr 16 2005;330(7496):879.

33. Rowe-Murray HJ, Fisher JR. Operative intervention in delivery is associated with compromised early mother-infant interaction. *Br J Obstet Gynaecol*. Oct 2001;108(10):1068-1075.

34. Ryding EL, Wijma K, Wijma B. Psychological impact of emergency cesarean section in comparison with elective cesarean section, instrumental and normal vaginal delivery. *J Psychosom Obstet Gynaecol*. Sep 1998;19(3):135-144.

35. Press JZ, Klein MC, Kaczorowski J, Liston RM, von Dadelszen P. Does cesarean section reduce postpartum urinary incontinence? A systematic review. *Birth*. Sep 2007;34(3):228-237.

36. Nelson RL, Westercamp M, Furner SE. A systematic review of the efficacy of cesarean section in the preservation of anal continence. *Dis Colon Rectum*. Oct 2006;49(10):1587-1595.

37. MacLennan AH, Taylor AW, Wilson DH, Wilson D. The prevalence of pelvic floor disorders and their relationship to gender, age, parity and mode of delivery. *Br J Obstet Gynaecol*. Dec 2000;107(12):1460-1470.

38. Mollison J, Porter M, Campbell D, Bhattacharya S. Primary mode of delivery and subsequent pregnancy. *BJOG*. Aug 2005;112(8):1061-1065.

39. Bhattacharya S, Porter M, Harrild K, et al. Absence of conception after caesarean section: voluntary or involuntary? *BJOG*. Mar 2006;113(3):268-275.

40. Jolly J, Walker J, Bhabra K. Subsequent obstetric performance related to primary mode of delivery. *Br J Obstet Gynaecol*. Mar 1999;106(3):227-232.

41. Maymon R, Halperin R, Mendlovic S, et al. Ectopic pregnancies in Caesarean section scars: the 8 year experience of one medical centre. *Hum Reprod*. Feb 2004;19(2):278-284.

42. Smith GC, Pell JP, Dobbie R. Caesarean section and risk of unexplained stillbirth in subsequent pregnancy. *Lancet*. Nov 29 2003;362(9398):1779-1784.

43. Kennare R, Tucker G, Heard A, Chan A. Risks of adverse outcomes in the next birth after a first cesarean delivery. *Obstet Gynecol*. Feb 2007;109(2 Pt 1):270-276.

44. Gray R, Quigley MA, Hockley C, Kurinczuk JJ, Goldacre M, Brocklehurst P. Caesarean delivery and risk of stillbirth in subsequent pregnancy: a retrospective cohort study in an English population. *BJOG*. Mar 2007;114(3):264-270.

45. Vendittelli F, Riviere O, Crenn-Hebert C, Rozan MA, Maria B, Jacquetin B. Is a breech presentation at term more frequent in women with a history of cesarean delivery? *Am J Obstet Gynecol*. May 2008;198(5):521 e521-526.

46. Chattopadhyay SK, Kharif H, Sherbeeni MM. Placenta praevia and accreta after previous caesarean section. *Eur J Obstet Gynecol Reprod Biol*. Dec 30 1993;52(3):151-156.

47. Lydon-Rochelle M, Holt VL, Easterling TR, Martin DP. First-birth cesarean and placental abruption or previa at second birth(1). *Obstet Gynecol.* May 2001;97(5 Pt 1):765-769.

48. Kacmar J, Bhimani L, Boyd M, Shah-Hosseini R, Peipert J. Route of delivery as a risk factor for emergent peripartum hysterectomy: a case-control study. *Obstet Gynecol.* Jul 2003;102(1):141-145.

49. Sheiner E, Levy A, Katz M, Mazor M. Identifying risk factors for peripartum cesarean hysterectomy. A population-based study. *J Reprod Med.* Aug 2003;48(8):622-626.

50. Habek D, Becarevic R. Emergency peripartum hysterectomy in a tertiary obstetric center: 8-year evaluation. *Fetal Diagn Ther.* 2007;22(2):139-142.

51. Royal College of Obstetricians and Gynecologists. *Birth after previous cae-sarean birth 2007.* Green-top Guideline No. 45.

52. Annibale DJ, Hulsey TC, Wagner CL, Southgate WM. Comparative neonatal morbidity of abdominal and vaginal deliveries after uncomplicated pregnancies. *Arch Pediatr Adolesc Med.* Aug 1995;149(8):862-867.

53. Hook B, Kiwi R, Amini SB, Fanaroff A, Hack M. Neonatal morbidity after elective repeat cesarean section and trial of labor. *Pediatrics.* Sep 1997;100(3 Pt 1):348-353.

54. Kolas T, Saugstad OD, Daltveit AK, Nilsen ST, Oian P. Planned cesarean versus planned vaginal delivery at term: comparison of newborn infant outcomes. *Am J Obstet Gynecol.* Dec 2006;195(6):1538-1543.

55. Richardson BS, Czikk MJ, daSilva O, Natale R. The impact of labor at term on measures of neonatal outcome. *Am J Obstet Gynecol.* Jan 2005;192(1):219-226.

56. Hernandez-Diaz S, Van Marter LJ, Werler MM, Louik C, Mitchell AA. Risk factors for persistent pulmonary hyper-tension of the newborn. *Pediatrics.* Aug 2007;120(2):e272-282.

57. Levine EM, Ghai V, Barton JJ, Strom CM. Mode of delivery and risk of respiratory diseases in newborns. *Obstet Gynecol.* Mar 2001;97(3):439-442.

58. MacDorman MF, Declercq E, Menacker F, Malloy MH. Infant and neonatal mortality for primary cesarean and vaginal births to women with "no indicated risk," United States, 1998-2001 birth cohorts. *Birth.* Sep 2006;33(3):175-182.

59. Smith JF, Hernandez C, Wax JR. Fetal laceration injury at cesarean delivery. *Obstet Gynecol.* Sep 1997;90(3):344-346.

60. Wiener JJ, Westwood J. Fetal lacerations at caesarean section. *J Obstet Gynaecol.* Jan 2002;22(1):23-24.

61. Lao TT, Panesar NS. Neonatal thyrotro-phin and mode of delivery. *Br J Obstet Gynaecol.* Oct 1989;96(10):1224-1227.

62. Franklin RC, Carpenter LM, O'Grady CM. Neonatal thyroid function: influence of perinatal factors. *Arch Dis Child.* Feb 1985;60(2):141-144.

63. Hagnevik K, Faxelius G, Irestedt L, Lagercrantz H, Lundell B, Persson B. Catecholamine surge and metabolic adaptation in the newborn after vaginal delivery and caesarean section. *Acta Paediatr Scand.* Sep 1984;73(5):602-609.

64. Fujimura A, Morimoto S, Uchida K, Takeda R, Ohshita M, Ebihara A. The influence of delivery mode on biological inactive renin level in umbilical cord blood. *Am J Hypertens.* Jan 1990;3(1):23-26.

65. Sangild PT, Hilsted L, Nexo E, Fowden AL, Silver M. Vaginal birth versus elective caesarean section: effects on gastric function in the neonate. *Exp Physiol.* Jan 1995;80(1):147-157.

66. Franzoi M, Simioni P, Luni S, Zerbinati P, Girolami A, Zanardo V. Effect of delivery modalities on the physiologic inhibition system of coagulation

of the neonate. *Thromb Res.* Jan 1 2002;105(1):15-18.

67. Agrawal S, Agrawal BM, Khurana K, Gupta K, Ansari KH. Comparative study of immunoglobulin G and immunoglobulin M among neonates in caesarean section and vaginal delivery. *J Indian Med Assoc.* Feb 1996;94(2):43-44.

68. Thilaganathan B, Meher-Homji N, Nicolaides KH. Labor: an immunologically beneficial process for the neonate. *Am J Obstet Gynecol.* Nov 1994;171(5):1271-1272.

69. Gronlund MM, Nuutila J, Pelto L, et al. Mode of delivery directs the phago cyte functions of infants for the first 6 months of life. *Clin Exp Immunol.* Jun 1999;116(3):521 526.

70. Gronlund MM, Lehtonen OP, Eerola E, Kero P. Fecal microflora in healthy infants born by different methods of delivery: permanent changes in intestinal flora after cesarean delivery. *J Pediatr Gastroenterol Nutr.* Jan 1999;28(1):19-25.

71. McKinney PA, Parslow R, Gurney KA, Law GR, Bodansky HJ, Williams R. Perinatal and neonatal determinants of childhood type 1 diabetes. A case-control study in Yorkshire, U.K. *Diabetes Care.* Jun 1999;22(6):928-932.

72. Patterson CC, Carson DJ, Hadden DR, Waugh NR, Cole SK. A case-control investigation of perinatal risk factors for childhood IDDM in Northern Ireland and Scotland. *Diabetes Care.* May 1994;17(5):376-381.

73. Dahlquist G, Kallen B. Maternal-child blood group incompatibility and other perinatal events increase the risk for early-onset type 1 (insulin-dependent) diabetes mellitus. *Diabetologia.* Jul 1992;35(7):671-675.

74. DiBaise JK, Zhang H, Crowell MD, Krajmalnik-Brown R, Decker GA, Rittmann BE. Gut microbiota and its possible relationship with obesity. *Mayo Clin Proc.* Apr 2008;83(4):460-469.

75. Sullivan A, Edlund C, Nord CE. Effect of antimicrobial agents on the ecological balance of human microflora. *Lancet Infect Dis.* Sep 2001;1(2):101-114.

76. Penders J, Thijs C, Vink C, et al. Factors influencing the composition of the intestinal microbiota in early infancy. *Pediatrics.* Aug 2006;118(2):511-521.

77. Wang BS, Zhou LF, Zhu LP, Gao XL, Gao ES. [Prospective observational study on the effects of caesarean section on breastfeeding]. *Zhonghua Fu Chan Ke Za Zhi.* Apr 2006;41(4):246-248.

78. Nissen E, Uvnas-Moberg K, Svensson K, Stock S, Widstrom AM, Winberg J. Different patterns of oxytocin, prolactin but not cortisol release during breastfeeding in women delivered by caesarean section or by the vaginal route. *Early Hum Dev.* Jul 5 1996;45(1-2):103-118.

79. Soltesz G, Patterson CC, Dahlquist G. Worldwide childhood type 1 diabetes incidence—what can we learn from epidemiology? *Pediatr Diabetes.* Oct 2007;8 Suppl 6;6 14.

80. Hakansson S, Kallon K. Caesarean section increases the risk of hospital care in childhood for asthma and gastroenteritis. *Clin Exp Allergy.* Jun 2003;33(6):757-764.

81. Bager P, Melbye M, Rostgaard K, Benn CS, Westergaard T. Mode of delivery and risk of allergic rhinitis and asthma. *J Allergy Clin Immunol.* Jan 2003;111(1):51-56.

82. Xu B, Pekkanen J, Hartikainen AL, Jarvelin MR. Caesarean section and risk of asthma and allergy in adulthood. *J Allergy Clin Immunol.* Apr 2001;107(4):732-733.

83. Renz-Polster H, David MR, Buist AS, et al. Caesarean section delivery and the risk of allergic disorders in childhood. *Clin Exp Allergy.* Nov 2005;35(11):1466-1472.

84. Eggesbo M, Botten G, Stigum H, Nafstad P, Magnus P. Is delivery by cesarean section a risk factor for food allergy? *J Allergy Clin Immunol.* Aug 2003;112(2):420-426.

85. Eggesbo M, Botten G, Stigum H, Samuelsen SO, Brunekreef B, Magnus P. Cesarean delivery and cow milk allergy/intolerance. *Allergy.* Sep 2005;60(9):1172-1173.

86. Li Y, Caufield PW, Dasanayake AP, Wiener HW, Vermund SH. Mode of delivery and other maternal factors influence the acquisition of *Streptococcus mutans* in infants. *J Dent Res.* Sep 2005;84(9):806-811.

87. Smith GC, Pell JP, Cameron AD, Dobbie R. Risk of perinatal death associated with labor after previous cesarean delivery in uncomplicated term pregnancies. *JAMA.* May 22-29 2002;287(20):2684-2690.

88. Landon MB, Hauth JC, Leveno KJ, et al. Maternal and perinatal outcomes associated with a trial of labor after prior cesarean delivery. *N Engl J Med.* Dec 16 2004;351(25):2581-2589.

89. Lydon-Rochelle M, Holt VL, Easterling TR, Martin DP. Risk of uterine rupture during labor among women with a prior cesarean delivery. *N Engl J Med.* Jul 5 2001;345(1):3-8.

90. Royal College of Obstetricians and Gynecologists. *Birth after previous caesarean birth* 2007. Green-top Guideline No. 45.

91. Cahill AG, Stamilio DM, Odibo AO, Peipert JF, Stevens EJ, Macones GA. Does a maximum dose of oxytocin affect risk for uterine rupture in candidates for vaginal birth after cesarean delivery? *Am J Obstet Gynecol.* Nov 2007;197(5):495 e491-495.

92. ACOG Committee Opinion No. 342: induction of labor for vaginal birth after cesarean delivery. *Obstet Gynecol. Aug 2006;108(2):465-468.*

93. American College of Obstetricians and Gynecologists. ACOG Practice Bulletin #54: vaginal birth after previous cesarean. *Obstet Gynecol.* Jul 2004;104(1):203-212.

94. Latendresse G, Murphy PA, Fullerton JT. A description of the management and outcomes of vaginal birth after cesarean birth in the homebirth setting. *J Midwifery Womens Health.* Sep-Oct 2005;50(5):386-391.

95. Lieberman E, Ernst EK, Rooks JP, Stapleton S, Flamm B. Results of the national study of vaginal birth after cesarean in birth centers. *Obstet Gynecol.* Nov 2004;104(5 Pt 1):933-942.

96. Wagner M. *Pursuing the Birth Machine.* Sydney: ACE Graphics; 1993.

97. Viswanathan M, Visco AG, Hartmann K, Wechter, ME, Gartlehner G, Wu JM, Palmieri R, Funk, MJ L, LJ, Swinson T, Lohr KN. *Cesarean Delivery on Maternal Request. Evidence Report/Technology Assessment No. 133.* Rockville, MD: Agency for Healthcare Research and Quality.; 2006. AHRQ Publication No. 06-E009.

98. Rooks JP, Weatherby NL, Ernst EK, Stapleton S, Rosen D, Rosenfield A. Outcomes of care in birth centers. The National Birth Center Study. *N Engl J Med.* Dec 28 1989;321(26):1804-1811.

99. Lydon-Rochelle M. Cesarean delivery rates in women cared for by certified nurse-midwives in the United States: a review. *Birth.* Dec 1995;22(4):211-219.

100. Johnson KC, Daviss BA. Outcomes of planned home births with certified professional midwives: large prospective study in North America. *Br Med J.* Jun 18 2005;330(7505):1416.

101. National Institute for Clinical Excellence. *Caesarean Section Clinical Guidelines.* London: National Collaborating Centre for Women's and Children's Health; 2004.

102. Declercq ER, Sakala C, Corry MP, Applebaum S. *Listening to Mothers II: Report of the Second National U.S. Survey of Women's Childbearing Experiences.* New York: Childbirth Connection; October 2006. 2006.

103. Gamble JA, Creedy DK. Women's request for a cesarean section: a critique of the literature. *Birth.* Dec 2000;27(4):256-263.

104. Gamble JA, Creedy DK. Women's preference for a cesarean section: incidence and associated factors. *Birth.* Jun 2001;28(2):101-110.

105. Gamble J, Creedy DK, McCourt C, Weaver J, Beake S. A Critique of the Literature on Women's Request for Cesarean Section. *Birth.* Dec 2007;34(4):331-340.

106. Fisher J, Astbury J, Smith A. Adverse psychological impact of operative obstetric interventions: a prospective longitudinal study. *Aust N Z J Psychiatry.* Oct 1997;31(5):728-738.

107. Arms S. *Immaculate Deception II: Myth, Magic and Birth.* Berkeley CA: Celestial Arts; 1996, p 92.

108. American College of Obstetricians and Gynecologists. ACOG Committee Opinion No. 340. Mode of term singleton breech delivery. *Obstet Gynecol.* Jul 2006;108(1):235-237.

109. Doyle NM, Riggs JW, Ramin SM, Sosa MA, Gilstrap LC, 3rd. Outcomes of term vaginal breech delivery. *Am J Perinatol.* Aug 2005;22(6):325-328.

110. Alarab M, Regan C, O'Connell MP, Keane DP, O'Herlihy C, Foley ME. Singleton vaginal breech delivery at term: still a safe option. *Obstet Gynecol.* Mar 2004;103(3):407-412.

111. Royal College of Obstetricians and Gynaecologists Clinical Effectiveness Support Unit. *The Management of Breech Presentation.* London: RCOG; 2006.

112. Smith J, Plaat F, Fisk N. The natural caesarean: a woman-centred technique. *BJOG.* July 2008;115(8):1037-1042.

Chapter 10: **CHOOSING HOMEBIRTH**

1. De Costa CM. "The contagiousness of childbed fever": a short history of puerperal sepsis and its treatment. *Med J Aust.* Dec 2-16 2002;177(11-12):668-671.

2. whomamedit.com. Ignaz Philipp Semmelweis. Available at: http://www.whonamedit.com/doctor.cfm/354.html. n.d.

3. Declercq E, Sakala C, Corry M, Applebaum S, Risher P. *Listening to Mothers: Report of the First U.S. National Survey of Women's Childbearing Experiences.* New York: Maternity Center Association; October 2002.

4. Declercq ER, Sakala C, Corry MP, Applebaum S. *Listening to Mothers II: Report of the Second National U.S. Survey of Women's Childbearing Experiences.* New York: Childbirth Connection; October 2006.

5. Durand AM. The Safety of Home Birth: The Farm Study. *Am J Public Health.* Mar 1992;82(5):450-453.

6. Parratt J, Johnston J. Planned homebirths in Victoria, 1995-1998. *Aust J Midwifery.* 2002;15(2):16-25.

7. Janssen PA, Lee SK, Ryan EM, et al. Outcomes of planned home births versus planned hospital births after regulation of midwifery in British Columbia. *CMAJ.* Feb 5 2002;166(3):315-323.

8. Johnson KC, Daviss BA. Outcomes of planned home births with certified professional midwives: large prospective study in North America. *Br Med J.* Jun 18 2005;330(7505):1416.

9. Martin JA, Hamilton BE, Sutton PD, et al. *Births: Final data for 2005 National Vital Statistics Reports.* Hyattsville, MD: National Center for Health Statistics; 2007; vol 56 no 6

10. Olsen O, Jewell MD. Home versus hospital birth. *Cochrane Database Syst Rev.* 2000(2):CD000352.

11. Wiegers TA, Keirse MJ, van der Zee J, Berghs GA. Outcome of planned home and planned hospital births in low risk pregnancies: prospective study in midwifery practices in The Netherlands. *Br Med J.* Nov 23 1996;313(7068):1309-1313.

12. Tew M, Damstra-Wijmenga SM. Safest birth attendants: recent Dutch evidence. *Midwifery.* Jun 1991;7(2):55-63.

13. Tew M. Place of birth and perinatal mortality. *J R Coll Gen Pract.* Aug 1985;35(277):390-394.

14. Tew M. *Safer Childbirth? A critical history of maternity care.* 3rd ed. London: Free Association Books; 1998.

15. Tew M. Do obstetric intranatal interventions make birth safer? *Br J Obstet Gynaecol.* Jul 1986;93(7):659-674.

16. Hatem M, et al. Midwife-led versus other models of care for childbearing women. *Cochrane Database Syst Rev.* 2008(4): CD004667.

17. MacDorman MF, Singh GK. Midwifery care, social and medical risk factors, and birth outcomes in the USA. *J Epidemiol Community Health.* May 1998;52(5):310-317.

18. Smulders B. *The Place of Birth: Its impact on midwives and mothers.* Brisbane, Australia: Birth International; 1999.

19. National Institute for Clinical Excellence. *Caesarean Section Clinical Guidelines.* London: National Collaborating Centre for Women's and Children's Health; 2004.

20. Department of Health. *Changing Childbirth, Part 1: the Report of the Expert Maternity Group.* London: HMSO; 1993, p 23.

21. Home Birth Aotearoa. Available at: http://www.homebirth.org.nz/statistics.html.

22. Martin JA, Hamilton BE, Sutton PD, et al. *Births: Final data for 2005.* Hyattsville, MD: National Center for Health Statistics; 2007. vol 56 no 6.

23. Wickham S. *Sacred Cycles. The Spiral of Women's Well-Being.* London: Free Association Books; 2004.

Chapter 11: LOVE, ATTACHMENT, AND YOUR BABY'S BRAIN

1. Trevathan WR. Evolutionary obstetrics. In: Trevathan WR, Smith EO, McKenna JJ, eds. *Evolutionary Medicine.* New York: Oxford University Press; 1999: 92-99.

2. Klaus MH, Klaus PH. *Your Amazing Newborn.* Second revised ed. Cambridge MA: Da Capo Press; 1998.

3. Chamberlain D. *The Mind of Your Newborn Baby.* Berkeley CA: North Atlantic Books; 1998.

4. Teicher MH, Andersen SL, Polcari A, Anderson CM, Navalta CP. Developmental neurobiology of childhood stress and trauma. *Psychiatr Clin North Am.* Jun 2002;25(2):397-426, vii-viii.

5. Schore AN. Back to basics: attachment, affect regulation, and the developing right brain: linking developmental neuroscience to pediatrics. *Pediatr Rev.* Jun 2005;26(6):204-217, p 204.

6. Mennella JA, Jagnow CP, Beauchamp GK. Prenatal and postnatal flavor learning by human infants. *Pediatrics.* Jun 2001;107(6):E88.

7. Talge NM, Neal C, Glover V. Antenatal maternal stress and long-term effects on child neurodevelopment: how and why? *J Child Psychol Psychiatry.* Mar-Apr 2007;48(3-4):245-261.

8. Bergstrom A, Okong P, Ransjo-Arvidson AB. Immediate maternal thermal response to skin-to-skin

care of newborn. *Acta Paediatr.* May 2007;96(5):655-658.

9. Christensson K, Siles C, Moreno L, et al. Temperature, metabolic adaptation and crying in healthy full-term newborns cared for skin-to-skin or in a cot. *Acta Paediatr.* Jun-Jul 1992;81(6-7):488-493.

10. Winberg J. Mother and newborn baby: mutual regulation of physiology and behavior—a selective review. *Dev Psychobiol.* Nov 2005;47(3):217-229.

11. Barbas H, Saha S, Rempel-Clower N, Ghashghaei T. Serial pathways from primate prefrontal cortex to autonomic areas may influence emotional expression. *BMC Neurosci.* Oct 10 2003;4:25.

12. Hariri AR, Bookheimer SY, Mazziotta JC. Modulating emotional responses: effects of a neocortical network on the limbic system. *Neuroreport.* Jan 17 2000;11(1):43-48.

13. Carter CS, Altemus M, Chrousos GP. Neuroendocrine and emotional changes in the post-partum period. *Prog Brain Res.* 2001;133:241-249.

14. Uvnas-Moberg K. *The Oxytocin Factor.* Cambridge MA: Da Capo Press; 2003.

15. Febo M, Numan M, Ferris CF. Functional magnetic resonance imaging shows oxytocin activates brain regions associated with mother pup bonding during suckling. *J Neurosci.* Dec 14 2005;25(50):11637-11644.

16. Storey AE, Walsh CJ, Quinton RL, Wynne-Edwards KE. Hormonal correlates of paternal responsiveness in new and expectant fathers. *Evol Hum Behav.* Mar 1 2000;21(2):79-95.

17. Wynne-Edwards KE. Hormonal changes in mammalian fathers. *Horm Behav.* Sep 2001;40(2):139-145.

18. Roberts RL, Jenkins KT, Lawler T, et al. Prolactin levels are elevated after infant carrying in parentally inexperienced common marmosets. *Physiol Behav.* Apr 2001;72(5):713-720.

19. Nissen E, Gustavsson P, Widstrom AM, Uvnas-Moberg K. Oxytocin, prolactin, milk production and their relationship with personality traits in women after vaginal delivery or cesarean section. *J Psychosom Obstet Gynaecol.* Mar 1998;19(1):49-58.

20. Winnicott DW. *The Child, the Family and the Outside World.* Harmondsorth: Penguin; 1964.

21. Uvnas-Moberg K. Physiological and psychological effects of oxytocin and prolactin in connection with motherhood with special reference to food intake and the endocrine system of the gut. *Acta Physiol Scand Suppl.* 1989;583:41-48.

22. Anisfeld E, Casper V, Nozyce M, Cunningham N. Does infant carrying promote attachment? An experimental study of the effects of increased physical contact on the development of attachment. *Child Dev.* Oct 1990;61(5):1617-1627.

23. Mason WA, Berkson G. Effects of maternal mobility on the development of rocking and other behaviors in rhesus monkeys: a study with artificial mothers. *Dev Psychobiol.* May 1975;8(3):197-211.

24. Teicher MH, Andersen SL, Polcari A, Anderson CM, Navalta CP. Developmental neurobiology of childhood stress and trauma. *Psychiatr Clin North Am.* Jun 2002;25(2):397-426, vii-viii, p 410.

25. Prescott J. America's lost dream: 'life, liberty and the pursuit of happiness': current research and historical background on the origins of love & violence. Paper presented at: Tenth Congress of the Association for Prenatal and Perinatal Psychology and Health, 2001; San Francisco.

26. Prescott J. Only more mother-infant bonding can prevent cycles of violence. *Cerebrum.* 2001;3(1):8-9 & 24.

27. Liedloff J. *The Continuum Concept: In Search of Happiness Lost.* Reading MA: Perseus Books; 1997.

28. Helliwell JF, Putnam RD. The social context of well-being. *Philos Trans R Soc Lond B Biol Sci.* Sep 29 2004;359(1449):1435-1446.

29. Schore AN. Attachment and the regulation of the right brain. *Attach Hum Dev.* Apr 2000;2(1):23-47.

30. Henry JP. Psychological and physiological responses to stress: the right hemisphere and the hypothalamo-pituitary-adrenal axis, an inquiry into problems of human bonding. *Integr Physiol Behav Sci.* Oct-Dec 1993;28(4):369-387; discussion 368.

31. Schore AN. *Affect Regulation and the Origin of the Self.* Hillsdale NJ: Lawrence Erlbaum Associates Inc.; 1994.

32. Schore AN. Back to basics: attachment, affect regulation, and the developing right brain: linking developmental neuroscience to pediatrics. *Pediatr Rev.* Jun 2005;26(6):204-217, p 209.

33. Schore AN. Effects of a secure attachment relationship on right brain development, affect regulation, and infant mental health. *Infant Mental Health Journal.* 2001;221(1-2):7-66.

34. Champagne F, Meaney MJ. Like mother, like daughter: evidence for non-genomic transmission of parental behavior and stress responsivity. *Prog Brain Res.* 2001;133:287-302.

35. Champagne F, Diorio J, Sharma S, Meaney MJ. Naturally occurring variations in maternal behavior in the rat are associated with differences in estrogen-inducible central oxytocin receptors. *Proc Natl Acad Sci USA.* Oct 23 2001;98(22):12736-12741.

36. Meinlschmidt G, Heim C. Sensitivity to intranasal oxytocin in adult men with early parental separation. *Biol Psychiatry.* Dec 1 2006.

37. Gordon I, Zagoory-Sharon O, Schneiderman I, Leckman JF, Weller A, Feldman R. Oxytocin and cortisol in romantically unattached young adults: associations with bonding and psychological distress. *Psychophysiology.* May 2008;45(3):349-352.

38. Suomi SJ. Early determinants of behaviour: evidence from primate studies. *Br Med Bull.* Jan 1997;53(1):170-184.

39. Schore AN. The effects of early relational trauma on right brain development, affect regulation, and infant mental health. *Infant Mental Health Journal.* 2001;221(1-2):201-269.

40. Milad MR, Rauch SL. The role of the orbitofrontal cortex in anxiety disorders. *Ann N Y Acad Sci.* Dec 2007;1121:546-561.

41. Drevets WC. Orbitofrontal cortex function and structure in depression. *Ann N Y Acad Sci.* Dec 2007;1121:499-527.

42. Schore AN. Attachment and the regulation of the right brain. *Attach Hum Dev.* Apr 2000;2(1):23-47, p 30.

43. Dalai Lama. Open Arms, Embracing Kindness (talk). Dalai Lama 2007 Australian Tour; 13 June, 2007; Brisbane Entertainment Centre.

44. Schore AN. Effects of a secure attachment relationship on right brain development, affect regulation, and infant mental health. *Infant Mental Health Journal.* 2001;221(1-2):7-66, p 21.

45. Kaffman A, Meaney MJ. Neurodevelopmental sequelae of postnatal maternal care in rodents: clinical and research implications of molecular insights. *J Child Psychol Psychiatry.* Mar-Apr 2007;48(3-4):224-244.

46. Dieter JN, Field T, Hernandez-Reif M, et al. Maternal depression and increased fetal activity. *J Obstet Gynaecol.* Sep 2001;21(5):468-473.

47. Feldman R, Weller A, Sirota L, Eidelman AI. Skin-to-skin contact (Kangaroo care) promotes self-regulation in premature infants: sleep-wake cyclicity, arousal modulation, and sustained exploration. *Dev Psychol.* Mar 2002;38(2):194-207.

48. Teicher MH, Andersen SL, Polcari A, Anderson CM, Navalta CP. Developmental neurobiology of childhood stress and trauma. *Psychiatr Clin North Am.* Jun 2002;25(2):397-426, vii-viii, p 415.

49. Perry BD, Pollard R. Homeostasis, stress, trauma, and adaptation. A neurodevelopmental view of childhood trauma. *Child Adolesc Psychiatr Clin N Am.* Jan 1998;7(1):33-51, viii.

50. Gunnar MR, Quevedo KM. Early care experiences and HPA axis regulation in children: a mechanism for later trauma vulnerability. *Prog Brain Res.* 2008;167:137-149.

51. Gunnar MR, Morison SJ, Chisholm K, Schuder M. Salivary cortisol levels in children adopted from romanian orphanages. *Dev Psychopathol.* Summer 2001;13(3):611-628.

52. Teicher MH, Andersen SL, Polcari A, Anderson CM, Navalta CP. Developmental neurobiology of childhood stress and trauma. *Psychiatr Clin North Am.* Jun 2002;25(2):397-426, vii viii, p 401.

53. Bugental DB, Martorell GA, Barraza V. The hormonal costs of subtle forms of infant maltreatment. *Horm Behav.* Jan 2003;43(1):237-244.

54. Gunnar MR, Quevedo KM. Early care experiences and HPA axis regulation in children: a mechanism for later trauma vulnerability. *Prog Brain Res.* 2008;167:137-149, p 141.

55. Solter A. *Tears and Tantrums.* Goleta CA: Shining Star Press; 1998.

Chapter 12: **BREASTFEEDING**

1. Chen A, Rogan WJ. Breastfeeding and the risk of postneonatal death in the United States. *Pediatrics.* May 2004;113(5):e435-439.

2. Hanson LA. Breastfeeding stimulates the infant immune system. *Science and Medicine.* 1997;4(6).

3. Hanson LA, Korotkova M, Telemo E. Breast-feeding, infant formulas, and the immune system. *Ann Allergy Asthma Immunol.* Jun 2003;90(6 Suppl 3):59-63.

4. Hanson LA, Korotkova M. The role of breastfeeding in prevention of neonatal infection. *Semin Neonatol.* Aug 2002;7(4):275-281, p 278.

5. Uvnas-Moberg K. The gastrointestinal tract in growth and reproduction. *Sci Am.* Jul 1989;261(1):78-83.

6. Oddy WH. The impact of breastmilk on infant and child health. *Breastfeed Rev.* Nov 2002;10(3):5-18.

7. Gartner LM, Morton J, Lawrence RA, et al. Breastfeeding and the use of human milk. *Pediatrics.* Feb 2005;115(2): 496-506.

8. Gillman MW, Rifas-Shiman SL, Camargo CA, Jr., et al. Risk of overweight among adolescents who were breastfed as infants. *JAMA.* May 16 2001;285(19):2461-2467.

9. DiBaise JK, Zhang H, Crowell MD, Krajmalnik-Brown R, Decker GA, Rittmann BE. Gut microbiota and its possible relationship with obesity. *Mayo Clin Proc.* Apr 2008;83(4):460-469.

10. Montgomery SM, Ehlin A, Sacker A. Breast feeding and resilience against psychosocial stress. *Arch Dis Child.* Dec 2006;91(12):990-994.

11. Kramer MS, Aboud F, Mironova E, et al. Breastfeeding and child cognitive development: new evidence from a large randomized trial. *Arch Gen Psychiatry.* May 2008;65(5):578-584.

12. World Health Organization. *Global Strategy for Infant and Young Child Feeding.* Geneva: World Health Organization; 2003 http://www.who .int/child-adolescent-health/New_ Publications/NUTRITION/gs_iycf.pdf.

13. World Health Organization. *The Optimal Duration Of Exclusive Breastfeeding: Report Of An Expert Consultation.* Geneva: World Health Organization; 2001.

14. Labbok MH, Clark D, Goldman AS. Breastfeeding: maintaining an irreplaceable immunological resource. *Nat Rev Immunol.* Jul 2004;4(7):565-572.

15. Collaborative Group on Hormonal Factors in Breast Cancer. Breast cancer and breastfeeding: collaborative reanalysis of individual data from 47 epidemiological studies in 30 countries, including 50302 women with breast cancer and 96973 women without the disease. *Lancet.* Jul 20 2002;360(9328):187-195.

16. Labbok MH. Effects of breastfeeding on the mother. *Pediatr Clin North Am.* Feb 2001;48(1):143-158.

17. Huo D, Lauderdale DS, Li L. Influence of reproductive factors on hip fracture risk in Chinese women. *Osteoporos Int.* Aug 2003;14(8):694-700.

18. Gunderson EP, Lewis CE, Wei GS, Whitmer RA, Quesenberry CP, Sidney S. Lactation and changes in maternal metabolic risk factors. *Obstet Gynecol.* Mar 2007;109(3):729-738.

19. Groer MW, Davis MW. Cytokines, infections, stress, and dysphoric moods in breastfeeders and formula feeders. *J Obstet Gynecol Neonatal Nurs.* Sep-Oct 2006;35(5):599-607.

20. Stuebe AM, Rich-Edwards JW, Willett WC, Manson JE, Michels KB. Duration of lactation and incidence of type 2 diabetes. *JAMA.* Nov 23 2005;294(20):2601-2610.

21. Ram KT, Bobby P, Hailpern SM, et al. Duration of lactation is associated with lower prevalence of the metabolic syndrome in midlife—SWAN, the study of women's health across the nation. *Am J Obstet Gynecol.* Mar 2008;198(3):268 e261-266.

22. World Alliance for Breastfeeding Action. LAM: The Lactational Amenorrhea Method. Available at: http://www.waba .org.my/specialpages/lam/lam.htm.

23. Kippley SK, Kippley JF. The relation between breastfeeding and amenor-rhea. *J Obstet Gynecol Neonatal Nurs.* 1972;1(4):15-21.

24. Schore AN. *Affect Regulation and the Origin of the Self.* Hillsdale NJ: Lawrence Erlbaum Associates Inc; 1994.

25. Uvnas-Moberg K. Physiological and psychological effects of oxytocin and prolactin in connection with motherhood with special reference to food intake and the endocrine system of the gut. *Acta Physiol Scand Suppl.* 1989;583:41-48.

26. World Health Organisation. *Global Strategy for Infant and Young Child Feeding.* Geneva: World Health Organisation; 2003 http://www.who .int/child-adolescent-health/New_ Publications/NUTRITION/gs_iycf.pdf.

27. American Academy of Family Physicians. AAFP Policy Statement on Breastfeeding. 2005. Available at: http://www .aafp.org/x6633.xml.

28. Dettwyler K. A Time to Wean: the hominid blueprint for the natural age of weaning in modern human populations. In: Stuart-Macadam P, Dettwyler K, eds. *Breastfeeding; Biocultural Perspectives.* New York: Aldine de Gruyter; 1995.

29. Filds V. The Culture and Biology of Breastfeeding: an historical review of Western Europe. In: Stuart-Macadam P, Dettwyler K, eds. *Breastfeeding; Biocultural Perspectives.* New York: Aldine de Gruyter; 1995.

30. Cunningham AS. Morbidity in breast-fed and artificially fed infants. *J Pediatr.* May 1977;90(5):726-729.

31. Dewey KG, Heinig MJ, Nommsen-Rivers LA. Differences in morbidity between breast-fed and formula-fed infants. *J Pediatr.* May 1995;126(5 Pt 1):696-702.

32. van den Bogaard C, van den Hoogen HJ, Huygen FJ, van Weel C. The relationship between breast-feeding and early childhood morbidity in a

general population. *Fam Med.* Sep-Oct 1991;23(7):510-515.

33. Onyango AW, Receveur O, Esrey SA. The contribution of breastmilk to toddler diets in western Kenya. *Bull World Health Organ.* 2002;80(4):292-299.

34. Fisher JO, Birch LL, Smiciklas-Wright H, Picciano MF. Breast feeding through the first year predicts maternal control in feeding and subsequent toddler energy intakes. *J Am Diet Assoc.* Jun 2000;100(6):641-646.

35. As Good As Chocolate And Better Than Ice-cream: Study Asks Aussie Tots About Breastfeeding. *Science Daily.* August 5 2005.

36. Lawrence RA, Lawrence RM. *Breastfeeding: A guide for the medical profession.* 5th ed. Sydney: Mosby; 1999.

37. Hatherley P. *The Homeopathic Physician's Guide to Lactation.* Brisbane: Luminoz; 2004.

Bees, Baboos, and Boobies

1. Bumgarner N *Mothering Your Nursing Toddler.* Schaumburg IL: La Leche League International; 2000. www.myntoddler.com

Chapter 13: BABIES, MOTHERS, AND THE SCIENCE OF SHARING SLEEP

1. Shore R. *Rethinking the Brain: New Insights into Early Development.* New York: Families and Work Institute; 1997, p 15.

2. Christensson K, Siles C, Moreno L, et al. Temperature, metabolic adaptation and crying in healthy full-term newborns cared for skin-to-skin or in a cot. *Acta Paediatr.* Jun-Jul 1992;81(6-7):488-493.

3. Moore ER, Anderson GC, Bergman N. Early skin-to-skin contact for mothers and their healthy newborn infants. *Cochrane Database Syst Rev.* 2007(3):CD003519.

4. Richard CA. Increased infant axillary temperatures in non-REM sleep during mother-infant bed sharing. *Early Hum Dev.* Jun 1999;55(2):103-111.

5. Richard CA, Mosko SS. Mother-infant bedsharing is associated with an increase in infant heart rate. *Sleep.* May 1 2004;27(3):507-511.

6. Scragg RK, Mitchell EA, Stewart AW, et al. Infant room-sharing and prone sleep position in sudden infant death syndrome. New Zealand Cot Death Study Group. *Lancet.* Jan 6 1996;347(8993): 7-12.

7. Christensson K, Cabrera T, Christensson E, Uvnas-Moberg K, Winberg J. Separation distress call in the human neonate in the absence of maternal body contact. *Acta Paediatr.* May 1995;84(5):468-473.

8. Bergman NJ. Skin-to-Skin Contact and Perinatal Neuroscience. Paper presented at: Capers Breastfeeding Seminar: Breastfeeding A Lifelong Investment; May 13 2006, 2006; Brisbane, Australia

9. Teicher MH, Andersen SL, Polcari A, Anderson CM, Navalta CP. Developmental neurobiology of childhood stress and trauma. *Psychiatr Clin North Am.* Jun 2002;25(2):397-426, vii-viii.

10. McKenna JJ, McDade T. Why babies should never sleep alone: a review of the co-sleeping controversy in relation to SIDS, bedsharing and breast feeding. *Paediatr Respir Rev.* Jun 2005;6(2):134-152.

11. McKenna JJ, McDade T. Why babies should never sleep alone: a review of the co-sleeping controversy in relation to SIDS, bedsharing and breast feeding. *Paediatr Respir Rev.* Jun 2005;6(2):134-152, p142.

12. Thevenin T. *The Family Bed.* New York: Perigee Trade; 2002.

13. American Academy of Family Physicians. AAFP Policy Statement on Breastfeeding. 2005 http://www.aafp.org/x6633.xml.

14. Small M. *Our Babies, Ourselves.* New York: Random House; 1998.

15. Nelson EA, Taylor BJ, Jenik A, et al. International Child Care Practices Study: infant sleeping environment. *Early Hum Dev.* Apr 2001;62(1):43-55.

16. Barry H, Paxson LM. Infancy and childhood: cross-cultural codes. *Ethology.* 1971;10:466-508.

17. Mahendran R, Vaingankar JA, Mythily S, Cai YM. Co-sleeping and clinical correlates in children seen at a child guidance clinic. *Singapore Med J.* Nov 2006;47(11):957-959.

18. Welles-Nystrom B. Co-sleeping as a window into Swedish culture: considerations of gender and health care. *Scand J Caring Sci.* Dec 2005;19(4):354-360.

19. Willinger M, Ko CW, Hoffman HJ, Kessler RC, Corwin MJ. Trends in infant bed sharing in the United States, 1993-2000: the National Infant Sleep Position study. *Arch Pediatr Adolesc Med.* Jan 2003;157(1):43-49.

20. Ball HL. Breastfeeding, bed sharing, and infant sleep. *Birth.* Sep 2003;30(3):181-188.

21. McKenna JJ, Mosko S, Richard C. Breast-feeding and Mother-Infant Cosleeping in Relation to SIDS Prevention. In: Trevathan WR, Smith E, McKenna JJ, eds. *Evolutionary Medicine.* New York: Oxford University Press; 1999.

22. Nelson EA, Chan PH. Child care practices and cot death in Hong Kong. *N Z Med J.* Apr 26 1996;109(1020):144-146.

23. Schore AN. *Affect Regulation and the Origin of the Self.* Hillsdale NJ: Lawrence Erlbaum Associates Inc; 1994.

24. Nakamura S, Wind M, Danello MA. Review of hazards associated with children placed in adult beds. *Arch Pediatr Adolesc Med.* Oct 1999;153(10):1019-1023.

25. Drago DA, Dannenberg AL. Infant mechanical suffocation deaths in the United States, 1980-1997. *Pediatrics.* May 1999;103(5):e59.

26. Scheers NJ, Dayton CM, Kemp JS. Sudden infant death with external airways covered: case-comparison study of 206 deaths in the United States. *Arch Pediatr Adolesc Med.* Jun 1998;152(6):540-547.

27. Blair PS, Fleming PJ, Smith IJ, et al. Babies sleeping with parents: case-control study of factors influencing the risk of the sudden infant death syndrome. CESDI SUDI research group. *BMJ.* Dec 4 1999;319(7223):1457-1461.

28. Mitchell EA, Tuohy PG, Brunt JM, et al. Risk factors for sudden infant death syndrome following the prevention campaign in New Zealand: a prospective study. *Pediatrics.* Nov 1997;100(5):835-840.

29. Hauck FR, Herman SM, Donovan M, et al. Sleep environment and the risk of sudden infant death syndrome in an urban population: the Chicago Infant Mortality Study. *Pediatrics.* May 2003;111(5 Part 2):1207-1214.

30. Carpenter RG, Irgens LM, Blair PS, et al. Sudden unexplained infant death in 20 regions in Europe: case control study. *Lancet.* Jan 17 2004;363(9404):185-191.

31. Tappin D, Ecob R, Brooke H. Bedsharing, roomsharing, and sudden infant death syndrome in Scotland: a case-control study. *J Pediatr.* Jul 2005;147(1):32-37.

32. Wailoo M, Ball H, Fleming P, Ward Platt MP. Infants bed sharing with mothers. *Arch Dis Child.* Dec 2004;89(12):1082-1083.

33. Ostfeld BM, Perl H, Esposito L, et al. Sleep environment, positional, lifestyle, and demographic characteristics associated with bed sharing in sudden infant death syndrome cases: a population-based study. *Pediatrics.* Nov 2006;118(5):2051-2059.

34. Gessner BD, Porter TJ. Bed sharing with unimpaired parents is not an important

risk for sudden infant death syndrome. *Pediatrics.* Mar 2006;117(3):990-991; author reply 994-996.

35. Gessner BD, Ives GC, Perham-Hester KA. Association between sudden infant death syndrome and prone sleep position, bed sharing, and sleeping outside an infant crib in Alaska. *Pediatrics.* Oct 2001;108(4):923-927.

36. UNICEF UK Baby Friendly Initiative with the Foundation for the Study of Infant Deaths. *Sharing a bed with your baby: A guide for breastfeeding mothers* 2005.

37. The Academy of Breastfeeding Medicine. *Guideline on co-sleeping and breastfeeding 2003.* Protocol #6.

38. Royal Australian and New Zealand College of Physicians Paediatrics and Child Health Division. *Breastfeeding.* June 2007.

39. Ostfeld BM, Perl H, Esposito L, et al. Sleep environment, positional, lifestyle, and demographic characteristics associated with bed sharing in sudden infant death syndrome cases: a population-based study. *Pediatrics.* Nov 2006;118(5):2051-2059, p 2052.

40. McKenna JJ, McDade T. Why babies should never sleep alone: a review of the co-sleeping controversy in relation to SIDS, bedsharing and breast feeding. *Paediatr Respir Rev.* Jun 2005;6(2):134-152, p 145.

41. Moon RY, Fu LY. Sudden infant death syndrome. *Pediatr Rev.* Jun 2007;28(6):209-214.

42. McKenna JJ, Mosko SS, Richard CA. Bedsharing promotes breastfeeding. *Pediatrics.* Aug 1997;100(2 Pt 1):214-219.

43. McKenna JJ, McDade T. Why babies should never sleep alone: a review of the co-sleeping controversy in relation to SIDS, bedsharing and breast feeding. *Paediatr Respir Rev.* Jun 2005;6(2):134-152, p 135.

44. Ball H. Parent-Infant Bed sharing Behavior: Effects of Feeding Type and Presence of Father. *Human Nature.* 2006;17(3):301-318.

45. Baddock SA, Galland BC, Taylor BJ, Bolton DP. Sleep arrangements and behavior of bed sharing families in the home setting. *Pediatrics.* Jan 2007;119(1):e200-207.

46. Ball HL. Breastfeeding, bed sharing, and infant sleep. *Birth.* Sep 2003;30(3):181-188, p 185-186.

47. Lewis RJ, Janda LH. The relationship between adult sexual adjustment and childhood experiences regarding exposure to nudity, sleeping in the parental bed, and parental attitudes toward sexuality. *Arch Sex Behav.* Aug 1988;17(4):349-362.

48. Forbes F, Weiss DS, Folen RA. The co-sleeping habits of military children. *Mil Med* 1992;157:196-200.

49. Mosenkis J. *The effects of childhood co-sleeping on later life development* [MSc]. Chicago: Department of Cultural Psychology, University of Chicago; 1998.

50. Okami P, Weisner T, Olmstead R. Outcome correlates of parent-child bedsharing: an eighteen-year longitudinal study. *J Dev Behav Pediatr.* Aug 2002;23(4):244-253.

51. Barrett A. X-treme Breastfeeding. Paper presented at: Breastfeeding: Making a Difference; March 2, 2006; Brisbane, Australia.

52. Lennig M. *The Curly Pyjama Letters.* Melbourne: Penguin Books Australia; 2001.

INDEX

A

Abandonment, 125

Abnormalities
diagnosing by ultrasound, 82–84, 93
termination and, 93

Acoustic streaming, 85–86

ADHD, 28, 230

Adrenalin, 26, 106, 134, 139, 228. *See also*
Epinephrine and Catecholamines

Affect synchrony, 223

Aggression, 160
and mother-infant carrying, 222
and mother-infant separation, 160

Aggressive-defensive maternal behavior, 103

Amniocentesis, 83

Amniotic fluid, 84

Amygdala, and early mother-infant interactions, 225–226

Anemia, newborn and cord clamping, 166–67

Antibiotics for group B strep
allergy to, 57
and newborn gut flora, 57–58, 60, 61

Arginine vasopressin (AVP) and newborn, 226

ARM (artificial rupture of membranes), 73–74

Artwork, benefits in pregnancy, 17

Attachment, mother-infant
affect synchrony and, 223
building, 231–33
importance of, 42–43, 222–25
lack of, 124–25, 227–31

Attunement, 224

Augmentation of labor, risks of, 110

Autism, 104, 114, 230

Autonomic nervous system (ANS), 225

B

Babies
attachment and, 222–25, 227–33. *See also*
Attachment
brain development of, 218, 221, 222–27, 248
capabilities of newborn, 217–18
carrying, 221–22
and prolactin, 109
cesarean risks to, 119–21, 165–66, 196–98

circumcision of, 161, 191, 222, 233
communicating with, before birth, 31
early clamping and, 163–65
emotional regulation of, 224, 225–26
epidurals' effects on, 141–48
healing for, 269–70
ideal environment for, 220–22
induction's effects on, 70–71, 75, 113–14
instrumental deliveries of, 136–37
LGA (large for gestational age), 49, 67
and gestational diabetes, 49
and overdue, 67
mutual regulation and, 219–20, 249
neglect and, 227–31
overdue, 66–70
perinatal mortality of, 41–42, 43–44, 66
resuscitation of newborn, 169–70
skin-to-skin contact with, 124–25, 158, 219, 226, 249
sleep patterns of, 248–49
synthetic oxytocin and, 170
temperature regulation system of, 147–48

Baby-Friendly Hospital Initiative (BFHI), 125, 152

Baker, Jeannine Parvati, 25, 30, 126, 192, 270

Balaskas, Janet, 16

Banks, Maggie, 19

Bed sharing. *See* Cosleeping

Beech, Beverley, 79

Bergman, Nils, 159, 160

Beta-endorphin
brain development and, 238
breastfeeding and, 105, 126
effects of, 104–5
epidurals and, 116–17
hormonal imprinting and, 116
induction and, 131
in labor, 104–5, 134
reward and, 115
production of, 104

Bilirubin, benefits of, 168

Birth. *See also* Cesareans; Homebirth; Hospital birth; Labor; Undisturbed birth
breech, 201
choosing helpers for, 18
dance of, 19

depression after, 10
ecstasy of, 25, 96–97
energy and, 17–18
evolution of, 42, 97–98
first, making choices for, 20
hormones of, 99–109
impact of obstetric procedures on, 110–19
informed-choice approach to, 10–11
instinctive, 12–19
lotus, 34, 131, 183, 189–91
love and, 28–29, 131
medical approach to, 8–9, 25
meditation as, 100
memories triggered at, 268
as multifaceted crystal, 12
passion and, 26–28
physically preparing body for, 15–16
power of, 8, 11, 25, 30–31
sacred cycle and, 212
safety and, 18, 19
satisfaction with, 152–53
surrender and, 29–30
transformation and, 32–36
unassisted, 18, 129
unwelcome outcomes at, 267–68
water-, 212–15
Birth stories
Emma's, 20–24
Jacob's, 185–92, 212–15
Maia's, 128–31
Zoe's, 32–36
Brain
development of, 218, 221, 222–27, 248
emotional, 99
neglect and, 227–31
BRAN model for decision making, 39–40,
44, 45
Brazelton Neonatal Behavioral Assessment
Scale (NBAS), 118, 145–46
Breastfeeding
bed sharing and, 257–59, 266
benefits of, 123–24, 234–38
cesareans and, 122–23, 198
child spacing and, 238
early separation and, 122, 126
epidurals and, 149–52
evolutionary importance of, 42–43
full-term, 239–40
gut flora and, 123–24

hormones and, 103, 105, 108–9, 126, 221,
238–39
importance of, 42–43
love and, 126, 238, 240–41
as second chance, 126
Breech birth, 201
C
Cardiovascular disease, 104
Catecholamines (CAs), 106–8, 134–35,
156–58
Cavitation, 85
Cervix, short, 84
Cesareans, 119–123, 193–203
breastfeeding and, 122–23
costs of, 194
cord clamping and, 165–66, 185
effects on mothers 122–23, 195–96,
201–2
effects on offspring 198, 119–121, 165–66,
196–98
elective repeat, 198–99
epidurals' effects on, 137
good, 202–3
good reasons for 201–2
gut flora and, 120
history of, 193–94
hormones and, 119–20
planning a good, 202–3
rate of, 9, 194
reasons for unnecessary, 193, 200, 201
risks and adverse effects of, 119–23,
165–66, 195–98, 200–201
unnecessary, 200
vaginal birth after, 198–200
WHO recommendations, 194
Childbirth Connection, 205
Children. See also Babies
cosleeping and, 260–61
following lead of, 270
healing for, 269–70
memories of, of birth and early life, 270
Choice, informed, 10–11, 40–41, 77
Circumcision, 160, 191, 222, 233
Cochrane Collaboration, 11, 79, 177, 182, 206
COMET (Conventional Obstetric Mobile
Epidural Trial), 136
Compassion, development of, 226
Contractions
in induced labor, 71, 110–12

oxytocin and, 101, 102, 156
Contractions, *continued*
    in third stage of labor, 156–57
Cord blood banking, 170–75
Cord clamping. *See also* Lotus birth
    cord blood gas analysis and, 164–65
    delayed, 173, 182–83
    early, 163–65, 166–67, 169–70
    feto-maternal hemorrhage and, 179–81
    iron and, 166–67
    jaundice and, 167–69
    nuchal cord and, 165
    polycythemia and, 167–68
    postpartum hemorrhage and, 163,
        177–79
Cord traction, 176, 181
Corning, J. Leonard, 132
Cortisol, and infant brain 228, 229, 230, 250
Cosleeping. *See also* Sleeping
    advantages of, 259–60
    breastfeeding and, 257–59, 266
    definition of, 251
    frequency of, 252–53
    history of, 251–52
    international survey of, 252–53
    long-term, 260–61
    safety of, 254–57
    studies of, 253–54
CRH (corticotrophin-releasing hormone),
    99, 104
Crying, 124, 250–51
CSE (combined spinal epidural), 133
Cytotec. *See* Misoprostol
D
Dalai Lama, 226
Darwin, Erasmus, 166–67
Day, Clair Lotus, 191
Decision-making in pregnancy and birth,
    37–41
Demerol, 104, 114, 169. S*ee also* Opiates
Depression
    after birth, 10, 25, 27, 43
    cesareans and, 195
    early trauma and, 225, 227, 230
    oxytocin and, 104
    prevalence of, 25–26
DES (diethylstilbestrol), 38
Despair-dissociation response 159, 228–29,
    233, 250

Diabetes, gestational, 45–54
Dissociation, 228–29
Doppler ultrasound, 80, 85, 87, 88, 89
Down syndrome, 81, 82, 83
Drug addiction, 104, 115–16
Drugs. *See* Antibiotics; Epidurals; Opiates;
    Pitocin; *individual drugs*
Due date, estimating, 64–65, 82. *See also*
    Induction; Overdue babies
Dunn, Peter, 165
E
Earth, connecting with, 14–15
Emotional brain. *See* Limbic system
Emotional regulation, 224, 225–26
Enkin, Murray, 11
EOGBS disease, 54–57
Epidurals, 116–19, 132–53
    animal studies of, 148–49
    birth satisfaction and, 152–53
    breastfeeding and, 149–52
    definition of, 132–33
    effects of, on labor, 117–18, 135–38
    fathers' presence and, 10
    frequency of, 9
    history of, 132
    labor hormones and, 28, 116–17, 133–35
    maternal fever and, 140, 143
    mothering behavior and, 118–19
    side effects from, 118, 138–48, 178–79
    walking, 133, 138–39
Epinephrine, 26, 106, 134–35, 139, 228. *See*
    also Catecholamines
Ergometrine (ergonovine), breastfeeding
    and, 176–77
Estrogen, 100
EDD (expected date of delivery) 64–65. *See*
    also Overdue
F
Father, baby's
    effects of birth on, 32, 43
    energy between mother and, 17
    presence of, at birth, 10
    prolactin and, 109
    role in decision-making 5, 44
    support for 10, 127
Fear-terror, 159, 228, 229, 230
Feminism and birth, 8
Fentanyl (Sublimaze), 104, 114
Ferguson reflex, 102, 106

Feto-maternal hemorrhage (FMH), 179–81
Fetus ejection reflex, 102, 106–7
Fever, 140, 143
FHR (fetal heart rate)
    epidural, effects of, 137, 142–43, 144
    epinephrine, effects of, 106
    opiate drugs, effects of, 115
    Pitocin, effects of, 111, 137
Fight-or-flight response, 104, 106, 156, 160,
    228. *See also* Catecholamines
Forceps deliveries, 136–37
Frye, Anne, 47–48, 61

G
Gaskin, Ina May, 17
Gestational diabetes mellitus (GDM), 45–54
Greer, Germaine, 92
Group B strep (GBS)
    disease, early onset 54–57
    screening, 54–63
Gut flora
    antibiotics and, 58–60
    breastfeeding and, 123–24
    importance of, 60, 236

H
Haire, Doris, 111
HCG (human chorionic gonadotropin), 186
Healing from trauma
    for children, 269–70
    choosing paths for, 268–69
Homebirth, 204–12. *See also* Midwives
    by country, 208–9
    history of, 204
    interventions and, 205–6
    lack of support for, 207–8
    reasons for choosing, 207
    sacred cycle and, 212
    safety of, 205–7
    setting up, 209–10
    support groups for, 208, 211
Homeostasis, 219, 225
Hormonal imprinting, 116, 148, 160, 170, 224
Hormones. *See also individual hormones*
    breastfeeding and, 103, 105, 108–9, 126,
        221, 238–39
    cesareans and, 119–20
    epidurals and, 28, 116–17, 133–35
    labor and, 13, 17, 26–29, 99–109, 121,
        133–35
    of love, 28–29, 101

mothering and, 108, 219, 221
of paternity, 109
stress and, 228
Hospital birth
    history of, 204–5
    risks of, 205, 206–7
Hyperarousal, 159, 228
Hypothalamic-pituitary-adrenal (HPA) axis,
    160,125, 229, 230
Hypothalamus, 226

I
ICH (intracranial hemorrhage), 73–74
Induction for "going overdue," 63–77
    alternatives to, 74–77
    benefits of, 66–68
    prostaglandins and, 73
    rates of, 64
    risks of, 70–74
    studies of, 69–70
    with synthetic oxytocin, 110–14
Infant Breastfeeding Assessment Tool
    (IBFAT), 150
Infants. *See* Babies
Informed choice, 10–11, 40–41, 77
Informed refusal 40, 41
Instincts
    birth and, 12–19
    energy and, 17–18
    trusting, 18–19
Instrumental deliveries, 136–37
Iron stores, and cord clamping, 166–67
IVH (intraventricular hemorrhage) and cord
    clamping, 167

J
Jaundice, 167–69
Journal, keeping in pregnancies, 16–17

K
Kangaroo care, 124
Kitzinger, Sheila, 15, 20
Kloosterman, G., 126–27
Kynurenine, as neuroprotective factor, 121

L
Labor. *See also* Birth; Induction; Third stage
    of labor
    benefits of, for baby, 119–21
    epidurals' effects on, 135–38
    hormones and, 13, 17, 26–29, 99–109,
        121, 133–35
    opiates and, 114–16

Lactational amenorrhea method (LAM), 238
Lactoferrin, 234
Learning disorders, 28
Leidloff, Jean, 222
Leukemia, 170, 171
LGA (large for gestational age) babies, 49, 67
Limbic system, 99, 224, 225
LOGBS disease, 54, 57
Lotus birth, 183, 189–91
Love
    birth and, 28–29
    breastfeeding and, 240–41
    hormone of, 28–29, 101
    importance of, 222–27
    lack of, 227–31
Lucas, Peter, 22–23, 35
M
Macrosomia. *See* LGA
Maternal circuit, 220–21
Maternal subroutine, and prolactin, 109
Maternity Center Association, 205
McCracken, Leilah, 18
McKenna, James, 253
Meperidine (Demerol), 104, 114, 169
Mesocorticolimbic dopamine reward system,
    104, 221, 239
Methylergonovine, 163, 176
Metabolic syndrome, early separation and,
    160
Midwives. *See also* Homebirth
    accreditation of, 209–10
    finding, 210
    quality of care from, 208
    questions to ask, 210–11
    resurgence of, 209
    role of, 29
Misoprostol (Cytotec), 38, 73, 177
Morphine, 104
Mortality rates
    infant, 9, 41–42, 43–44, 66
    maternal, 9
Motherbaby, concept of, 220
Mother-infant relationship. *See* Attachment
Mothers
    breastfeeding's benefits to, 237–38
    energy between baby's father at birth
        and, 17
    energy between daughters at birth and, 18
    interactions of, with baby, 222–25,

227–33
    mutual regulation and, 219–20, 249
    self-esteem of, by delivery method, 122
    skin-to-skin contact between baby and,
        124–25, 158, 219, 226, 249
    sleep for, 261–62
Mutual regulation, 219–20, 249
N
Naish, Francesca, 14–15
Nalbuphine (Nubain), 104, 114
Naloxone (Narcan), 169–70
National Institute for Clinical Excellence, 56,
    69, 201, 209
Neglect, effects of, 227–31
Neurologic and Adaptive Capacity Score
    (NACS), 145–47
Nocebo effect, 40, 44–45
Nonviolent Communication (NVC), 271
Noradrenaline (norepinephrine), 26, 106,
    134, 139, 228. *See also* Catecholamines
Nothing, doing, 40, 53, 62–63, 76–77
Nuchal cord, 165
Nuchal translucency (NT) test, 81
O
Occipitoanterior (OA) position, 97–98
Odent, Michel, 13, 43, 44, 53, 75, 101, 106,
    160
OGTT (oral glucose tolerance test), 47
Opiate drugs, 104, 114–16, 138, 140, 144, 149
    breastfeeding and, 149, 150
    epidurals and spinals, 133, 138, 139, 140,
        142, 144
    exposure at birth and drug addiction,
        115-16
Orbitofrontal cortex (OFC), 225–26, 238
Overdue, babies going, 66–70
Oxytocin
    breastfeeding and, 103, 122, 126, 238
    cardiovascular disease and, 104
    effects of natural, 102–4
    epidurals and, 117, 133–34, 135, 149
    half-life of, 101
    as hormone of love, 17, 26, 28–29, 101
    in labor, 101–2, 133, 156–57
    mothering behavior and, 219, 221
    pheromonal transmission of, 103
    in postnatal period, 102–3
    production of, 101, 102
    stress reduction and, 103, 221, 226

synthetic, 110–14, 170, 177

P

Parasympathetic nervous system (PNS), 219, 228

Parent Effectiveness Training (PET), 271

Parenting
  mistakes in, 271
  path of, 270–71
  techniques for, 270–71

Passion, in birth, 26–28

Pearce, Joseph Chilton, 125, 160

Penicillin, 57–58, 61

Perinatal mortality (PNM), 41–42, 43–44, 66

Perry, Bruce, 228

Pethidine, 104, 114, 169. *See also* Opiate drugs

PGF2 alpha, 117

The Pink Kit, 13–14, 16

Pitocin (Syntocinon), 28, 73, 110–14, 137, 170. *See also* Induction
  autism and, 114
  desensitization of uterus and, 28, 72,112, 179
  effects on autonomic nervous system, 113–14
  effects on baby, 73,110–11,113, 145,
  effects on labor, 28, 71, 110–14,
  epidurals and, 137, 153
  FHR, effects on 111, 137, 142
  hormonal imprinting and, 114, 170
  hyperstimulation, and, 111–12, 142
  in third stage
    effects on baby, 170
    placental transfusion and, 163

Placenta
  beliefs and rituals surrounding, 191–92
  burial of, 191–92
  cesareans and, 196
  development of, 185–86
  lotus birth and, 189–91
  previa (low-lying), 83–84
  role of, 185–92
  symbolism of, 192
  transfusion from, 161–63

Polycythemia, 167–68

POP (persistent occipito-posterior) position, 135–36

Post-traumatic stress disorder (PTSD), 229, 230

PPH (postpartum hemorrhage), 140, 155, 177–79

Pregnancy
  cesarean risks to future, 196
  connection to Earth and, 15
  decision-making in, 37–41
  dreams during, 16–17
  internal work during, 16–17
  journals, 16–17
  medicalization of, 37
  smoking during, 264–65
  as social experience, 37
  stress during, 103, 218, 232
  weight gain during, 52

Prescott, James, 221

Progesterone, 100, 108

Prolactin
  breastfeeding and, 108–9, 122, 126, 221, 238
  effects of, 27, 108–9, 156, 158
  production of, 108

R

Rachana, Shivam, 14

Refusal, informed, 41

Reist, Melinda Tankard, 93

RhD sensitization, 180–81

Risk, concept of, 41–43

Rothman, Barbara Katz, 93

RPU. *See* Ultrasound

Russell, Bedford, 59

S

Schizophrenia, 104, 230

Schore, Allan, 218, 224

Semmelweis, Ignaz, 205

Separation
  distress cry of, 124
  early, 123–26, 159–61, 229
  stress and, 231, 249–51

Sex
  as induction alternative, 74
  power of, 26

Shanahan, Christine, 22–23, 35

Shanley, Laura, 18

Shore, Rima, 248

SIDS (sudden infant death syndrome), 236, 249, 252, 253–57, 263, 265, 266

Skin-to-skin contact, 124–25, 158, 219, 226, 249

Sleeping, 247–66. *See also* Cosleeping
  bedding for, 263
  breastfeeding and, 266

clothing for, 264

Sleeping, *continued*
  concerns about, 247–48
  evolutionary perspective on, 249
  modern arrangements for, 251–53
  for mothers, 261–62
  mutual regulation and, 249
  through the night, 247, 248
  position for, 263
  safety and, 254–57
  safe bedding for, 263
  separation and, 249–51
  studies of, 253–54
  tips for, 263–66
Smell, mother-infant bonding and, sense of,
    103
Smoking, risks of SIDS, 264–65
Soft markers, relevance in ultrasound, 83
Somato-sensory affectional deprivation
    (S-SAD), 222
Spanking, 230
Spinals. *See* Epidurals
Stadol, 104, 114
Stillbirth, risks when overdue, 66, 68, 70, 76
Stress
    effects on infants of, 228–29
    during pregnancy, 103, 218, 232
    resiliency to, 227
    separation and, 124, 159–610, 249–51
Sublimaze, 104, 114
Sullivan, Michael, 171
Surrender, 29–30
Sweep and stretch, 75–76
Sympathetic nervous system (SNS), 228
Syntocinon. *See* Pitocin
Syntometrine, 163

T
Tactile stimulation. *See* Touch, importance of
Tests. *See also* Ultrasound
    gestational diabetes, 45–54
    Group B strep, 54–63
    nocebo effect of, 40, 44–45
    nuchal translucency (NT), 81
Tew, Marjory, 206
Third stage of labor. *See also* Cord blood bank-
    ing; Cord clamping; Cord traction
    active management of, 155–56, 163,

175–81
    choosing natural, 183–85
    definition of, 154
    hormones in, 156–59
    postpartum hemorrhage and, 177–79
    potential of, 183
    recent thinking about, 181–83
Touch, importance of, 124–25, 158, 219, 226,
    249

U
Ultrasound, 78–94
    biological effects of, 84–90
    definition of, 80–81
    Doppler, 80, 85, 87, 88, 89
    exposure and dose for, 90, 92
    history of, 79–80
    human studies of, 88–90
    information gained from, 81–84
    nonmedical, 81
    recommendations for, 94
    record of, 91
    vaginal, 80–81
    women's experiences of, 92–93
Undisturbed birth
    nature of, 95, 126–27
    obstacles to, 96–97
    pain and, 98
    suggestions for, 127–28
Uvnas-Moberg, Kerstin, 103, 104

V
VBAC (vaginal birth after cesarean),
    198–200

W
Waterbirth, 212–15
Weeks, Andrew, 166, 169–70
Weight gain, 52
Wickham, Sara, 181
Winnicott, D. W., 231

X
X-rays in pregnancy, 38

Y
Yoga, 14, 16